Also by Kenneth Bock, M.D.

THE ROAD TO IMMUNITY
NATURAL RELIEF FOR YOUR CHILD'S ASTHMA
THE GERM SURVIVAL GUIDE

Also by Cameron Stauth

BRAIN LONGEVITY
(with Dharma Singh Khalsa)

WHAT HAPPY PEOPLE KNOW
(with Dan Baker)

MEDITATION AS MEDICINE
(with Dharma Singh Khalsa)

ONE BODY, ONE LIFE
(with Gregory Joujon-Roche)

THE PAIN CURE
(with Dharma Singh Khalsa)

THE NEW APPROACH TO CANCER

HEALING
THE NEW
CHILDHOOD
EPIDEMICS:

AUTISM, ADHD, ASTHMA,
AND ALLERGIES

KENNETH BOCK, M.D.
AND CAMERON STAUTH

Special Contributions by Korri Fink

HEALING
THE NEW
CHILDHOOD
EPIDEMICS:

AUTISM, ADHD, ASTHMA,
AND ALLERGIES

*The Groundbreaking Program
for the 4-A Disorders*

Ballantine Books   New York

Published in the United States by Ballantine Books, an imprint of The Random House
Publishing Group, a division of Random House, Inc., New York.

BALLANTINE and colophon are registered trademarks of Random House, Inc.

ISBN 978-0-345-49450-4

Library of Congress Cataloging-in-Publication Data
Bock, Kenneth
Healing the new childhood epidemics: autism, ADHD, asthma, and allergies: the
groundbreaking program for the 4-A disorders/by Kenneth Bock and Cameron Stauth;
special contributions by Korri Fink.
p. cm.
ISBN-13: 978-0-345-49450-4 (hc: alk. paper)
ISBN-10: 0-345-49450-4
1. Autism in children.   2. Attention-deficit hyperactivity disorder.   3. Asthma in
children.   4. Allergy in children.   I. Stauth, Cameron.   II. Fink, Korri.   III. Title.

RJ506.A9B63 2007
618.92'85882—dc22   2006050415

Printed in the United States of America on acid-free paper

www.ballantinebooks.com

2 4 6 8 9 7 5 3 1

First Edition

Book design by Carol Malcolm Russo

For Marjorie Harvey,
a wonderful mother, wife, sister, and aunt,
with love.

CAMERON STAUTH

For Bernard Rimland, Ph.D.,
the father of the biomedical approach to autism,
who paved the way for the recoveries of thousands of children.

For Elizabeth "Liz" Birt
who dedicated her life to recovering her child from autism,
and to uncovering the truth behind the autism epidemic.

and

For my children, Alicia and Jordan,
and for all children and parents,
and the love between them,
which is the ultimate healing force.

KENNETH BOCK, M.D.

ACKNOWLEDGMENTS

THE AUTHORS GRATEFULLY ACKNOWLEDGE THE HELP OF THE MANY people who played critically important roles in the creation of this book.

Caroline Sutton, Senior Editor of Ballantine Books, was the perfect editor for this project. She was completely in tune with all that we wished to accomplish, and made our highest hopes for this book into reality. Thanks also to her able assistant, Christina Duffy.

Agent Matthew Guma conceived this project, and brought every element of it together. His vision, commitment, and effort lie at the heart of the book.

Richard Pine, of Inkwell Management, was incredibly supportive, as he has been for so many years. Thanks also to Inkwell's David Forrer.

Korri Fink, our director of research, was vitally important in the interviewing and document evaluation process of the book, and her work, under difficult circumstances, added a depth and dimension to the book it would otherwise have lacked.

Sandra Stahl, once again, was extraordinarily valuable as the word and information processor of the book. As usual, she worked with the ethic of excellence that has enabled her to excel in so many areas.

Gabriel Stauth helped a great deal with research and was the lead technical and computer advisor in the production of the manuscript. His assistance was invaluable, and deeply appreciated.

Bonnie Sgarro was extremely helpful in literature research, and her assistance and timeliness were much appreciated.

Melissa Starnes was exceptionally helpful in bringing together the many diverse elements that result in a finished book, and the authors are grateful for her acumen and good cheer.

A large number of patients, parents, other family members, doctors, and therapists offered their insights and personal accounts, with remarkable candor and perception. Without their help, this book would not exist. More than that, the work and courage of these kids and families inspired not just a book, but a new way of saving children's lives.

DR. BOCK'S PERSONAL ACKNOWLEDGMENTS

In addition to the terrific help that we received from the people who were most intimately involved with the creation of this book, most notably Caroline Sutton and Matthew Guma, I wish also to thank those who have been vitally important in the development of the biomedical approach to autism and the other 4-A disorders.

The knowledge I have gained evolved out of years of meetings with researchers, clinicians, and many dedicated parents, all of whom were looking for answers to the puzzle of autism. Many of these encounters came in the form of think tanks and conferences that were organized by the Defeat Autism Now organization, which is sponsored by the Autism Research Institute. I am deeply grateful to DAN, ARI, and to the parents, patients, and colleagues with whom I have worked.

Although I generally refer to my individualized rendition of the DAN protocol as my own approach, or as the Healing Program, I believe that many other DAN physicians could have written this book, based upon their own similar clinical approaches, experiences, and ideas. These physicians include dedicated, caring, experienced DAN doctors such as Sid Baker, Stephanie Cave, Jane El-Dahr, Anju Usman, Jeff Bradstreet, John Green, Jaquelyn McCandless, Liz Mumper, Nancy O'Hara, Andrew Levinson, Stuart Freedenfeld, James Neubrander, Cindy Schneider, Paul Hardy, Mary Megson, Jerry Kartzinel, Derrick Lonsdale, Bryan Jepson, and Marvin Boris.

Jaquelyn McCandless has already written a very helpful book about autism, *Children with Starving Brains,* and Sid Baker, in concert with the brilliant nutritional biochemist, Jon Pangborn, has written a comprehensive treatment manual entitled *Autism: Effective Biomedical Treatments,* a book that I recommend if you are looking for additional details. Although biochemically complex, many parts of the book are written in that incredible, reader-friendly Sid Baker style.

I particularly wish to thank Sid Baker for being my mentor in the early 1980s, after I finished my residency. He and I were part of a group of approximately twenty-five physicians in the Northeast who met regularly to advance our own knowledge, and to help further the approaches of nutritional biochemistry, clinical nutrition, and integrative medicine. Sid's approach to caring for patients contributed strongly to my becoming what we both now refer to as a "medical detective." Sid taught me to never cease investigating the complex issues that comprise medical problems. When I reunited with him in the late 1990s, as part of the DAN movement, it was intellectually rewarding and emotionally satisfying.

I must also acknowledge the researchers who have provided us with the scientific backbone that is the basis of our clinical work. These incredible people include Jill James, who is one of the smartest and loveliest people one might ever meet, as well as my estimable colleagues Richard Deth, Martha Herbert, Tim Buie, Arthur Krigsman, and Andrew Wakefield. Thanks also to Paul Shattock, who is so dedicated to helping spread the message that autism is treatable, and is one of the funniest and most likable people I have ever met.

Special thanks go to Lauren Underwood for her work in our early collaboration on healing autism. She was also instrumental in bringing together the group of people who brought this book to fruition.

With great admiration, I also thank Bernie Rimland, the father of the biomedical approach to the treatment of autism, who initially stood up alone for what he knew to be true. I am also grateful to his assistant, Steve Edelson, whose continued support of Bernie has helped this movement grow.

Maureen McDonnell, of Wellness Associates, has produced some of the most amazing conferences that I have ever had the good fortune to be part of, and was extremely supportive of me early on, as I became part of the DAN family, and I wish to thank her for that.

Many thanks also go to my partner and brother, Steven Bock, as well as to our associate, Michael Compain, for supporting our medical practice while I was away so frequently. Thanks, too, to my cousin, neurologist Jay Lombard, for teaching me so much about the clinical use of neurobehavioral medications.

I am also appreciative of my colleagues in the American College for Advancement in Medicine, which is my other medical "home." I have been honored to serve as president of ACAM over the past year, as I have long been keenly aware of the value that the physicians in this group do to advance education and research in the field of integrative medicine.

Most important, I give my thanks and my love to my family, who too often have had to bear the effects of my absence. My medical practice, my lecturing, clinical research, think-tank activities, responsibilities for ACAM, and my work on this book have often left me with too little time for those I wish most to be with. Marian, Alicia, and Jordan, I love you all, and I thank you for your understanding and support. I know it's not easy.

And lastly, my love and thoughts go to my deceased parents, Fred and Nora Bock, whose loving support throughout the years contributed to my ability to make projects like this manifest.

CONTENTS

HEALING
THE NEW
CHILDHOOD
EPIDEMICS:
AUTISM, ADHD, ASTHMA, AND ALLERGIES

PART ONE

NEW
PROBLEMS, NEW
SOLUTIONS

CHAPTER ONE

THE
CHILDREN

New Haven, Connecticut

IT WAS THE MOST ORDINARY OF FAMILY MOMENTS. THE BABY WAS just starting to talk, and Mom wanted a video of it.

Lynne Avram handed the video camera to her husband, and he started shooting the playful interactions between Lynne and the baby–chubby little Paul, with his bright eyes beaming–focusing almost entirely on his son, instead of his wife, as new fathers are prone to do. To him, and to Lynne, too, the baby–and every ordinary thing the baby did–was absolutely *unprecedented*. It was as if no child had ever before taken so majestic a first step, or burped so remarkably.

Dad narrated as he filmed. "This is the day before Paul's very first birthday," he said, getting a close-up of gleeful Paul, tottering around barefoot in his red-striped shirt. "Can you say hi, Paul?"

"Ha-ee! Ha-ee!" Paul responded, waving at the camera.

"Hi, sweetie!" said Lynne. "Hi-hi!"

Paul grinned at Lynne, and his face was lit with love, easy to read, in that striking nonverbal way that toddlers have of telling the world how they feel.

"Ha-ee, da-duh!" said Paul.

"Can you say, 'Hi Mama?'" Lynne asked.

Paul gazed happily at his mother, and brushed at his nose. His nose was a little runny. It had been runny for several days. Lately, he was picking up every cold that came around.

"Pauly," said Lynne, "can you say ma-ma? Ma-ma?"

"Da-duh!"

"You think this is pretty funny, huh?" Lynne said, laughing.

"*Uh*-uh!" said Paul, shaking his head emphatically. "*Uh*-uh!"

What a unique child! What an extraordinary family moment!

Truth be told, of course, it was all quite ordinary.

In the years to come, though, Lynne and her husband would watch this video many times.

It was a video of one of their last ordinary family moments.

Paul's runny nose lingered for several days. Then he started to get better, but caught something else. Paul seemed to have a bad case of the common malady that parents call the day-care flu–catching every germ in town–even though Paul stayed at home with Lynne.

Paul, in fact, still had his cold on the day he was due for his next-to-last round of immunizations, at fourteen months. He needed a measles-mumps-rubella shot, and a booster to protect him against a form of meningitis.

Just before the appointment, Lynne called Paul's doctor and asked if it was safe to give vaccines to kids when they were sick. The doctor told her not to worry–it happened all the time. If parents waited for perfect health in their toddlers, he said, the kids would *never* get all their shots. These days, he said, there were more shots than ever, and they were all important. Whole epidemics had been wiped out!

But Lynne still felt uneasy. Jittery. Couldn't shake it. She was a registered nurse at a prominent hospital near the Yale University campus, and it seemed to her that it went against medical common sense to provoke a powerful immune response in a child whose immune system was already battered by illness. But she told herself that her fear was just garden-variety parental paranoia. After all, she worked with some of the finest physicians in America, and she had a flint-hard faith in their expertise. As a nurse in one of the world's best coronary intensive care units, she regularly saw doctors snatch patients' lives back from the shadow of death. They worked miracles.

So Paul got his shots, and everything was back to normal. Lynne and Paul went home and played. Later, Lynne made dinner for her husband, Wesley–who was a Communications professor at Yale Divinity School–even though she was exhausted. Getting simple chores done was tough with a baby in the house. But she knew it wouldn't last. Kids grow up. Easier times were ahead.

Over the next few days, though, Paul's nose and eyes grew disturbingly red, against his now ghostly skin. Dark circles began to droop under his inflamed eyes. Patches of scaly skin grew on his soft face. He no longer wanted to play. He was always tired and congested, irritable—not himself. Lynne told herself that she would have to wait a little longer for the easier days.

One evening, a couple of weeks after the immunizations, while waiting for Paul's latest bout with a cold-bug to end, Lynne took him to the window and started to play a familiar game, in which she would point at something and say, "I see a *tree*"–prompting Paul to repeat "tree."

"I see *grass*," she said. But Paul didn't seem interested.

"I see the *sky*." No response.

"I see *car-car. Car-car!*" Nothing.

"Pauly?"

Paul was changing. Lynne didn't want to believe it, but it was undeniable. The changes, frighteningly, did not seem to be just predictable responses to pervasive symptoms of colds and flu. Paul's whole personality was changing. More precisely, it was just evaporating. His trademark mannerisms, his unique facial expressions, his words, his eye contact, his hugs and kisses, his lopsided grin: gone. His playfulness was gone. His child's joy was gone. Replaced by nothing.

Paul couldn't sleep through the night. He woke up screaming. His digestion and elimination suddenly soured, as if his belly were now filled with a wet, noxious mix of food and poison. It soaked his diapers and burned little lesions into his bottom, no matter how often Lynne changed him. His new nickname was Poopy Pauly.

He started to suffer from almost constant ear infections. The pain and the crying never seemed to let up. Wesley and Lynne took the relatively drastic step of having plastic tubes inserted into Paul's ears to drain the congestion, but the infections just shifted to other areas, including his throat, lungs, and buttocks.

Instead of playing with his toys, Poopy Pauly started rambling around the house in a strange state of stupor that was punctuated by sudden meltdowns. He ignored everyone. Nothing penetrated–not love, not a raised voice, not constant attention. As Paul stumbled around the house, he would often bruise himself, but he didn't seem to notice. Lynne could only follow in his wake, cleaning up his messes and keeping him safe.

Sometimes Paul drifted into what seemed to be his own mental purgatory, standing for hours in front of a running faucet on his spindly, weak legs, mesmerized by the water, acting almost as if he were high on drugs. Lynne and Wesley began to alternate on what they called Paul Duty. One would work or do chores while the other was on Paul Duty, then they'd switch, fall into bed, and wait for Paul to wake up screaming. Another month crept by, then another.

Lynne made a video approximately eight weeks after Paul's immunizations, and it portrayed a child who was vastly different from the child in Paul's first-birthday video. In the new video, Lynne coaxed Paul to interact, but he just sat mutely on the floor, drooling and wooden, his eyes vacant. At one point in the video, Wesley entered the room and said, "Hi, Paul." But his voice sounded very different in this video. He spoke to Paul in a sad monotone, as if he expected no reply, the way one might speak to a person in a coma. After that, there weren't many more videos.

Summer came and went, as Lynne embarked on a pilgrimage to the medical world. But no doctor offered a diagnosis or proposed a treatment. None would even confirm Lynne's certainty that something dreadful was happening, and that her child should *not* be trying to drink from the toilet, or eat dryer lint, or chew on electrical cords, or play with his own dirty diapers, or smash his head into mirrors. She was told that kids developed at different paces. She was told that toddlers were a handful. She discovered that the medical world was much different for the patient than it was for the professional.

A year somehow crawled past, with Lynne constantly searching for signs of improvement, but never finding any. Family outings dwindled to trips to just one playground, which had a high enough fence to keep Poopy Pauly, still in diapers, safe.

After another exhausting summer, the holidays came. Theoretically. But there was no way to have a holiday in the Avram home. At Halloween, Paul–almost three now–was completely oblivious to the costumes and candy. Kids would come to the door and he wouldn't even look up, so Lynne turned off the lights. Thanksgiving dinner, of course, was completely impossible with Paul in the house, and at Christmas Paul just tore open everyone's packages, with no interest whatsoever in their contents. Normal activities ceased. Bike rides? Not possible. The movies? No way. The mall? Out of the question. Church, where Wesley was the minister? No—Lynne and Paul sat outside on the curb. Play dates? With *whom*? Paul Duty didn't consist of play dates.

Ordinary family life was over, practically before it had begun.

Then one night Wesley was channel-surfing and came across a scene of a child staring hypnotically at water running out of a faucet—like Paul! It was a segment on Cable News Network. The moment it was over, Wesley hurried to his computer, dialed-up the relatively new Internet, and typed in A-U-T-I-S-M.

"Lynne. You've gotta look at this! I think Paul has autism."

"Autism?"

Lynne vaguely recalled hearing about autism in nursing school. Back then, in the late 1980s and early 1990s, autism was considered a very rare mental disorder, not nearly common enough to merit much study. Lynne hadn't heard about it since. None of Paul's doctors had ever mentioned it.

Lynne sat next to Wesley and they paged through the painfully slow Internet.

When they finished, Lynne felt sick. The symptoms of autism applied to Paul. Uniformly. Why had no one *mentioned* this?

Autism: incurable. Cause unknown. No medical treatments. Inability to communicate. Emotional sterility. Halfway houses. Institutionalization.

It was as if Paul, right then and there, had died. It was really that bad. Or—God help Paul—maybe even worse.

Lynne became, in her own words, The Crazy Mom. She began to confront doctors about why no medical treatments were available. They responded that some treatments actually were available, but that they were all psychological therapies, not biomedical treatments. Standard therapy consisted mostly of just behavior modification. Besides, the doctors said, Paul had not yet been formally diagnosed as autistic. That could not happen until he was slightly older, and by then he might outgrow his quirky behaviors, and learn to speak, look at people, and use the toilet. Remember, they said, Albert Einstein was a late bloomer!

What about the physical symptoms, Lynne asked—the digestive disorders, the diarrhea, the persistent eczema, the recurrent infections, the poor muscle tone? The doctors said that none of that was pertinent.

Autism, they reiterated, was a *psychiatric* disorder, defined by behavioral characteristics. They assured Lynne, though, that she shouldn't blame herself, because poor parenting had recently been ruled out as a cause. For many years, they said, doctors had thought that kids became autistic because their mothers were emotionally frigid—"refrigerator mothers," in the psychiatric lexicon. In these more sophisticated times, they said, it had become apparent that autism was simply genetic, and therefore inevitable for a tiny percentage of children.

But if it were strictly genetic, Lynne argued, Paul would presumably have been born with some of its symptoms, when in fact he had been quite normal his first year. To which the doctors responded, in effect: No, he was *never* normal, but Crazy Moms who can't handle the reality of this tragedy just see what they need to see.

One thing they did recommend was that Lynne carry a card, the size of a business card, that briefly explained autism, and could be handed to people in public situations when Paul went wild.

Lynne sometimes broached the subject of immunizations causing autism—which was mentioned on the Internet—but most doctors patiently explained that this theory was a myth, invented by distraught parents. Other doctors were quite condescending about the theory to Lynne, even though she was a medical professional who could speak their language. A few doctors, particularly pediatricians, got angry about it. Pediatricians administer most immunizations, and some of them seemed to take it personally when Lynne raised doubts. It's *not* the *shots,* they insisted.

Then why, Lynne asked, did there now appear to be a virtual epidemic of autism—with rates soaring far beyond those of her nursing school years? And why did that epidemic appear to start right around 1991, when a whole new batch of vaccinations had been mandated? The answer was quite simple, most of the doctors replied. There was no epidemic. Just better diagnosis.

Their essential message was: Give up. Accept it. Move on. But Lynne kept swallowing her pride and plugging away. She and Wesley spent over $100,000 on behavioral and educational therapies, which decimated their finances, and did little good.

Then one day, through a network of parents who had autistic kids, Lynne heard about a dietary approach. It consisted of eliminating most grains, along with milk products.

It sounded rather simplistic to Lynne. But what did she have to lose?

She tried it. A few days later she woke up–and it was *morning*. Paul had slept through the night.

The next day, while they were riding on a bus, Paul looked at Lynne–right in her eyes–and said, "I hungry." He was *there*.

"Paul? What? *Hungry?*"

He was gone again.

Lynne turbocharged her efforts to find a medical treatment for autism, and discovered a nurse in New Jersey who knew more about the disease than anyone Lynne had ever met. "There's a doctor you should consult," the nurse said. "He's in a little town called Rhinebeck, up in New York. His name is Ken Bock."

"Does he have a treatment?"

"He has *recoveries*."

Syracuse, New York

When the ugly rash on Kevin Densak's head and back hit the one-year mark, his mother knew she needed to find a new doctor. She had already seen a dozen doctors about Kevin's rash, and his other problems, including hyperactivity and chronic diarrhea, but nobody knew what to do. The dermatologist had given Kevin a cream for the rash, the pediatric gastroenterologist had prescribed a thick white liquid for the diarrhea, and the family doctor had given Kevin medication for the hyperactivity, but nothing had achieved lasting results. The treatments for some problems had even made others worse.

The doctors had put two diagnostic labels on Kevin: ADHD, and Asperger's syndrome, which is a type of autism. But the labels hadn't helped him heal.

Kevin's rash of red, circular welts blanketed his back, and was starting to migrate to his neck and head. It was making his hair fall out, and was creeping into the corners of his eyes. His preschool teacher told Kevin's mom, Denise, that if it got worse, Kevin would have to leave school.

But Denise knew that Kevin *needed* the structure of that school. Two years earlier–right after his measles shot–he had suddenly become almost uncontrollable. He now careened around in whirlwinds of pointless motion, destroying things, angering people, not listening, and losing his temper. He was a *wreck,* and he was getting worse as he grew older, not better. Lately, he was waking up at 4:00 A.M. every night, laughing hysterically. It was chilling to be awakened in the dark by that laugh.

One weekend, Denise drove all the way to Boston to attend a conference on hyperactive kids.

At registration, Denise asked a coordinator which speeches she would suggest.

"You should definitely go to this one," the coordinator said. "It's by Dr. Kenneth Bock. You'll hear things you've never heard before."

Livingston, New York

It was the worst night ever for little Keri O'Mara, and that meant it was the worst night ever for her mom, too. To Keri's mom, Donna, the only thing worse than the suffering of a child was the pain of the parent who had to watch it.

Keri's eyes were wide with fear and hurt as she fought for air. Donna held her, trying to somehow absorb some of Keri's pain into herself, and trying to transfer some of her own strength into her little girl.

For the past hour, ever since Keri had awakened in the middle of the night wheezing, she had been struggling to force enough breath into her lungs to keep from passing out. If she blacked out, there was always the chance, with asthma as severe as hers, that she would die. Keri's diaphragm and chest were exhausted, and exhaustion is the leading cause of death from asthma.

To Keri, it felt to her as if someone were smothering her with a wet pillow. Keri felt the shock of this slow drowning all over her body, even in her toes and face, which were beginning to turn purple. The pain in her chest—the one that she called the zipper pain, because it felt as if her lungs were zipped shut—was worse than ever. It was even worse than it had been during the times when her chronic lung infections had flamed into full-blown pneumonia, causing her chest to gurgle with algae-colored mucus.

Was it time to rush Keri to the hospital? Donna didn't know. The doctors there couldn't do much more than she could do here, with the nebulizer, the inhaler, and the standard meds.

Donna shepherded Keri to the bathroom and blasted hot steam into the bathtub as Keri hunched over the sink. Keri vomited from the congestion in her throat and from the spasms that choked her chest. Her red, curly hair stuck to her chalky face.

When Keri's stomach was empty the vomiting subsided, and she started getting a few gulps of air. Then a few more.

.   When it was over, Donna lay in bed with her eyes open, listening to Keri's room with the baby monitor. It was quiet, but Donna kept getting up to check. Quiet might not be good.

The next morning, Keri's pediatrician, a doctor Donna genuinely loved for the times he'd saved Keri from acute crisis, looked sad and bewildered.

"I can't help anymore," he said. "I need to refer you to a colleague. He seems to help kids that nobody else can. He mostly works with autism, but he gets results with asthma, too. And he's close. Up in Rhinebeck."

Rhinebeck, New York

I arrived at my office early in the morning, as usual, but by the time I got there, the waiting room was a scene of controlled chaos, as it often is, with autistic kids and hyperactive kids bouncing around, heedless of their mothers' admonitions, and asthmatic and allergic kids coughing and wheezing.

"Dr. Bock," my receptionist said, "your first patient is ready. It's Paul Avram. He's here with his mother, Lynne."

Little Paul Avram was very withdrawn when he and Lynne sat down in my office for his first visit. He wouldn't look at me. His eyes were dead as marbles.

This was a few years ago. It was at the same time that I also met Keri O'Mara and Kevin Densak. I recall that it seemed slightly unusual to be seeing only kids from my own part of the country, because I tend to treat children from all over America and throughout the world. When I first opened my clinic with my brother Steven, about twenty years ago, I would never have predicted that we would someday have an international clientele, but that's how it's turned out. Families come from afar to see me because, over the years, I have developed a very special treatment program: *a biomedical program for autism. This same program has also been extremely successful for children with ADHD, asthma, and life-threatening allergies.*

These four disorders–the 4-A disorders–are the new childhood epidemics. All four can destroy children's lives.

Just when modern medicine had almost eradicated the traditional childhood epidemics of measles, mumps, rubella, diphtheria, polio, and tetanus, these even more insidious new disorders began to haunt our children with unprecedented occurrence.

The end of one set of epidemics and the beginning of the other was not a coincidence. The medical technology that defeated the old epidemics was created by America's burgeoning industrialism, and this industrialism also created the ubiquitously toxic environment that has indirectly triggered the new epidemics.

Furthermore, the immunizations that were directly responsible for ending the old epidemics were also directly responsible for helping to create the new ones. The newspaper reports and parents' accusations that you may have heard are true: *Vaccinations, administered with toxic levels of mercury in them, helped cause an epidemic of autism.* They also contributed to the new epidemics of ADHD, asthma, and allergies.

The tragic irony of this would be overwhelming, except for a single, salient fact: *The new epidemics can be defeated. They are epidemics of metabolic dysfunction and toxicity, and they can be overcome by rebalancing the metabolism, and reversing that toxicity.*

Most doctors don't yet realize this. Some doctors, however, do realize it, and I have worked with these doctors to develop a new pediatric Healing Program, which has had unprecedented success. By reversing metabolic dysfunction and reducing toxicity, I have helped a robust percentage of my young patients to achieve remarkable improvement, and even full recoveries.

Treating these four new epidemics is quite complex, and can often be baffling. However, in plain English:

- **Autism can be reversed,** especially in young children who regress after a period of apparent normalcy. The conventional belief that it is biomedically untreatable is wrong. Children with other disorders on the autism spectrum, including Asperger's syndrome, can also greatly benefit.

- **ADHD can be reversed** in many children, without Ritalin or other drugs that may have significant risks of adverse effects, and be required throughout life.

- **Asthma can be reversed,** even when it is so severe that it's potentially fatal. Asthma is generally caused by many of the same factors that cause autism and ADHD.

- **Allergies can be reversed,** relieving kids of terrible symptoms that make them miserable, stunt their development, and sometimes even kill them. Allergies also contribute to full-blown autism, ADHD, and asthma.

I *know* that these reversals can occur, because I have helped to *make* them occur a great many times.

As I developed my Healing Program, I also became aware of another fact that is still unknown to the majority of physicians: There is a powerful link–of both cause and recovery–among autism, ADHD, asthma, and allergies. To most casual observers, and even to most doctors, these 4-A conditions appear to be largely unrelated. However, beneath the surface there is an unmistakable, unshakable web of interrelationship among the 4-A disorders, characterized primarily by toxicity in the brain and body, which causes metabolic dysfunction. For example, food allergies–which can profoundly affect the brain–can grossly exacerbate not just autistic symptoms, but also ADHD symptoms, and also asthma. In addition, severe ADHD can so closely mimic autism that I personally have come to consider severe ADHD as part of the autism spectrum. Also, simple deficiencies in brain nutrition, caused by our unhealthy and often toxic food supply, can contribute to the onset of not only full-blown autism, but also ADHD, allergies, and asthma.

The causal links among these disorders go on and on. These links even extend, to a significant degree, to other modern childhood epidemics, including those of learning disabilities, depression, teen suicide, substance abuse, speech pathologies, diabetes, childhood obesity, and recurrent ear infections. It is not your imagination: All of these problems are on the rise, some are running wild, and many are intimately related.

Because there is such a strong common denominator of toxicity and metabolic failure among the 4-A disorders, there are many common traits and experiences among the children who suffer from these disorders. When I first meet these children and their parents, they often seem to feel completely isolated, as if their ordeals are cruelly unique. But even during that first visit, they usually begin to see that *they are not alone.*

If a child you love has one of these problems, this program can probably help your family, too. We're *all* in this together. We all love our children. And we *can* defeat the disorders that are limiting their lives.

CHAPTER TWO

THE HEALING PROGRAM

Finding Paul

I LIVE MY PROFESSIONAL LIFE IN AN ATMOSPHERE PERMEATED BY pain, working with families who are still often shocked by the depths of their own suffering. But I also work in an atmosphere that is charged with the most generous and powerful form of love that exists, the love of a parent for a child. The moms and dads I meet, like so many parents, would gladly take on *all* of their children's pain, if only it were possible. Love is the only thing that brings children to my office. The parents I meet are extraordinary.

When I break through the barrier of aloneness that surrounds these parents, I never forget the experience. I still remember Lynne Avram's first visit quite distinctly.

She and I began to go through my standard work-up. It covers the fundamental physical aspects of autism, which have traditionally been ignored in conventional autism treatment.

"Has Paul had bowel problems? Chronic diarrhea?"

"Yes, chronic diarrhea."

"When did this begin?"

"Right after his MMR shot, March before last."

"Was he sick when he had that immunization?"

"He had a cold. They said it didn't matter."

"And did he get sick more frequently after that?"

"Much more."

"Does he often show signs of inflammation?"

"*Yes*, in his ears, his skin, and his bottom."

"Food allergies? Food cravings?"

"Definitely allergic to dairy and wheat. *Loves* his chicken nuggets. *Is all this common?*"

"It seems to be."

She told me more about Paul's life—the story I told you—and by the end of it I was certain that Paul had a clear case of regressive autism, a disorder in which children begin to develop normally, but then regress severely after a sudden assault upon their vulnerable, undeveloped systems. Regressive autism is the type of autism that has soared in incidence over the past twenty years. It now accounts for the vast majority of all current cases. The incidence of kids actually being born with autistic symptoms, which is known as classic autism, is still extremely rare.

In Paul's case, as in those of many autistic kids, one of the primary assaults on his system was probably from vaccinations that contained high levels of toxic mercury. This assault appeared to have harmed his brain and the rest of his body. The net result was chronic physical distress, accompanied by profound, secondary psychiatric symptoms. Autism is still classified as strictly a psychiatric disorder, but that's a diagnostic error. It certainly doesn't start from emotional problems. It starts from physical harm to the brain. Therefore, it's actually a *neurological* disorder. More specifically, it's a *neurotoxic* disorder, because it's caused primarily by the presence of destructive elements that injure the brain:

- Toxic chemicals.
- Viruses.
- Incomplete proteins.
- Inflammation.
- Immune cells that attack the brain.

These harmful forces wreak havoc upon the brain, and also cause terrible damage to the rest of the body. They are especially damaging to the very sensitive gastrointestinal systems and immune systems of young children. That is why I consider autism to be a three-faceted illness, with direct damage to:

The immune system.
The gastrointestinal system.
The nervous system.

After these three systems have been damaged, they begin to further injure one another, in a vicious spiral of interwoven destruction. This destruction includes:

- Inflammation of the brain and gut.
- Viral infiltration of the brain and gut.
- Severe nutritional deficiencies.
- Food reactions that have neurological consequences.
- Autoimmune attacks upon the brain and body.
- Immune system overactivity and underactivity.
- Undernourished muscle tissue.

Unfortunately, most of these problems can not be easily observed. All that can be readily seen is the behavior that they cause.

I have trained myself to be a medical detective, however, and to see beneath the surface of this behavior, and solve the underlying root problems that result in the misclassified, misunderstood, dooming diagnosis of autism.

As Lynne and I talked, Paul stared off into space, oblivious to us and to the toys that are in my office. He kept repeating the same gesture with his hands again and again, an autistic trait that's called stimming, because it stimulates these children's brains. He also kept saying the same sound repeatedly, which is known as perseveration. Doing this seems to bring some sense of order to the chaos in these kids' minds. His belly was bloated, his eyes were watery, and he had poor muscle tone. But other than that, he was an adorable-looking little kid, with a sweet face, and I took an immediate liking to him, as I do to most kids. I believed I could help him, because his problems were so similar to those of other kids I've helped. Of course, by conventional medical standards, his recovery would be an absolute impossibility. However, the kids I work with often seem to achieve the impossible, no matter how hard it is for them. They're great kids.

Paul–the real Paul–was in that tortured little body somewhere, lost and alone, sad, scared, with an inflamed belly, a sore throat, a raw butt, aching muscles, a stuffy nose, a confused mind, and no way to tell his mom. He lived in a world of pain. But he lived in a world of love, too. That was easy to see. Lynne watched him tenderly, then looked at the floor and said softly, more to herself than me, "How did this *happen?*"

How It Happened

Contrary to conventional medical wisdom, the cause of autism is not primarily genetic, but is a complex combination of genetics and environment. Genetics, so to speak, load the gun, and environment pulls the trigger.

Genetics alone don't cause epidemics. Genetics are essentially constant from one generation to the next. Epidemics occur when genetic vulnerabilities are assaulted by *environmental changes*–introductions of a new virus, a new bacteria, or a new toxin.

The current rates of autism and the other 4-A disorders are now undeniably epidemic.

Autism has increased, according to most estimates, from approximately one in every 2,500 to 10,000 births to *one in every 150–166 births,* over just the past twenty years. This is a fifteen-fold to sixty-fold increase: 1,500 percent to 6,000 percent. Now at least a half-million American children have autism-spectrum disorders, and some experts believe it to be as high as 1.5 million. Better diagnosis does not account for this, because the diagnostic criteria have not changed significantly for many years. Besides, if this epidemic were just a matter of more accurate diagnosis during childhood, where are all the thirty-year-old autistics?

ADHD has increased by at least 400 percent over the same twenty years. Now, 3.5 million children suffer from it. The very worst symptoms of ADHD are similar to those of children on the autism spectrum. American kids now consume 90 percent of the world's Ritalin, the most popular ADHD medication.

Asthma has increased by 300 percent over the same time period, and asthma deaths have increased by 56 percent, despite improvements in acute crisis care. Now 6 million American kids have asthma.

Allergies have increased by 400 percent over this period. Now approximately 20 percent of all kids have some type of allergy. Peanut allergy, one of the most common fatal food allergies, has more than doubled since 1997. Two hundred people, many of them children, now die from food allergies every year.

Add together all of the children who have these disorders, and it comes to 20 million kids, or almost *one-third of all American children.* Of these 20 million, at least 10 million have serious problems: autism-spectrum disorders, ADHD, asthma, or severe allergies. These conditions limit their lives, define their identities, and haunt their families.

These new childhood epidemics were caused primarily by four fundamental, catastrophic changes in the environments of American children. I am convinced that I now know what these changes were, because of the clinical successes I have achieved by addressing the damage done by the changes.

THE FOUR CATASTROPHIC CHANGES

1.   Toxins Proliferated. Over the past 20 years, our water has become so increasingly polluted with hydrocarbons, pathogens, and waste that many people now buy it in bottles. Our air has been saturated with mercury from coal-burning plants, with IQ-damaging lead, with diesel exhaust (which is particularly linked to autism), and with other pollutants. In some cities, such as Leominster, Massachusetts, open smokestacks have created "autism clusters" of extremely high incidence. Furthermore, our oceans are so full of poison, especially mercury, that it's now unsafe to eat more than one can of tuna per week. Also, our foods have been fouled with chemicals, hormones, and antibiotics to a level that was unheard of twenty years ago. The total toxic burden on the average American is measurably higher than it was even ten years ago.

2.   Nutrition Deteriorated. The average intake of essential nutrients has steadily declined since the 1980s, and the eating of unhealthy foods has increased. Children, significantly more than adults, have been lured into the seductive sump of fast foods and processed foods. Obvious results, including obesity, are less destructive than subtle metabolic damage, which contributes to the 4-A disorders. Without the right nutrients, the body can't properly protect, detoxify, or restore itself.

3.   Vaccinations Increased. They *doubled* in number since 1991, which increased the load of toxic mercury, increased the frequency, and increased the probability of children receiving multiple vaccines in a single injection. Mercury has now been removed from most vaccinations. Many integrative physicians believe, however, that damage has already been done, although this perspective is controversial.

4. Ability to Detoxify Dwindled. The toxins that entered children's bodies over the past ten to fifteen years became more likely to *stay* there, due particularly to damage among millions of children to two important detoxification processes known as methylation and sulfation, which are responsible for removing mercury and other toxins. Ironically, a gross overload of mercury *debilitates* the process of methylation. Therefore, the increased presence of mercury, from the environment and vaccinations, has robbed many children of this protective process. My colleagues and I have learned how to restore it, though, and to help kids once again experience what I call the miracle of methylation.

These four catastrophic changes created a veritable perfect storm of physical and neurological insult, which struck hardest at our society's most vulnerable members: our children.

Adults have suffered, too, as is apparent in the rising rates of cancers linked specifically to toxins, such as bladder cancer and lymphoma. But kids, with their smaller bodies and immature metabolisms, have absorbed a disproportionate blow. As evidenced by the new childhood epidemics, children are our society's proverbial canaries in the coal mine, the probable harbingers of increased, widespread illness among all Americans in the future.

If any one of these four deadly changes had been avoided, the epidemics might not have occurred. The most easily avoidable, and therefore the most tragic, was the increase in immunizations, and the way these immunizations were administered. This was a classic example of a horrific mistake that seemed like a good idea at the time.

In 1991 the federal government, with seemingly good intentions, recommended inauguration of a new series of immunizations, for hepatitis-B, to begin on a child's day of birth. A year later the government added three new shots for a potent form of meningitis. In response to these recommendations, the medical profession and the pharmaceutical industry began to increase the use of multiple vaccinations in single injections to save time and money, and to ensure better compliance. Later, the government began to recommend annual flu shots containing mercury to all children who were six months or older, and to pregnant women.

This doubled the number of immunizations from eleven to twenty-two in a child's first eighteen months, and crammed them much closer together, which increased the vaccinations' toxic burden.

Most of these vaccinations contained a form of mercury called thimerosal, which is a preservative. It's long been known that mercury is the second most toxic substance on earth, after uranium, and is especially damaging to the human nervous system, because it tends to selectively lodge in brain tissue.

These extra vaccinations gave kids too much mercury. Even just the three vaccinations given to two-month-old infants contained *99 times* more mercury than the Environmental Protection Agency regards as safe. The amount of mercury given to newborns on their first day of life was *36 times* too much.

In addition, the viral material in the vaccinations can be toxic by itself, when immunizations are given in excess, or over too short of a time period, or to a child with an already compromised immune system. The viruses, plus the mercury, combine to create a double hit against the immune system, which can skew its normal function, making it too inactive to respond properly to even weakened viruses, or so overactive that it attacks healthy cells, including brain cells.

Astonishingly, no one in a position of authority, it now appears, ever made these simple observations about toxicity, or added the cumulative totals of mercury. Furthermore, no one made allowances for important extraneous factors, such as a child's illness at the time of vaccination, or the presence of other toxins that the child may have been exposed to.

The risks of the new vaccination programs were not brought to the attention of the public until years later, when journalists and public health advocates, including David Kirby, Dr. Stephanie Cave, Dr. Sidney Baker, and Robert Kennedy Jr., began to write about them.

By that time, terrible damage had been done. This lack of recognition by the medical authorities had caused a medical tragedy of historic proportions, which may even exceed other tragedies that have been caused by pharmaceutical medication, including the recent deaths of thousands of people from arthritis drugs and pain medications.

When legions of parents began to complain that their children had become ill soon after their vaccinations, while still controversial, the government studied the situation and in 2001 began to gradually phase thimerosal out of the vaccinations. Even with this gradual removal, however, the damage was done. Now there are countless new cases of autism, with more emerging every day, and there are also millions of other children with very serious cases of the other 4-A disorders, which are also partly due to the unsafe vaccinations.

Furthermore, the government *still* allows thimerosal to be put into flu vaccines, and still recommends these vaccines be given to children and pregnant women. In addition, health authorities still cling to the accelerated schedule of immunizations.

Despite all this, I am absolutely *not* anti-vaccination. I am simply in favor of *safer* vaccinations, administered properly, to healthy children, without thimerosal, over an extended time period. In this book, I will tell you about safer ways to have your children vaccinated. Please see Appendix #1 for more information.

The vaccinations, though, are by no means the only reason for the onset of the autism epidemic, or the other 4-A epidemics. The widespread exposure to environmental toxins from food, water, and air are a huge part of our current problem. Genetics are also partly responsible, and so is inadequate intake of detoxifying nutrients. All of these factors, working together, created this problem.

The problem, though, is not the focus of this book. The focus is the *solution:* the Healing Program.

THE HEALING PROGRAM

The Healing Program creates recoveries by:

- **Eliminating** further exposure to toxins.

- **Flushing** existing toxins out of the system, primarily by detoxification, and by restoring the miracle of methylation.

- **Healing** the damage that the toxins have triggered.

- **Restoring** proper function of the nervous system, the immune system, and the gastrointestinal system.

All of these goals must be met for recovery to occur, and only a comprehensive program can achieve this. Because my Healing Program is so multifaceted, it can help kids recover from not just autism, but also ADHD, Asperger's, asthma, and allergies, all of which have so many causal links.

Not all kids, however, need to follow every element of the program to recover. If a child's condition is relatively mild—such as a single food allergy or occasional asthma—the program can be simple. It might consist of just eliminating a particular food and taking some supplements. If the problem is more critical—such as autism, severe asthma, or life-threatening food allergies—the child may need to strictly follow a detailed program. That's what little Paul Avram had to do. But Paul and his parents, like so many of the families I work with, were fantastic about following the program.

The Healing Program consists of four synergistic elements. Following is a shorthand version of it. I'll give you all the details later.

THE HEALING PROGRAM

1. Nutritional Therapy

- **Whole, organic, nutrient-dense foods** must be eaten. Children must exclude tuna; avoid any meats that have been treated with arsenic, hormones, and antibiotics; and restrict foods with pesticides and herbicides. Wholesome foods have an extraordinary ability to restore proper metabolic function.

- **No allergenic foods** may be eaten. This includes foods that cause the sometimes more subtle reactions of food sensitivities and food intolerances. These allergenic foods can wreak havoc upon the brain.

- **Yeast-proliferating foods** must be avoided by some children, because excess yeast, or candida, acting as a fungus in the intestines, harms digestion and sends toxins to the body and brain.

• **Gluten-free, casein-free foods** must be eaten by the children who react to gluten and casein. This means no wheat, and no dairy products. In some kids, these foods cause horrible neurological and gastrointestinal problems.

• **Carbohydrates** are limited for some kids, to stabilize their blood sugar, and to improve the health of their gastrointestinal systems. Low blood sugar can trigger some autistic and ADHD symptoms.

2. Supplementation Therapy

• **Detoxifying supplements,** such as methyl-B-12, folinic acid, and dimethylglycine, are tremendous for restoring the detoxifying process of methylation.

• **Metabolism-supporting supplements,** such as multivitamins, antioxidants, and essential fatty acid supplements, kick-start the body's repair.

• **Energizing supplements,** such as carnitine and coenzyme Q-10, stimulate the proper function of energy-deprived cells in the body and brain, and help overcome autistic and ADHD symptoms.

• **Herbal supplements** help kill the fungi, parasites, and bacteria that attack the gastrointestinal tract and nervous system.

• **Probiotics,** such as acidophilus, restore proper digestion, and control yeast overgrowth.

• **Brain-supporting supplements,** such as phosphatidylcholine and amino acids, improve cognition and mood.

3. Detoxification

• **Chelation therapy,** an FDA-approved procedure for removing some heavy metals, has triggered many recoveries by eliminating excessive mercury and lead.

• **The miracle of methylation,** once restored, rescues innumerable children from severe problems. It can be boosted not only by supplements, but also by subcutaneous and intravenous administration of specific substances. So can the similar process of sulfation.

• **Stimulating the organs of detoxification and elimination,** including the liver, kidneys, colon, and skin, is very important, and can be achieved with uncomplicated lifestyle techniques, such as drinking extra fluids, and increasing a child's degree of sweating and detoxification with far-infrared saunas. As toxins exit the body, changes in behavior and cognitive ability frequently occur.

4. Medication

• **Antifungals,** such as fluconazole, kill the yeast and other fungi that can harm digestion and send disruptive partial-proteins and other toxins from the gut to the brain.

• **Antibiotics** can help kill the bacteria lodged in the gut that can impair immunity, and can trigger autoimmune responses. Certain antibiotics also kill neurotoxic bacteria.

• **Antivirals** can help overcome the various viruses that disrupt proper neurological, gastrointestinal, and immune function.

• **Anti-inflammatories** can directly fight inflammation in the brain, and also can decrease gastrointestinal tract inflammation, which can strongly contribute to impaired cognitive function.

• **Highly individualized medications** help various patients. These can include drugs ranging from psychoactive medications to antihistamines. There is no single magic bullet for any of the 4-A disorders, but a carefully chosen and monitored medication program can be a valuable contributor to healing.

This Healing Program, along with behavioral and educational interventions, are the treatments most kids need in order to recover, except for one other thing: their parents' love. Love—and all the attention, talking, teaching, helping, and work that comes with it—is the final element that brings these recovering children out of darkness, into light.

It was love, ultimately, that held the key to Paul Avram's recovery.

CHAPTER THREE

THE RESULTS

I KNEW PAUL AVRAM WAS LOST IN THE UNLIT CHAOS OF HIS OWN mind, but I didn't know quite how lost until I studied his lab work—work that no other doctor had yet performed. His mercury level was literally off the charts. He also had high levels of arsenic, as well as elevated cadmium, aluminum, and tin. In addition, he had enough lead to significantly lower his IQ. People often seem to think that kids need to eat paint chips to have high levels of lead, but that was only true in the long-ago days of fewer environmental pollutants.

Previous testing had shown that even though Paul mostly avoided dairy products, he still had enough maldigested partial-proteins from milk in his system to create pseudo-morphines, which can be so intoxicating that they make kids space-out into their own inner worlds, and become fascinated by mundane things, such as running water or the movements of their own hands.

Paul's overall metabolism was just a mess. He had numerous food allergies, gross deficiencies of many nutrients, and excesses of others. All of this was combining to bombard his brain and his body in endless cascades of related dysfunction. Despite the roundness of his yeast-infested, allergy-inflamed belly, the cells in his body and brain were starving. It was a wonder that he had any energy at all, or any ability to focus.

However, these were all problems that could be *fixed*.

Not easily, though. That was up to Lynne, and the strength of her love. She later told me that when she left my office that day, she felt totally overwhelmed by the changes she would have to make. She said that on the way home she felt like having a nervous breakdown. But then Paul would be stranded. She postponed it.

Gradually, though, the changes in diet, supplementation, detoxification, and medication began to take traction, as they generally do when moms, dads, and kids start fighting this disorder as if it were death itself. A few isolated words came. Touches. Looks. Play. Paul was *still Paul,* struggling to stay alive inside the solitary confinement of his own mind—and he was beginning to occasionally come outside of himself.

Paul had first seen me in the summer, when he was three, and by Halloween he was cognizant enough to go to the door and hand out candy. Lynne was thrilled by this simple act of normalcy. Shortly after that she and Paul drove up for another office visit.

He still looked lost, and he couldn't converse. His belly was bloated, and his diarrhea, which had abated, was back. He was fidgety, stimmy, and his eyes wandered aimlessly. But Lynne was buoyant about his improvement, and that was encouraging. Moms *know.*

I adjusted his program once again, adding several new nutrients, some of which are known to significantly boost the detoxifying process of methylation. Methylation is so powerful! I also recommended the use of chelation therapy, in which a substance called DMSA is administered, to help flush out heavy metals. In addition, I began to give Paul the medication known as secretin, which is a neurohormone that has many receptors in the brain's amygdala, a primary memory center that is closely linked to fear and to understanding facial expressions. In the late 1990s, a doctor had achieved some amazing results with secretin, and had promoted it as a magic bullet against autism. However, when studies were done, they were understandably inconclusive, since there *is* no single, isolated substance that can overcome this complex disorder.

More changes! More words. Better eye contact. Better behavior. More emotion. Increasingly complex thought processes began to occur, as Paul's educational therapy finally began to penetrate his mind.

On Paul's fourth Halloween, he dressed up in a costume and went trick-or-treating for the first time. It was a magical night for Lynne and Wesley. After so many years of Paul Duty, they were beginning to feel as if they had the chance to have a normal son. A normal family. A normal life.

Lynne brought Paul to see me right after Halloween, about eighteen months after his first visit. Paul was very introverted, emotionally flat, and evasive. He still had some skin problems, he had significant abdominal bloating, he suffered from poor digestion, and he had a tendency to tantrum. But before he left, Paul spoke to me. He pointed to the room in which he'd first had secretin administered, and said, haltingly, "I wanna *feel* better. In *that* room." Lynne was so proud of him. I was proud of both of them.

Right after Christmas, though, Lynne called in a panic. Paul was regressing, she said. He was losing his newfound ability to converse. He was turning into the old Paul. He threw fits. His stomach was grossly distended. He was pale, with dark circles under his eyes. Lynne and Wesley were back on Paul Duty.

It was bad news. The worst. What was happening? Had he just eaten more Christmas candy than he could handle? Or had something more threatening happened? I couldn't be certain.

Lynne made it very clear, though, that even with this setback, she considered Paul's treatment to have been extremely successful. Prior to it, he had been largely vacant from his own life, and now he *had* a life. Helping severely autistic children to at last reach out of their painful haze and be part of the world is always a blessing to the kids and their families. Even just helping a twelve-year-old autistic boy to finally get out of diapers can make a huge difference in the lives of that boy and his mom and dad.

I always hope for complete recovery, of course. That's the goal. But I'm always grateful for whatever degree of recovery the kids achieve. And their parents are invariably even *more* grateful.

Keri and Kevin

When you're a clinician, as I am, you can't allow yourself to become overly preoccupied with just one case, even one as important as Paul's, because too many other people depend upon you. Keri O'Mara and Kevin Densak were, during this same time, depending completely on me to help them recover from their respective cases of severe asthma and ADHD. Compared to Paul's situation, these kids' problems were less clinically complex, but to these children and their families, recovery meant *everything*.

Keri, whose asthma was so severe that it was life threatening, went on the Healing Program right around the time Paul did. Keri, of course, didn't have an autism-spectrum disorder, but labels like autism, Asperger's, and ADHD don't describe the real, root problems that most kids have. The real root causes of most of the 4-A disorders are metabolic dysfunction and elevated toxicity. At first, Keri had many of these same metabolic and toxic problems as Paul, though they had manifested themselves as asthma, instead of autism. Keri, I discovered, had food allergies that were so severe that they clogged her lungs with mucus. At one point the congestion was so out of control that Keri was tested for cystic fibrosis. The test was negative, but the doctors who administered it neglected to test her for the much more common condition of allergy. Modern medicine is often myopic, with doctors seeing the world only through the lens of their own specialty. Unfortunately, the new childhood epidemics are invariably caused by multiple factors, and require generalism, not specialism.

Keri's other problems included poor digestion, which was linked to her allergies. She also had a deficit of calcium, which was related to both poor digestion and to allergies. Furthermore, she suffered from severe inflammation, which was related to *everything*.

The key to treating Keri, as it is with practically every child I see, was to treat the whole person. Doctors need to treat the person that has the disease, not the disease that has the person.

After less than a year on the Healing Program, Keri's asthma went away almost *entirely*. It never came back, except for one minimal episode when she had bronchitis. Her health is now excellent, and she's finally free of the fear that just catching a cold could kill her.

I'm still in touch with Keri's mom, Donna, who says that Keri only vaguely remembers the crying at night, the choking, the vomiting, the "zipper pain," the gasping, and the burning feeling in her lungs. But Donna remembers every moment of it, and that makes every moment now that much better.

Kevin Densak, who'd been labeled with ADHD and Asperger's, was somewhat harder to treat. When he first saw me, he was still waking up in the middle of the night laughing hysterically, which was very disturbing to his mother, Denise. It was hard to even run simple tests on him, because he was always bouncing off the walls.

Kevin had many of the same problems that affect most of the kids I treat. He was very sensitive to wheat, gluten, corn, soy, and dairy. His previous testing had missed these sensitivities, though, because it had consisted of a standard allergy test that I consider incomplete for food reactions.

In addition, Kevin had a streptococcus bacterial infection, which was triggering an attack upon his brain. The name of the infectious disorder was PANDAS, which stands for Pediatric Autoimmune Neuropsychiatric Disorder Associated with Streptococcus. Many doctors are not familiar with it, but I've treated a number of kids who've had it. I gave Kevin the antibiotic Zithromax, followed by a long-term course of preventive antibiotics, and it really helped quell the infection and calm him down. I had to do this very carefully, though, because antibiotics are often harmful for kids with ADHD, Asperger's, and autism, because they kill healthy bacteria and promote yeast overgrowth in the gastrointestinal tract. They can also increase mercury toxification. In fact, it's not uncommon for kids to first show symptoms of autism-spectrum disorders after they've gone on a long course of antibiotics. To prevent the possibility of the antibiotics causing yeast overgrowth, or intestinal candidiasis, I gave Kevin the antifungal drug nystatin.

Kevin also went on a low carbohydrate diet, and took a form of B-12 called methylcobalamin, or methyl-B-12, which revives the miraculous process of methylation.

The last time I saw Kevin, he gave me a dazzling grin, sat down, and said, "Hi, Dr. Bock." I had a nice conversation with him, as one might with any well-behaved child. He was delightful to be around.

His mother, Denise, recently told me that Kevin still has to watch his diet, but that he never fights her about it, or sneaks food. On Halloween, he goes trick-or-treating, hands his candy to Denise, and says, "Give this to my brothers." How could you not love a kid like that?

Paul

I was right, thank God, about Paul's Christmastime regression. It was due to candy and cookies. Autistic kids are so sensitive.

Lynne redoubled her efforts, and the changes came faster and faster, and built upon one another. There is a terrible, powerful synergy to the causation of disease, but there is an even more dynamic synergy—driven by the positive force of life itself—to the process of healing.

As Paul continued his chelation, the mercury in his body decreased considerably, allowing the process of methylation to charge into overdrive. His gastrointestinal problems vanished. His skin became clear and his eyes glowed. His own metabolism was no longer his worst enemy. He played with other children, talked to his parents, and even started school in a mainstream classroom. He was still a little emotionally fragile, though, and would sometimes cry when Lynne left for work.

One day, though, as she was leaving, expecting the usual insecurity from him, he came to her and said, "Mama, when you go to work, I'm lonely. And when you're lonely, it means you love someone. I love you, and you will always be right here, in my heart. And you love me, and I will always be in yours."

Lynne felt as if she could not breathe.

Rhinebeck, New York

As the Healing Program has become increasingly effective over the past few years, I have become ever more busy, seeing kids from many different states and countries. I also now travel extensively, speaking about the program, and about the new childhood epidemics.

I consider myself one of the most blessed physicians in America, due to the success I have had in adapting the new approach of integrative medicine to our devastating new childhood epidemics. Just yesterday, I saw three autistic kids who had recovered: *three*–in one day! That's what can happen when you're a good medical detective, and keep looking for root causes. But I get tired. Sometimes, exhausted.

I was bone-tired the last time that I saw Paul Avram. A long day was waning, and with it, my energy.

Paul came in with Lynne. He looked great–pink and vibrant with health. He was in Little League, he skated, played hockey, played the strategy game Pokemon with his friends, and was a great student. He was doing all those boy-things that boys remember for all of their lives.

Soon he would be a fine young man, off on his own, and his suffering would seem like another life, long ago. Would he even remember me?

The second he saw me, he ran across the room and threw his arms around me. He held on for dear life, and didn't seem to want to let go. I didn't want to, either.

It was hard for me to believe that this was the same little Paul, who just two years before had been unable to give of himself at all. What a miracle he was! Tears burned at my eyes, but I blinked them back and swallowed. I tried to say something to Lynne, but failed and swallowed again. I could feel Paul's vast child's energy flow right into me. As Lynne stood above, I could also feel the powerful, flowering force of her mother's love.

These are the moments for which I now live. These moments, these mothers, these children: We all have so much, when finally connected, that we can give.

PART TWO

THE FOUR NEW CHILDHOOD EPIDEMICS AND THEIR CONNECTIONS

1. AUTISM

CHAPTER FOUR

MYSTERIES
AND MIRACLES

FLASHBACK: A DETECTIVE STORY

Milwaukee, Wisconsin, 2000

IT WAS ONE OF THOSE SLUSHY, SHINY MARCH DAYS IN WISCONSIN that was trapped between seasons, with hot sun casting cold shadows, and Megan decided to take Kyle out of the basement onto the porch, even though he might try to scream and run away. Megan usually stayed down in the basement with Kyle, because it was secluded enough to focus his mind and muffle his cries for help, but the basement could drive you mad as a hatter if you were down there long enough. Megan needed a change of scenery.

Out on the porch, little Kyle squinted against the yellow glint. He wanted to stay out and play all day, like a regular kid, instead of work, work, work, down in the basement. Years later, he would have no recollection of what it had been that he had wanted to play that day–maybe, hide 'n' seek, his favorite game. *Anything.* He just wanted to feel good, for once.

So he started formulating his request to stay outside. He knew he should ask nicely, because this was no time to get ignored by speaking in baby talk or bad-boy talk–and besides, he loved Megan. She was his teacher. He framed his ideas carefully, paused thoughtfully: Hauled off and smashed his fist into the side of Megan's head.

Kyle felt good. He was finally learning to express himself! Grown-ups *loved* that. Now, play-time!

Megan felt her temple turn hot and hurt but she kept a poker-face, because rule number-one of Applied Behavior Analysis was, *Don't reward negative behavior,* not even with negative attention.

"Time to go downstairs and work," Megan said calmly.

Kyle couldn't believe it. Now *he* was the bad guy?

"Time to go downstairs and work, Kyle."

Kyle was still mystified. Megan gave him his third directive, as per proper ABA procedure, then picked him up and lugged his dead-weight body down to the basement for what ABA called positive practice, which in this situation meant ordering Kyle to stand up and then sit down approximately one hundred times, in hopes that Kyle might associate his hitting her with this negative consequence. It was not punishment. Punishment was a concept Kyle couldn't begin to understand. This was just behavioral reinforcement, and in the year 2000–back in the Olden Days of autism treatment–ABA behavioral therapy was the absolute pinnacle of therapy: expensive, cutting-edge, medically approved, and fraught with promise.

But noisy. Kyle's shrieks–"*Mommy! Momeeee!*"–knifed through the floors and walls into just about every room in the house, and Megan was thinking, "Oh, God, poor Eric and Elizabeth"–Kyle's parents–"they must be thinking there's bloody murder going on down here." In fact, though, the whole positive practice exercise was as hard on Megan as it was on Kyle, because of course he wasn't cooperating, so every time she said "Stand up," she had to physically hoist his heavy little body–despite the fact that she was built along the lines of a chickadee–and it was like pumping sixty-pound weights for a half hour, except that the weights were squirming, and screaming at you.

Eric heard the commotion and got a familiar, sick feeling: Here we go again, another therapist bites the dust! Eric was paying a fortune for this therapy, but even from inside the house he had heard Kyle's fist crack into Megan's head, and he knew that nobody could be expected to take that kind of abuse forever. Except parents.

Eric's wife, Elizabeth, in another room, alone, doing laundry, felt desolate. What more could she *do?* The whole family already revolved around Kyle. Elizabeth had quit her job as an interior designer, and Eric's career was in tatters. He was a pro golfer, and had once had quite a glamorous future gleaming before him, but a golf career couldn't withstand the 24/7 demands of having an autistic son. So Eric had given up the only thing he'd ever loved doing–the sport that might have made him famous, just as it had made his mother famous—and now he managed a shoe store. Their daughter, a couple of years younger than Kyle, spent her days running away from Bully Brother. Family life now orbited around watching Kyle scream, melt down, hit people, and space out.

As the ruckus in the basement died down, Kyle realized that he'd lost another battle, for some mysterious reason. But he didn't feel sad, because he *never* felt sad. He had only one consistent, overriding emotion. Later on in his life, when he was asked to describe that emotion, he couldn't put it into words, because he hadn't had words to express it back when he'd experienced it. To describe the old feeling, he went, "*Grrrrr!*," making the sound of a snarling dog.

Elizabeth, folding clothes upstairs, trying to block the sound of her son's anguish, was on the cusp of desperation. ABA held some hope, but the greater reality was that nobody really had a *clue* about autism. It was just a mystery, they all said.

When Kyle Olson had first been tentatively diagnosed, during a thirty-minute evaluation back in late 1998, shortly before his third birthday, Elizabeth had assumed that the medical system would somehow solve the situation, if it happened to persist. Elizabeth believed in the medical system, and just about every other system. After all, she was successful, attractive, educated, Republican, well-bred, charming, and married to a handsome pro golfer. What system was *not* to believe in? How could her son—golden-haired, radiant, and preppy even as a toddler—*not* outgrow his delayed speech, emotional outbursts, and clumsiness?

That first diagnosis hit Eric harder, though, and right away. After it, he spent the next four days spontaneously erupting into tears. He had all the standard dad-dreams—of going fishing with his son, of teaching Kyle to play golf, and watching Kyle's first basketball game—but suddenly every dream was a torment. An image of him doing some guy-thing with Kyle would flash into his mind, and he'd collapse.

Then Elizabeth's mother was diagnosed with the autoimmune disease of scleroderma, and when it became clear that she was dying, Eric and Elizabeth back-burnered their despair and focused on the more immediate disaster. Scleroderma was a terrible way for Elizabeth's mom to have to die, as her immune system—already battered by rheumatoid arthritis and severe allergies—turned against her body, causing horrific inflammation, shrinkage of muscles, hardening of her skin, and multiple organ failure. The ordeal made Elizabeth start to worry about her family's genetics. Her grandfather had suffered a heart attack when he was only forty. Elizabeth didn't think any of this could have much to do with autism, but it still made her feel more vulnerable.

At about the same time, Eric's mother got sick. She began to experience the first symptoms of Parkinson's, the neurological disease characterized by muscle tremors, which was particularly cruel for her, since she'd been one of the great female golfers of her generation. She'd won the state championships of over half the states in the country, more than any other woman in history, but she was quickly being crippled by this terrible disease. Eric had to help out a lot with his mother's illness, because his father, understandably enough, wasn't dealing with it well. Eric's dad was a brilliant engineer—he could visualize things in his mind as if he were watching a computer simulation—but real-world people-problems weren't his forte.

Months passed. And Kyle wasn't outgrowing *anything*. They'd ask him if he'd prefer waffles for breakfast, or pancakes, and he'd reply, "Purple," if he replied at all. It was just as likely that he would struggle to answer, then freak out, smack everybody within range, and then hibernate into one of his obsessions, such as emptying the refrigerator of condiments, then filling it back up. Emptying, filling, emptying, filling, as Elizabeth watched in dismay. His memory was atrocious, and even though he was approaching his fourth birthday, he couldn't dress himself, and was so unresponsive to his name that they had him tested for deafness. Kyle could barely walk across the room without tripping over his own feet, and couldn't even hold on to a crayon. His flaccid little muscles couldn't begin to scale a jungle gym, and his neck seemed to have a hard time supporting his large head. His clumsiness was tough for Eric to watch, because Eric had been a physical savant—his mother's son!—blessed with grace even as a toddler.

Kyle often looked at his books—"reading in baby talk," as he later put it—but as soon as he got to the last page he'd hurl the book across the room, fetch it, read it again, throw it, read it, throw it, then finally hug it like a security blanket.

Eric and Elizabeth dreaded the specter of school, so to soften the blow they enrolled Kyle in an expensive, private preschool that was supposed to make extra accommodations for special children. Right away, though, Kyle went wild and bashed a bunch of kids over their heads with a broom handle, and got kicked out. Kyle was baffled by that. There he'd been, trying to make friends, by using the broom handle, but none of the kids had responded in an appropriate way at *all.* The teacher had *turned* on him. It made no sense. Everybody was against him.

He didn't really care, though. Whether people were nice to him or not, he still had that feeling of the snarling dog deep inside him all the time. *Nobody* understood that feeling. They all seemed to think it meant "mad." Mostly, though, it meant scared.

The only bright spot was that Kyle's health seemed to have stabilized. He'd been born ten days prematurely, and had been discolored with jaundice, apparently from an Rh blood type incompatibility, even though Elizabeth's doctors had tried to prevent the problem during her pregnancy by giving her an injection of the standard medication Rhogam, which contained mercury. As a baby, Kyle's immune system had seemed to be on permanent vacation. At four months, he'd started having ear infections, and had suffered through twelve of them, including three that had coincided with his scheduled childhood vaccinations. For years, he had practically lived on antibiotics. Lately, however, except for his muscle weakness, some eye problems, and some rather persistent diarrhea, he was a healthy kid. Thank God for that. In fact, Elizabeth and Eric, who shared a strong faith, thanked God for many things, including the strength of their marriage, which was somehow withstanding the stress. The divorce rate among parents of autistic kids, they had learned, was about 85 percent.

When Kyle reached age four, they scheduled him with the best pediatric neuropsychologist in the best hospital in the city. They had to wait three months to see her.

She looked professional, and tired. She ran a number of tests, including an IQ test, and finally called them into her office.

"Kyle is autistic," she said flatly.

"Is there a chance it's PDD?" Eric asked hopefully, referring to Pervasive Developmental Disorder, another diagnostic label.

"Autism *is* PDD."

"I thought PDD was milder."

"Some forms of PDD are milder, but autism is the most severe form of PDD." She was looking at Eric, he felt, as if he were The Idiot Dad.

"Whatever it is," said The Idiot Dad, "we want to beat it."

She replied something to the effect of, "Acceptance is always the best medicine." It sounded rehearsed. She smiled wanly at Eric, who now felt like The Idiot Dad In Denial.

"I read a study on the Internet that said Applied Behavior Analysis has helped some kids recover," said The Idiot Dad In Denial.

She didn't seem impressed, and essentially answered, "It's your money."

"What's his IQ?"

"Sixty-nine. Mild retardation."

"How high could it get with special education?"

"Sixty-nine."

"Is it at *all* possible to get it higher?" Eric asked.

"It would take a miracle." She stood.

Eric didn't bother to tell her that he believed in miracles, and in luck, too—and not just because of God. As the great golfer Ben Hogan once said, "Golf is a game of luck. And the harder I work, the luckier I get."

The neuropsychologist wished them luck, and ushered them out to her waiting room, which was crammed, mostly with kids she couldn't really hope to help. The autism tsunami was just beginning to crest, and it occurred to Eric that her career, like his, was probably taking a trajectory she'd never expected.

Eric didn't cry after that diagnosis. He was too pissed off. If there was *any* way he could save his son, he would do it. Elizabeth agreed absolutely. Other marriages were being destroyed by this, but theirs was being strengthened—purified and illumined by pain.

They quickly researched ABA and hired Megan to come in and work with Kyle a full forty hours every week, because the primary study on Applied Behavior Analysis with autistic children had indicated that the kids who got forty hours did better than those who only got twenty. That study was small, dated, and disputed, but at least it offered *some* hope. It had been done by UCLA psychologist Ivar Lovaas, who had created a system of teaching autistic children to do one tiny, little task at a time, a method he called Discrete Trial Training, and to reward the kids immediately upon every tiny, little achievement. The program was based on the concepts of the famous twentieth century behavioral psychologist B. F. Skinner, who'd created an approach he called operant conditioning, which said that people don't have to gaze into their navels and analyze their dreams to overcome negative behaviors, they just need to experience reward for good behavior and no reward for bad. Long before the year 2000, Skinner's approach had been eclipsed by the more popular Freudian-based school of Be Yourself psychology, but nonetheless, ABA seemed to be a good fit for four-year-old kids who couldn't speak and twelve-year-old kids who were still in diapers. Megan was great at the therapy—she had the patience of a saint, bruises and all—and she enlisted Eric and Elizabeth to uphold its consistency twenty-four hours a day. Elizabeth bought a three-ring binder and began to record every step with meticulous accuracy. The binder became the bible of Kyle's progress.

He slowly began to improve. The constant rewards for success— M&Ms, hugs, and high-fives—prompted more normalized behavior.

Even so, Eric would try to play catch with Kyle, and Kyle would just watch the ball bounce off his chest, with that funny, sideways glance of his. Eric would tell Kyle the story of Jonah and the Whale ten times in a row, then ask Kyle what the story was about, and get a response along the lines of, "Joe ate a fish. Candy lunch!"

The therapy was slow-going, and when it was time to establish consequences with the stand-up/sit-down routine, Eric worried that they were going off the deep end.

Then one day Elizabeth took Kyle to a McDonald's play area, a place she liked because he couldn't wander off. She was eating her hamburger when she heard a little girl start to wail, so she rushed over to see if her son had caused it. He had, of course—he'd smacked her right in the face—so Elizabeth went up to the girl's mother to offer the usual apology and endure the usual glare of what-kind-of-parent-are-you? She told the mom that Kyle had autism, as she generally did in these situations, and the mom looked startled. Her son had autism, too. They started talking, and the mom told Elizabeth that her son had improved on the gluten-free, casein-free diet.

Right away, Elizabeth stopped shopping just at Cub Foods, and for the first time in her life was going to health food stores, and being, like, a granola-mom—everything but the Birkenstocks. It felt weird. Then she told her doctor about it, and instead of him treating her like the long-suffering, good-Republican mom, as he usually did, he started treating her like The Crazy Mom.

It didn't matter. Kyle was getting better! It was hard to tell, because the changes were so subtle and slow, but Elizabeth's binder proved it. It showed that two months earlier Kyle had hardly been able to say one coherent word, and now he was stringing two words together in a relatively logical way.

But time was passing. Quickly.

In May of 2001, Elizabeth went to her first Defeat Autism Now conference, in Atlanta.

Shortly after that, she arrived in Rhinebeck.

Kyle still remembers the day of his first appointment.

He remembers: "In the morning, I was swimming underwater in the pool at the Holiday Inn. It was like that underwater scene in the fourth Harry Potter book, *Goblet of Fire,* where Harry walks into the lake at Hogwarts, looking stupid to everybody, while he waits for his magical powers to take effect."

He remembers: "Then mom and I went to the doctor's office. I'll always remember that. Because that was the day everything changed. *Everything.*"

Solving the Mystery

Okay, Detective, that's the story so far—right up until Kyle's first appointment with me in my Rhinebeck office—so how many clues about his condition did you notice? If you didn't pick up on too many of them, don't feel bad, because back in the dawning days of the new century, at Kyle's first appointment, when the Healing Program was in its earliest stages, I missed some of them myself.

Autism is baffling mostly because so *many* complex factors feed into it. It's not as if you can just isolate the autism germ and kill it.

Because of this complexity, if you have a child with autism or one of the other 4-A disorders, you're going to have to become a good medical detective and uncover your own child's unique clues, in order to help him or her heal. I'm going to help you, starting right now. In the next chapter, I'm going to show you how I uncovered the clues about autism that helped Kyle to recover, and that may help *your* child on his or her road to recovery. We'll do it systematically, step by step, the same way I did back then, with the help of brave and great kids like the amazing Kyle Olson.

Here are some of Kyle's clues that you may have noticed.

KYLE'S CLUES

- Kyle's family had a history of autoimmune disorders (scleroderma and rheumatoid arthritis), allergies, and neurological disease (Parkinson's).
- Kyle was exposed to thimerosal in utero, when Elizabeth was injected with Rhogam.
- Kyle had impaired immunity, as indicated by his vulnerability to ear infections.
- Kyle took multiple courses of antibiotics, which interfere with the excretion of heavy metals.
- Kyle got three vaccinations while he was ill with ear infections, and was taking antibiotics.
- Kyle had food allergies and bowel problems.

You probably missed other clues, though, just as I did when I first met Kyle. Here's the short version of the more obscure clues. I'll tell you more about them later, as together we unravel the mystery of autism.

THE HIDDEN CLUES OF AUTISM

• Kyle's family had a history of extremely early heart attacks, as do the families of about *one-third* of all autistic kids. The usual suspects in early heart disease are inflammation and impaired fatty acid metabolism, both of which also harm the brain.

• Kyle's vision was characterized by a sideways glance. Conventional wisdom says this is just avoidance of eye contact, a behavioral characteristic. However, if you keep sifting through the evidence, you'll find that this common sideways glance is also due to physical problems with vision, often caused by a gross deficiency of vitamin A, which is also a major immune system nutrient. Autistic kids are typically low in vitamin A.

• Kyle had chronic anxiety–the "snarling dog" feeling–which is extremely common among autistic kids. Most autistic kids aren't just emotionally numb, they're *hurting*. Frustration? It's more than that. It's also because of neurological imbalance: overstimulation of their brain's primary fear center, the amygdala, which is also associated with memory. Many of the annoying, compulsive acts of autistic kids are just physical expressions of their nervousness and anxiety. We must never forget that most of these kids don't behave well simply because they don't *feel* well.

• Kyle had a terrible memory, and it was *not* due to mild retardation, because his IQ did shoot up dramatically during his biomedical treatment. In my experience, most autistic children, contrary to popular dogma, do not have mental retardation, and can be quite intelligent. Again, the ringleader that hijacked Kyle's memory was probably his brain's amygdala, which was, in effect, too busy with fear and not busy enough with memory. This hijacking was, in all likelihood, aided and abetted by poor function of his brain's main neurotransmitter of memory, acetylcholine, which is manufactured from the nutrient choline. Interestingly, though, almost 10 percent of autistic kids have savant-level memories, like the movie character in *Rain Man*. This is yet another indication of neurological imbalance. Autism is not purely a matter of deficits, but also excesses. With proper biomedical treatment, however, some of these excesses can be alchemized into gifts. Kyle was—not incidentally—gifted, beneath his deceiving veneer of dysfunction.

• Kyle's grandfather had an extraordinary ability to visualize things. This trait is intimately associated with autism, and has a genetic component. Also, Kyle's grandfather was an engineer, and one of the aphorisms of autism is, "Look back a generation or two, and you'll find an engineer." This is not, of course, an indictment of high-tech people, but is an indication that special gifts often come at the cost of balance. Nonetheless, in a great many cases, as these kids begin to recover, the gifts they've gained become well worth the prices they've paid.

• Kyle had an unusually large head, a relatively frequent trait among kids on the autism spectrum, and one that some people think tends to confer intelligence. One theory about autism is that autistics have so *many* neuronal connections that they are easily overwhelmed. One of the most common physical characteristics of autistic people is that they tend to have larger brains than most other people.

• Kyle was unusually clumsy. That's a classic trait of Asperger's, not autism, but I'm convinced that the diagnostic labels of kids on the autism spectrum are often arbitrary. I see the autism spectrum as fluid, not fixed, because I've seen so many kids progress from frank autism, to mild PDD, and then to normalcy, as their metabolic functions stabilize. Furthermore, it's not at all uncommon for gifted kids, such as Kyle, to be uncoordinated. Once more, it's a matter of balance. A deficit in one area can cause a surplus in another. As health returns, this surplus can become the child's greatest source of satisfaction.

• Kyle was a boy, and boys suffer from autism approximately 400 percent more often than do girls. One theory is that male hormones tend to increase the toxicity of mercury.

. . . So many clues. . . . So much mystery. Where to begin? Where would it end?

At the beginning of that very first meeting Kyle tried to settle into his chair, but he was so tense that he just teetered on the edge of it, his arms clamped to his sides. He was a block of rigid muscles and right angles. Once in a while, I caught him glaring at me out of the corner of his eye.

CHAPTER FIVE

WORKING THE CLUES

Rhinebeck, New York

Kyle's First Appointment

"WHERE DO WE BEGIN?" ELIZABETH ASKED AS SHE OPENED HER three-ring binder.

"With tests," I said.

"We've already done most of them," Elizabeth replied, flipping through the binder for the results.

I explained that my tests were not the standard behavioral analyses, which are important in their own sphere, but limited. Those tests generally don't diagnose a medical problem that can be solved, but merely describe the behavior that the problem is creating. There's a tendency in psychiatry to isolate a problem, such as social anxiety, stick the word "disorder" behind it, and end up with a neatly packaged "diagnosis"– Social Anxiety Disorder–which explains *nothing* about the root cause. I believe in finding root causes. A good diagnostician is a good detective.

So I started Kyle's treatment by giving him a battery of basic tests– of his blood, urine, and stool. I monitored his liver enzymes, nutrient levels, detoxification ability, and gastrointestinal function. In medical jargon, I was looking for elements of co-morbidity–problems that existed at the same time as his autism, without necessarily being related to it. Autistic kids tend to have a number of co-morbidities. At least, that was my thinking back then, and that perception is still conventional wisdom among most physicians. However, if I'd known then what I know now, I would have realized that almost all of Kyle's ancillary problems were actually contributing to his autism.

It's still common these days for most doctors to overlook these contributory problems, because each problem by itself is usually insufficient to cause a major malfunction of the brain. However, my training–even at this early stage of my investigation of autism–had left me reluctant to ignore even small, seemingly unrelated problems.

Similarly to most doctors, my medical school training had emphasized the value of specialization, and of breaking down problems deductively, piece by piece, with Cartesian logic, until each part of the problem was separate and distinct, and thus ready for a very specific treatment. I found this way of looking at the human body to be an elegant and promising theoretical construct.

However, after I graduated, and began to try to heal real people in the real world, I found that even though I could suppress their isolated symptoms with highly specific medications and procedures, my patients' underlying conditions tended to remain. It became clear to me that to really heal people, I needed to address their entire biological systems, since each separate element of their bodies was intimately connected to the other elements, through vast and sometimes mysterious networks of nerves, ducts, blood vessels, genetic codes, feedback loops, nutrient channels, hormones, and neurotransmitters. The leg bone, as they say, is connected to the thigh bone.

I realized that I needed more education. For the next two years, I spent most of my time studying nutrition, immunity, metabolism, and the body's own astonishing healing mechanisms.

In these early days of my practice, in addition to prescribing standard medication, I began to apply comprehensive programs of dietary modification, nutritional supplementation, stress management, detoxification, and lifestyle alteration, and I started to get far better results. I was finally achieving notable clinical successes against complex, chronic, intractable conditions, such as fibromyalgia, asthma, recurrent infections, and chronic fatigue syndrome.

My work with modulating immunity attracted the attention of some of the doctors who were members of Defeat Autism Now, because these doctors believed that impaired immunity was a common trait among autistics. They invited me to speak at a DAN conference, and soon several parents came to me to treat their children. As these children began to show significant improvement, more parents brought their children. One of those parents was Elizabeth.

As Elizabeth and I talked, Kyle fidgeted fitfully, and began pulling things off my desk and examining them distractedly out of the corners of his eyes. He kept pressing his hands together compulsively, stressfully. Kyle seemed to be trapped somewhere between anxiety and oblivion. I spoke to him, but it was like talking to a television set that squawked back at you without registering a word you'd said.

These days, years later, Kyle can no longer recall exactly what he'd been thinking about during that first appointment, except that it had been during the time when he'd had "bad thoughts, all the time, that just kept coming, again and again and again."

Where do you *start* with a kid like that?

Elizabeth wanted to start with chelation. Like many mothers of autistic children at that time, she had heard rumors and reports that childhood vaccinations sometimes triggered autism by poisoning children with heavy metals, which could be removed by chelation.

I had read similar reports in the emerging biomedical literature on autism, and had begun to test that theory. But it wasn't appropriate for Kyle at this point. His lab work had revealed that he had significantly elevated fungal markers in his urine, indicating heavy overgrowth in his gut of yeast, or candida. All the antibiotics he'd taken had probably caused it, because they kill not only disease-causing bacteria but also healthy bowel bacteria, allowing yeast to take over. I knew that if I gave Kyle a standard chelating agent, such as DMSA, which contained sulfur, it would probably upset his GI tract even more. Chelation would have to wait.

Even so, I thought that just getting rid of the candida overgrowth would be a good place to start. In adult patients, I'd seen remarkable results from clearing candida overgrowth. It had helped some patients with chronic fatigue syndrome to quickly feel much better, and it had even helped some people overcome mental and emotional problems, such as depression, anxiety, lassitude, and impaired cognitive function. These problems can be caused when toxins created by yeast metabolism enter the bloodstream and invade the brain. They can also be triggered when yeast harms the walls of the intestines, and allows partially digested food molecules to enter the system, and create cerebral allergies.

If this was, indeed, happening to Kyle, it would not be an uncommon occurrence. Millions of people, often unknowingly, suffer serious problems due to yeast overgrowth—known as fungal dysbiosis. This happens not just because of antibiotic use, but also because many people consume large amounts of yeast-stimulating products, such as breads, sugar, and fermented foods. As you do your own detective work on your kids, look for the following clues, which reveal yeast overgrowth.

FUNGAL DYSBIOSIS
Caused by Yeast Overgrowth

Clinical clues:

- Recurrent infections.
- History of frequent antibiotic use.
- Chronic diarrhea.
- Constipation.
- Decreased cognitive function, or brain fog.
- Gas, bloating, and abdominal discomfort.
- Low energy.
- Depression or anxiety.
- Decreased cognitive function.
- Fatigue.
- Chronic sinus congestion.
- Itching in the vagina, anus, or in other mucosal membranes.

I prescribed Nystatin for Kyle's candida overgrowth. Another choice could have been Diflucan, as I'll describe in the chapter on medication. These meds are typically given in very short courses for simple vaginal yeast infections, but require more prolonged use for chronic candida overgrowth, with systemic symptoms. I also put Kyle on a yeast-free diet (see Chapter 17), along with probiotics and herbal antifungals (see Chapter 18).

In addition to this anti-yeast nutritional therapy, I boosted Kyle's intake of vitamin A, which his tests had indicated was extremely low. I also fine-tuned his diet, to help heighten his body's capacity for self-healing, through the natural mechanisms of restoration and balance, which some doctors refer to as "the wisdom of the body."

That was it: end of appointment. Elizabeth seemed a little disappointed that we hadn't taken more dramatic measures. However, I believe in introducing therapies one at a time, to keep from overwhelming the body with change, and to help me ascertain what is really working.

By the end of the appointment–during which Kyle had stayed completely disconnected–I was convinced of only one thing: His behavioral therapy, by itself, would never be enough to help him heal. He had already been through a year of ABA, and his improvements had been slow and inconsistent.

Even during this early period of my treatment of autism, I was growing increasingly convinced that *autism is not a psychological disorder, and can therefore not be reversed using only behavioral, psychological therapy.* As a stand-alone treatment, it is simply inadequate. Many psychologists and therapists think it is adequate on its own, but I must respectfully disagree.

Behavioral therapy can be of *great* value, though, when it's applied in conjunction with biomedical treatment. The biomedical treatment heals the brain's hardware, so to speak, while the behavioral therapies improve its software, or thinking processes. *Both must be addressed.* By the time that some kids' brains start to heal, they are years behind in social and intellectual development, and they need help to catch up. In many cases, their hardwiring is so damaged that they even need to forge whole new neuronal pathways—new ways of solving old problems. In a way, they're rather like some stroke victims—still capable of learning, but not in the damaged portions of their brains.

Here are the most common and helpful forms of nonbiomedical therapy.

BEHAVIORAL, DEVELOPMENTAL, AND CLINICAL THERAPIES

Applied Behavior Analysis, or ABA, uses positive reinforcement to teach kids new skills and better behaviors. Kyle was helped immensely by ABA, but much of the benefit came after his biomedical treatment had begun.

Floortime is a spontaneous, play-based therapy that capitalizes on each child's own favorite activities.

Occupational Therapy is not job-related, despite its name, but encourages kids to become well-rounded, and better at fine motor skills.

Speech and Language Therapy is essential for autistic children, due to their language delay and speech problems. This therapy also helps them to better recognize facial expressions and body language, which is hard for most autistic kids (probably because this brain function occurs primarily in the amygdala).

Sensory Integration Therapy uses games and exercises to help kids block extraneous sensory input, and focus on what's important.

Physical Therapy focuses exclusively on motor skills, such as eating and drawing, and on the development of coordination, balance, and strength. Kyle did a lot of physical therapy, and got a great deal of good out of it.

Relationship Development Intervention helps kids learn to relate better to other people, using specific games and exercises.

That first appointment was primarily a fact-finding mission. The appointment mostly just confirmed my belief that it is very difficult to heal autistic kids using only behavioral therapy.

I was optimistic, though, about Kyle's treatment. In fact, I was excited. Next time, if the yeast had cleared, I would start chelation, to try to reverse the condition that my colleagues and I consider to be one of the root causes of many cases of autism: heavy metal overload, including mercury toxification–part of it due to childhood vaccinations.

I couldn't wait to see what would happen. But what did happen caught me totally offguard–and not in a good way.

CHILDHOOD VACCINATIONS

Are We Poisoning Our Children?

The common heavy metal mercury has been employed industrially since the 1800s, when hat makers used it to manufacture felt. Many hat makers, however, were poisoned by inhaling mercury, which is more toxic than any substance on earth, except for uranium. They began to experience acute memory loss, poor cognitive function, speech problems, anxiety, irritability, loss of coordination, and depression; symptoms that gave rise to the phrase "mad as a hatter."

Mercury was first used medically in the 1800s by American dentists trying to avoid the expense of gold dental fillings. To save money, they used an amalgam of silver, combined with mercury, then commonly called quicksilver, or quacksilver. The early governing body of American dentists, however, disapproved of using this toxic quacksilver. They coined another new phrase of the era, by calling the dentists who used it "quacks."

Until around the mid-1900s, it was a popular practice among the general public to use minute amounts of mercury as an antibacterial agent, in products such as Mercurochrome and Merthiolate, but this fell out of favor, due primarily to issues of toxicity and the burning of the skin.

Mercury, however, has enjoyed its greatest success as a preservative used in vaccinations. It was first used this way in the 1930s, when a form of it known as thimerosal, which contains 49.6 percent mercury by weight, was produced by the Eli Lilly pharmaceutical company. There were, understandably, early signs of toxicity. In one of the first studies on thimerosal, twenty-two already ill patients were injected with it, and all twenty-two died within weeks. When used in smaller amounts, though, it appeared to cause no immediate harm to adults.

In a 1935 study, however, approximately half of a group of dogs injected with thimerosal died, leading company researchers to conclude that thimerosal was "unsatisfactory as a serum intended for use on dogs."

Thimerosal was used by the military as a vaccine preservative during World War II, but the government required Eli Lilly to label stocks of it as "Poison." In 1967, a study showed that thimerosal caused mice to die when it was added to their vaccines, and in 1977, ten babies died in a Toronto hospital when it was used as an antiseptic on their umbilical cords.

By 1982 so many reports of toxic reactions had surfaced that the Food and Drug Administration proposed that thimerosal be banned in over-the-counter products, and in 1991 the FDA considered banning it from animal vaccinations. Even so, it remained a standard in human vaccinations, because it was unquestionably effective as a preservative. American health authorities, still traumatized by the polio epidemic of the mid-1900s, embraced the concept of vaccination, and were willing to accept the negative aspects of thimerosal as a reasonable element of the risk/benefit ratio.

However, even as further evidence of thimerosal toxicity kept accumulating, children began to be exposed to increasing amounts of it in vaccinations. For example, baby boomers who were born before 1963 received only one vaccination for polio, and one other combination vaccine for diphtheria, tetanus, and pertussis (DTP). By 1989, children were still only receiving three different vaccinations.

In 1991, though, the Centers for Disease Control recommended that all infants receive the hepatitis-B vaccine and the vaccination for HIB (*Haemophilus influenzae* type B). By this point, the number of childhood vaccinations had increased to more than twenty, and by the age of six months children were receiving:

- 75 micrograms of thimerosal from three DTP injections.
- 75 micrograms from three injections of the HIB vaccine.
- 37.5 micrograms from three injections of hepatitis-B vaccine.

This added up to 187.5 micrograms of thimerosal. In retrospect, it appears to have been too much.

This meant that six-month-old infants who received their vaccinations on schedule would get a mercury dosage that was 87 times higher than the guidelines recommended to adults for the maximum daily consumption of mercury in fish. The amount given on the day of birth alone was 36 times higher than the safety threshold recommended by the Environmental Protection Agency. The amount given to two-month-old infants was 99 times higher than the standard EPA recommendations.

Even in 1991, at the beginning of the era of the increased dosage of thimerosal, many industry leaders were worried about the effects that this amount of mercury might have upon children's health. A memo from a leading executive at a drug company that was dispensing thimerosal warned that, "The mercury dose appears rather large."

By the end of the 1990s, when there was an explosion in the incidence of autism, many parents blamed it on the vaccinations, because their children's health had seemed to deteriorate shortly after they had been vaccinated. The type of autism that increased most dramatically in incidence during this time is known as regressive autism. Children with regressive autism have no apparent symptoms at birth, but begin to drastically deteriorate around the age of approximately eighteen months.

At almost exactly the same time that the autism epidemic was unfolding, so were epidemics of ADHD, asthma, and allergies. I now believe, as do many others, that these other 4-A epidemics are also related, in part, to the increase in childhood vaccinations, which can trigger subsequent skewing of the immune system.

Despite the current preponderance of evidence, many people still think it is safe to administer vaccinations with thimerosal. They note, for example, that a can of tuna fish contains an average of 17 micrograms of mercury, compared to 12.5 micrograms in a single dose of the hepatitis-B vaccine. However, as the prominent physician Stephanie Cave, M.D., has pointed out:

- Because infants and children are so much smaller than adults, their bodies are more sensitive to toxins.
- When mercury is consumed in food, such as tuna, it is partially detoxified by the liver, and does less damage than mercury that is injected into the bloodstream.
- When an infant receives an injection of mercury, his or her brain has not yet fully developed the protective membrane known as the blood-brain barrier, and is therefore more vulnerable to toxins.
- Even older children's brains and organs are still developing, and these children are therefore much more likely than adults to be harmed by toxins.

One strong indication that mercury has probably contributed to the autism epidemic is the similarity of symptoms that are shared by people with autism, and people with mercury poisoning.

Dr. Cave, who was one of the first clinicians in America to make the connection between autism and mercury (along with Sallie Bernard, Lyn Redwood, and a few others) has classified these shared symptoms as follows:

SYMPTOMS OF AUTISM
Compared with Those of Mercury Poisoning

Symptom	Autism	Mercury Poisoning
Movement Disorders	Clumsiness, slow physical development, and difficulty swallowing.	Clumsiness, impaired development, and difficulty chewing and swallowing.
Movement Characteristics	Arm flapping, repetitive movements, abnormal gait, and walking on the toes.	Arm flapping, rocking, and walking on the toes.
Sensory Problems	Sound sensitivity, touch avoidance, and distractibility.	Sound sensitivity, touch avoidance, and abnormal sensations in the mouth and limbs.

Speech and Language Problems	Delayed speech, tendency to be verbally inarticulate, and difficulty in being clearly understood.	Loss of ability to speak, tendency to be verbally inarticulate, and difficulty in being clearly understood.
Cognitive Pathologies	Inattentiveness, poor cognitive processing, inability to grasp abstraction, and poor concentration.	Decreased intelligence, poor cognitive processing, and difficulty understanding words.
Physical Disorders	Poor muscle strength, dermatitis, bowel disorders, allergies, asthma, and autoimmune disorders.	Poor muscle strength, dermatitis and skin problems, bowel disorders, allergies, asthma, and autoimmune disorders.

In addition to the toxic reactions that vaccinations with thimerosal appear to have caused, subsequent live-virus vaccinations may have also caused problems. These vaccinations, which contain small amounts of living viruses, may have directly created infections—through viral material—in children's gastrointestinal tracts. One such virus that seems to have been particularly damaging, according to the pioneering research of Andrew Wakefield, M.D., was the live (but weakened) measles virus that's found in the combination vaccination for measles, mumps, and rubella (MMR). Just as mercury tends to lodge in the brain and nerves, measles virus has an affinity for the gastrointestinal tract. Some doctors now believe that in the GI tract this virus can multiply and cause chronic, subacute measles infection. This infection can then trigger inflammation in the walls of the GI tract, making these walls porous and allowing harmful toxins from the gut to enter the system. Some of the toxins that escape from the gut are bacteria, some are viruses, and some are morphine-like molecules known as caseomorphin and gluteomorphin, which can cause a type of intoxication. Dr. Wakefield believes that many of the children who experience almost immediate deterioration after their MMR vaccinations have been infected with this measles virus. This very sudden onset of symptoms is known to happen most frequently to children after their MMR vaccinations.

Thus, the vaccinations that contained thimerosal may have created a double hit against the immune system. (1) They assaulted the immune system with toxic mercury. (2) This was followed by injection of combined live viruses, which could not be effectively handled by a mercury-altered immune system.

Furthermore, the best recent research has pointed out yet another terrible problem that mercury can cause: It directly inhibits the body's natural ability to detoxify itself, through the processes of methylation and sulfation. In effect, it poisons the body, and then prevents the poisons from being excreted.

Not all children, of course, have been harmed by the heavy schedule of vaccinations that contained mercury. A disturbingly high percentage, though, seem to have been. One in 150–166 children show signs of autism, and a great many more suffer from ADHD, asthma, and allergies. When all of these maladies are combined, in both their mild and virulent forms, they are present in almost half of all American children.

This still means, though, that about half of all children were not susceptible. The factors that are believed to influence susceptibility are:

- Genetic predisposition.
- Illness during a vaccination.
- Acceleration of the vaccination schedule beyond the norm, to compensate for missed vaccinations.
- Taking an antibiotic at the time of vaccination.
- Exposure to other environmental toxins, in combination with the vaccination toxins.
- Exposure to toxins in utero.
- Nutritional deficits, or excesses.
- Exposure to other viruses and bacteria.
- Presence of other health insults, including candida problems and allergy.
- A family history of autoimmunity and allergies.

In short, the children who suffer the most destructive forms of these assaults are usually those who are situated at an ugly, unlucky nexus of genetics and environment. Thus, as many of the DAN doctors now say, in a phrase originally attributed to Sudhir Gupta, M.D., "Genes load the gun, and environment pulls the trigger."

However, even most children who have genetic vulnerability would probably still be able to remain healthy, if they were *not* exposed to mercury. This is apparent from two revealing studies of large groups of children who did not get vaccinated, and remained free from regressive autism. One group was that of the Pennsylvania Amish, who don't vaccinate their children for religious reasons. Over many years, they have had virtually no incidence of autism. The CDC has rationalized this absence of autism by saying that the Amish have a "genetic connectivity" that protects them. However, there is another large group of children who also haven't been vaccinated, due to conservative Christian beliefs, and this group shares *no* common genetics. This group of approximately 35,000 children, who belong to a home-schooling organization, is centered in the Chicago area. This group, too, has no recorded cases of autism. Furthermore, incidence of asthma, allergies, and ADHD is extremely low among this group, and is low among the Amish.

In the late 1990s, when tens of thousands of parents began to claim that vaccinations had harmed their children, the federal government investigated the issue and decided, in the year 2000, to phase out thimerosal from all vaccinations, except for flu vaccinations, which are still recommended for pregnant women and infants. This removal of thimerosal was also mandated by the governments of Japan, Russia, Great Britain, and all of the Scandinavian countries.

Despite this removal, however, the American government has steadfastly denied that the vaccinations, and the mercury in them, have caused the autism epidemic, or the epidemics of the other 4-A disorders. The government, in minimizing thimerosal's harm, has primarily cited several epidemiological studies done in Europe that seemed to indicate that thimerosal can be safely used in vaccines. Many American researchers, however, found these European studies to be very unconvincing, for various reasons. For example, the studies were examinations of vaccinations that contained far less thimerosal than that found in American vaccinations, and incidence of autism in the groups that were studied appears to be underreported, due to unrealistically strict definitions of the disease. There were also questions regarding methodology.

Shortly after its brief investigation, the U.S. government embargoed its own research statistics, and refused to investigate the issue any further. One particularly unpopular tactic the government used was passing an act called "The Eli Lilly Protection Act," as part of a Homeland Security law, which prohibited parents from collecting damages for children who had suffered vaccine-related brain disorders. The justification for the law was that if Eli Lilly were put out of business by lawsuits, it could not protect America from biological attacks by terrorists.

Although such institutional denial of the right of families to seek a remedy for the harm they have suffered may seem self-serving, it is understandable public policy that government and health care business would work in concert to protect themselves from what could prove to be devastating consequences.

Even so, I am not anti-vaccination. I am pro–safe vaccination. Vaccinations, it still appears, can be done safely and effectively, if they are free of thimerosal, and if they are administered on a prudent schedule, to healthy children, who have no extra risk factors. If you are a parent who must make this decision, please read Appendix #1, on the safer administration of vaccinations.

Kyle's Second Visit–Seven Weeks Later

With great anticipation, I started Kyle on his first chelation treatment, using DMSA to help remove the mercury and other heavy metals from his body.

He responded almost immediately. His improvement was marked.

I was bewildered.

I was very, very happy for Kyle. *But improvement from heavy metal detoxification absolutely cannot occur instantaneously. It takes time.*

I did not *know* why Kyle had improved. And therefore I couldn't be certain it would last.

I was back to the drawing board.

So, Detective, what do you make of *that*?

CHAPTER SIX

THE END OF
THE BEGINNING

Rhinebeck, New York

Kyle's Third Visit–Thirteen Weeks After His First

THE FIRST THING I DEDUCED FROM KYLE'S IMMEDIATE IMPROVEMENT was how *little* I still really knew about the terrible mystery of autism.

By the process of elimination, all that I had thus far confirmed was that:

• Kyle's autism was not simply a psychological and behavioral disorder, because psychotherapies and behavioral therapies were not adequately healing him.

• His condition was not principally due to the neurological effects of nutritional deficiencies, because his careful diet and supplement program were not correcting it.

• His autism had not been triggered primarily by the neurological consequences of candida overgrowth, because solving that hadn't dramatically helped him.

• His illness wasn't strictly a matter of mercury poisoning from vaccinations, because he had begun to improve *before* he'd had time to eliminate much mercury.

Autism is so baffling. It's no wonder that most doctors have found it so difficult to treat.

Elizabeth, though, at this third appointment, was bright with hope. "He's not melting down so much," she said, stroking Kyle's golden helmet of hair as he squirmed in his chair. "He's talking better. His mood's better. I feel like his true personality is finally starting to shine through."

I smiled at Kyle and tried to engage him, but he was still remote and wary, as if he couldn't tell if I were smiling or scowling, friend or enemy. He was fidgeting and flopping around my office like a fish on the shore, but at least he was making occasional eye contact with me. Also, he was no longer looking at everything sideways, with his peripheral vision, possibly because his vitamin A supplementation was finally healing the function of his eyes' cones and rods, the parts of the eyes that are often damaged in autistic children. The clues to Kyle's healing were slowly coming together. I'd recently learned, for example, that night blindness is common in the families of autistic kids, because of genetic problems with vitamin A metabolism. Dr. Mary Megson taught me that. She was part of the group of doctors who were, at this time, inaugurating the concept of biomedical treatment for autism.

It was time to introduce a couple of new measures. The first was administration of phosphatidylcholine. Phosphatidylchlorine is the main ingredient in plain old lecithin–the common supermarket supplement that helps dissolve fat in the bloodstream. It is also, though, the primary nutritional building block, or precursor, of the main neurotransmitter in the brain that carries thought and memory: acetylcholine. It had been shown to help patients with Alzheimer's and other memory disorders by boosting levels of their thought neurotransmitter, so I believed that it might also help jump-start Kyle's very sketchy memory, which was improving only moderately. Elizabeth told me, with great pride, that Kyle had recently remembered that a big puddle in front of their house had been there the day before. That was a major achievement for him, so something was obviously still missing in his memory center.

I was also aware that phosphatidylcholine might help Kyle's entire nervous system, including his brain, to produce more myelin, the fatty substance that coats and insulates brain and nerve cell connections. There was, at this time, an embryonic body of evidence that said autistic people often had a deficit of myelin, which was presumably causing short circuits in their brains and nerves, just as it does with people who have the classic disease of myelin deficit, multiple sclerosis. It was reasonable to assume that more myelin might mean better function of Kyle's body and brain.

Additionally, I was aware that phosphatidylcholine might also improve the functioning of the cell membranes throughout Kyle's body and brain, allowing healthy nutrients to get in, and toxins to get out. When that happened, it might boost his nutritional therapy, and turbocharge his heavy metal detoxification, via DMSA. In addition, it could help his liver detoxify.

As you can see, I was counting on this single nutrient to have a four-pronged effect. Most of the best nutrients not only exert multiple actions, but also trigger reactions in other nutrients. This type of synergistic, metabolic therapy is complex, but that's why it works so much better than just knocking down symptoms one at a time with pharmaceutical drugs, which tend to have dramatic but isolated effects.

The second important measure I wanted to try was an intravenous injection of glutathione. Glutathione is now one of the Big Guns in the biomedical arsenal against autism, but back then it was largely unappreciated. It's a combination of three amino acids, comprising a partial protein, and is terrific for detoxification, particularly of heavy metals. I'd just done some further testing of Kyle's heavy metal excretion, and he didn't seem to be eliminating large amounts of mercury, or other heavy metals, but that was no reason to give up on the DMSA. Things don't always work predictably. If they did, I wouldn't need to be a good Doctor Detective, and you wouldn't need to be a good Parent Detective. Sometimes you need to keep peeling back layers of mystery one by one to reach the heart of reality.

I also knew that glutathione was an extremely powerful antioxidant, capable of preventing damage from free radicals—the destructive, inflammatory molecules that are by-products of metabolism. I had seen emerging evidence that inflammatory free radical damage was an important cause of Parkinson's disease, heart disease, cancer, and arthritis. Why not autism? Maybe free-radical related inflammation contributed to it. And . . . aha! . . . *maybe that's why the DMSA, a powerful antioxidant and sulfur-containing compound, had caused such immediate improvement!*

It made sense.

. . . If I'd known then what I know now. . . . Now almost all doctors realize that inflammation is an extraordinarily important element of most critical, chronic diseases. For example, about half the people who die of heart attacks don't have the classic heart disease risk factors, such as high cholesterol, but they do have arteries that are hard and thick with chronic inflammation.

Here's what we know *now* about autism and inflammation.

Autism: The Inflammation Factor

- Autism is closely linked to chronic, persistent inflammation of brain cells, or neuroinflammation.
- The immune system triggers this brain inflammation. It does it through abnormal production of immune system messengers called cytokines and chemokines.
- Inflammation can impair, and even destroy, brain cells.
- Inflammation can impede the function of neurotransmitters, particularly dopamine, the neurotransmitter closely associated with a positive mood and physical grace. The primary cause of Parkinson's is the decline of dopamine function. Dopamine disorders can also trigger ADHD.
- Inflammation in the brain makes brain cells less capable of excreting toxic material, which then causes even more inflammation. It creates a spiral of degeneration.

Needless to say, I decided to continue Kyle's treatment with the DMSA. I also tweaked his diet and supplement program, stayed with the anti-candida strategy, kept working on the heavy metals, bumped up the vitamin A even more, and recommended he continue ABA. In my prior success with persistent, stubborn adult diseases, such as chronic fatigue syndrome and fibromyalgia, I'd found that only a comprehensive program worked. Would autism, exotic as it was, really prove to be that much different?

At this time, conventional wisdom said that autism was essentially genetic, and would probably yield only to a dramatic genetic intervention, which was still on the horizon. I was too curious and too concerned, though, to settle for that piece of conventional wisdom. And Kyle, Elizabeth, and Eric were too desperate. I had to soldier on, undeterred by vagary and doubt.

Even so...I didn't know it yet, but my third appointment with Kyle—who endured his IV treatment with big, scared saucer-eyes—was a turning point. It was, to paraphrase Churchill, not the end of Kyle's victory over autism, nor even the beginning of the end. *But it was the end of the beginning.*

Milwaukee, Wisconsin

Three Weeks Later

"Just go stand next to him, Kyle," said Elizabeth, looking at a boy in the park about Kyle's age, who was standing by a slide.

Kyle grabbed the back of Elizabeth's coat and wrapped it around him like a blanket, stealing occasional glances at the boy by the slide.

"You don't have to try to talk to him, honey, just go stand over where he is, like you're waiting to go on the slide. You'll get your pri-i-ize!"

Kyle really wanted that prize. He can't remember anymore what it was, but he can remember he was dying to get it. Even more clearly, though, he can remember how afraid he was. "It was *so* scary when I was around little kids. I didn't know how to use words. I was always like, duhhh. . . . I was scared of kids laughing at me, and I just wanted to be with Mom."

Elizabeth stood there with him for a long time. Her patience was becoming extraordinary, but at a cost, of course. She had almost lost touch with the concept of living her *own* life. She hadn't read a novel in four years—just books about autism, one after another, every night when Kyle was in bed. They weren't even very helpful, except for one by Karyn Seroussi, the mother of an autistic child. Most of the rest just seemed to revolve around the theme of, "How Not to Go Crazy When Your Kid's Autistic."

After about an hour of Kyle hiding behind her, Elizabeth took his hand and trudged home. Kyle was droopy with disappointment. This was the third day in a row he'd lost that prize. Elizabeth was crestfallen, too. Kyle had seemed to be getting *better*, especially after his third appointment. Now what? As they walked, Kyle got some mud on his shoe and panicked, as he often did when he got even a speck of dirt or snow on him. He had so many phobias.

Would he live his whole *life* cold with fear, unable to make a friend?

Love and Fear

"Like a prey-species animal, many people with autism experience fear as the primary emotion. . . . Complex emotional relationships are beyond my comprehension."
Temple Grandin, an autistic woman
Thinking in Pictures

The eternal human struggle for happiness and meaning revolves around the battle between the two most primal and pivotal of all emotions: love and fear. At the heart of all life lie these two lords of mankind.

Love brings happiness. But fear fosters survival. And we need *both*. Therefore, most people spend their lives balancing love and fear, often trading away the happiness of today in drudgery, sacrifice, and sorrow, out of fear of not having enough of what they need to live and love tomorrow.

The brain has been constructed by evolution to help us achieve a healthy balance between love and fear, through a delicate mix of structures and secretions that separately support each of these two megalithic forces of emotion.

Feelings of love generally reside in the most advanced sections of the brain, primarily the frontal lobes of the neocortex, while fear is housed in a distant, more primitive, animalistic area of the brain, the amygdala.

The amygdala is a small, almond-shaped area of the brain that is part of the brain's center of memory and emotion, the limbic system. The main job of the amygdala is to make sure you remember all the scary things that you need to know in order to survive. For example, if you ever stepped on a snake and still remember it, it's because your amygdala told you to remember it.

It's fine to have a big, active amygdala, because it will help keep you safe and motivated. However, it's bad to have one that's too big, and too active. Unfortunately, many autistic people do appear to have abnormalities of size and activity in their amygdalas. This is probably a primary reason why autistic people have elevated anxiety. It's been shown, for example, that over 50 percent of all high-functioning autistic adults have severe anxiety and panic attacks. The excessive fear that's experienced by autistics tends to often emerge as social anxiety, but it can also take the form of phobias, generalized anxiety disorder, sleep disturbances, obsessive-compulsive disorder, lack of impulse control, anger, abusiveness, depression, suicidal ideation, substance abuse, and paranoia.

An overactive amygdala, therefore, can wreak havoc upon the rest of the brain. It's connected to the other areas of the brain primarily through the nearby structure called the thalamus, which is also often dysfunctional in autistics.

The thalamus is best known as the part of the brain that screens out the barrage of sensory information that constantly floods in to us from our eyes, ears, noses, taste buds, and skin. It blocks out enough of the extraneous sensations to allow us to focus on the important things. Autistics, however, appear to frequently suffer from reduced size and impaired function of the thalamus. This probably means that their brains are often bombarded with a confusing torrent of information. This torrent, along with their general anxiety, may account for their frequent desire to fixate on simple, repetitive activities.

The thalamus is also a primary processing center for memory, emotion, and attention, three brain activities that are often dysfunctional in autistics. In addition, the thalamus helps regulate motor control, which could partly account for the tendency of kids in the autism spectrum to be clumsy and uncoordinated.

Another job the thalamus does is to help regulate the proper levels of neurotransmitters, particularly the calming neurotransmitter serotonin and the pleasure neurotransmitter dopamine, which are often skewed in autistic people. Serotonin and dopamine levels can't be too high or too low, but in autistics they're often outside their proper bandwidths. These disordered levels of serotonin and dopamine typically cause heightened anxiety, distress, confusion, and aggression.

This increased distress, in turn, makes the endocrine system bathe the body in stress hormones, such as cortisol—which pushes the amygdala into an even further frenzy, creating a spiral of worry, dread, and doubt that never seems to cease.

This wreckage of structures and secretions can derange the brain all the way down to the single-cell level. In fact, the chaotic physical forces that batter the autistic brain appear to even cause abnormality in a special type of brain cell that may hold within it the very heart of love. This type of brain cell is called the mirror neuron.

Mirror neurons were discovered in a European brain laboratory in the late 1990s by a group of scientists who had wired a monkey's brain with electrodes, in order to track the monkey's brain activity as he performed various physical tasks. They noted, for example, that every time the monkey ate, brain cells in a certain, predictable area would cause a monitor connected to the monkey to make a sound: "Braaap... braaap... braaap!"

At one point, though, as the monkey was sitting passively, a researcher eating an ice cream cone walked over to him. "Braaap... braaap... braaap!"

The astonished scientists had just inadvertently discovered mirror neurons, a special class of brain cells that fire when an animal or a person registers awareness of what someone *else* is experiencing. These brain cells are essentially the physical sites of empathy, sharing, and caring.

Autistic people, however, appear to have malfunctioning systems of mirror neurons. This makes it very difficult for them to know how others feel, and therefore makes it hard for them to care. This malfunction was graphically revealed during a recent study of autistic children at UCLA using MRI scans. Compared to a control group of nonautistic children, the autistic kids registered very little activity in their mirror neurons when they observed photos of people who were making facial expressions of anger, fear, or happiness.

This failure of mirror neurons has two fundamental effects. *(1) It causes anxiety.* It's frightening to have, in effect, everyone around you wearing blank, indifferent masks. You can't tell how they're reacting to you, and you can't predict what they're about to do. *(2) It's an obstacle to love.* With no feedback from the interaction of facial expression and body language, autistics can be blind to love, even when it's right in front of their faces.

All of this damage and dysfunction in the autistic brain is now undoubtedly daunting to the neurological researchers who are trying to find valid treatments for autism. Do they focus on the amygdala? The thalamus? Serotonin? Dopamine? Mirror neurons?

My approach, of course, is to resist the temptation to focus too closely on any one area. The right amount of focus can be revealing, but too often, in the practice of specialty medicine, it ends in myopia.

My approach is based upon the medical principle of holism, which calls for addressing the human body as an integrated, interdependent, interrelated entity. Because every aspect of the brain interacts with every other aspect, I believe that the key to healing the autistic brain is to offer the brain every element of optimal neural metabolism that it requires, and then to step back, bow to the wisdom of the body, and allow self-healing to take its own natural, often miraculous course.

That was my approach to healing Kyle Olson's brain. And that is still my approach today.

Milwaukee, Wisconsin

Four Weeks Later

Elizabeth heard an unusual sound coming from Kyle's room. It sounded like conversation.

She peeked in, and Kyle was on the floor, by himself, with a *Star Wars* action figure in each hand. He had played with them before, making their arms move up and down, or making them fight. Now, he was having them *talk to each other.*

Elizabeth stood there, transfixed.

A few days later they were in the park again. Kyle was standing by the slide. The slide had always scared him, just as steep slopes and even stairs often frighten autistic people, who tend to have poor depth perception. He'd never gone down it, even with Elizabeth.

A boy came over.

Kyle looked at him. "You goin' down?" Kyle asked. The boy nodded. "Me, too," Kyle said. "Go together?"

"Sure."

The boy climbed the slide and Kyle followed. When the boy reached the bottom, Kyle called, "Watch!" and slid down.

Kyle ran to Elizabeth.

"I made a friend! Mommy! I gotta go!" He ran back to his friend.

Elizabeth took deep breaths.

Rhinebeck, New York

Kyle's Fourth Visit–Seven Months After the First

"Kyle's been so sweet lately," Elizabeth said, reaching for his hand, as he reached back.

"I heard you made a friend," I said to Kyle.

"On the slide," he said. "It wasn't scary, much. Then a *best* friend. And a bike, too. I ride it."

"You're talkin' better, too, kiddo." I gave him a big grin and he flashed it back. Boy, was I proud of this kid! He wasn't the only autistic child I was treating by this time, but he will always be special to me. He helped me figure out some things I thought I'd *never* understand, by sticking to his diet so well, swallowing all those pills, getting all those

needle pokes, putting up with all those ABA lessons—and by approaching a boy on a slide while his heart was still half-sick with fear.

The Healing Program was really coming together—and not because of
just the kids I was treating myself. A whole group of doctors was now actively coalescing around the issue of treating autism biomedically, and as
a team we were making new discoveries at a rapid pace, and sharing them.
These were brilliant and brave physicians—some with autistic kids of their
own—who weren't afraid to make waves and bust protocol to get to the
bottom of the terrible epidemic that was suddenly upon us. We were all
getting together in think-tank sessions a couple of days before every Defeat Autism Now conference, trading ideas around big conference tables.
The names of the people who sat at those tables might not mean much to
you now, but as this book progresses, you'll get to know them. I believe
that someday these names will be in books of medical history: Bernard
Rimland, Jon Pangborn, and Sid Baker (the founders of the biomedical approach); Stephanie Cave and Jeff Bradstreet (who pioneered the vaccination issue); Jaquelyn McCandless (who dedicated her own life to
recovering her granddaughter's life); Tim Buic, Arthur Krigsman, and Andrew Wakefield (who led the way on the gastrointestinal issues); Jill James,
Richard Deth, Boyd Haley, and Martha Herbert (whose scientific research laid the foundation of biomedical intervention); and other great researchers and clinicians, including Anju Usman, John Green, Andrew
Levinson, Jane El-Dahr, Jim Neubrander, Nancy O'Hara, Paul Hardy,
Marvin Boris, Alan Goldblatt, Amy Holmes, Lauren Underwood, Teresa
Binstock, Stuart Freedenfeld, Cindy Schneider, Lyn Redwood, Sallie
Bernard, Jerry Kartzinel, Bryan Jepson, Stan Kurtz, Susan Owens, and
Karyn Seroussi. None of them are big media names now, but they, and a
few others, will long be remembered as the people who gave back hope—
and gave back children—to families whose hearts had been broken.

At Kyle's fourth appointment, I helped him make another huge breakthrough.

I was happy with Kyle's progress, but he still had choppy language,
he had spells of staring off into space, he tended to state the obvious, he
had a tiny attention span, and he was pretty obsessive, mostly about *Star
Wars*. His balance was better, but he was still a fairly klutzy kid.

"There's something I'm really excited about, Elizabeth."

It was a new approach we'd just talked about at the most recent DAN think tank. Dr. James and Dr. Deth had discovered that many autistic children suffered from *a failure to naturally detoxify their own bodies*. Much of this failure was due to exposure to heavy metals–particularly mercury. Therefore, these kids were not only saddled with toxic heavy metals in their systems, but the metals themselves were preventing the kids from excreting them. In addition, the kids couldn't excrete other toxins–everything from pesticides, to allergens, to excess levels of stress hormones and neurotransmitters. Wow! We were getting close! And here was the best part: We believed there was a way to fix the problem.

The problem, in slightly more technical terms, was a failure to detoxify the body through the two natural processes of methylation and sulfation. These two processes help the body flush out toxins, primarily through the urine. Heavy metals put a biochemical headlock on these processes, but Jim Neubrander thought they could be restored by giving the kids very high dosages, generally subcutaneously, of a specific form of vitamin B-12 that's known as methylcobalamin.

This simple, harmless vitamin ushered in a *reversal* of the systemic toxification that caused metabolic and neurological degeneration. The therapy was uncomplicated, but often extraordinarily effective.

It was almost as if we had discovered a miracle: *The miracle of methylation!*

Okay, fine, I had a miracle treatment. Now–what else?

To paraphrase Ben Hogan, miracles did happen, but the harder I worked, the more miraculous they got.

I decided to give Kyle a transdermal application of a substance called TTFD (thiamine tetrahydrofurfuryl disulfide). This fat-soluble form of the B-vitamin thiamine can attach itself to heavy metals and help haul them out of the body. It also boosts the detoxifying process of sulfation. In addition, it improves the functioning of the cell's energy factories, the mitochondria.

I also gave Kyle some mild medications to help resolve his lingering bowel disorder. Many kids on the spectrum, I was finding, had bowel disorders, which created nutritional deficits, which created neurotransmitter deficits, which created . . . well, you know the drill by now. Everything is connected. That's why you have to treat the whole body.

I kept treating Kyle's candida problem, and also ran more tests to check him for allergy-type food reactions. Sure enough, he had some allergies, so we eliminated those reactive foods.

Shortly after that, I added one more protocol, an intravenous injection of the natural hormone secretin. I thought it might be able to help Kyle, even though most subsequent research has still not been able to confirm the ability of secretin to trigger early observed clinical improvements. Fortunately, Kyle did turn out to be one of those kids who responded to secretin almost immediately. Even on the way home from the treatment, he was talking to Elizabeth with better syntax, and was showing signs of a much improved memory. Although I generally don't use secretin, this instantaneous response does sometimes happen with it. It probably happens because secretin is a neurohormone, directly involved with cognition and particularly with normalization of amygdala function.

Over the next year, Kyle stuck with his Healing Program like a champ, and his improvements gained momentum and persistence. My gradual development of the Healing Program was virtually complete by this point. The Healing Program now addressed the three most fundamental elements of autism: dysfunctions of *(1) the immune system; (2) the gastrointestinal system;* and *(3) the nervous system.* Each of these three systems required multiple healing modalities, tailored to fit each child's unique needs. These modalities consisted of the four primary elements that I'll soon discuss in detail: *(1) nutritional therapy; (2) supplementation therapy; (3) detoxification;* and *(4) medication.*

I had also begun to employ the Healing Program for ADHD, asthma, and allergies, which all share so many of the same aspects of causation. It had become clear that America was not just in the midst of an autism epidemic, but a full-blown 4-A epidemic.

The Healing Program created changes in Kyle that were absolutely remarkable. He became a chatty, friendly, well-behaved grade school boy. He had sleepovers with his best friend, did a lot of swimming, and hated math. He loved to read books—*big* books: He devoured the entire *Harry Potter* series, C. S. Lewis' *The Chronicles of Narnia,* and whatever else piqued his growing imagination. His physical grace grew beautifully, as essential fatty acids, along with his improved dopamine metabolism, helped smooth out his coordination. His muscles also bulked up, as he began to more efficiently process the amino acid creatine, the muscle-building protein that's often low in autistics.

In 2004, when Kyle was eight, Eric and Elizabeth took him to the Mayo Clinic, to confirm what they felt they already knew: that Kyle was no longer autistic. Supposedly, even by this relatively late date in the development of the biomedical treatment of autism, that degree of full, robust recovery was still relatively uncommon. Even so, Eric and Elizabeth were certain it had occurred. *Parents know.*

After two days of intensive evaluation, the Mayo doctors issued their report. They said that Kyle did not suffer from any of the autism-spectrum disorders, and had only mild features of ADHD, which were so minor that he required no medication, nor any other treatment. They noted that he had a normal IQ, with areas of elevated intelligence, including a skill for reading. They did say, though, that he should probably be working harder at math.

For closure, Eric and Elizabeth took Kyle to the neuropsychologist who'd once said that it would take a miracle for him to be normal. "It's a miracle," she said. Eric resisted the urge to comment.

Elizabeth and Kyle came to see me shortly after that. Elizabeth brought me the Mayo Clinic report, the way a proud mom shows off a straight-A report card. The meeting felt more like a celebration than a medical appointment.

We'd been through so much together. Those early days . . . when Kyle only had ABA as a lifeline: "Stand-up-sit-down!" Hitting Megan on the porch. Bashing kids with a broom handle to try to make friends. The snarling dog feeling. The fear. The silence. Those first clues. . . .

As we all sat in my office, I realized that I had helped Kyle as much as I possibly could. So I put down my chart, stopped being a doctor, and just talked to Kyle like a friend. He launched on a discourse about the Harry Potter books, dissecting their plots and analyzing the characters. Boy, that Kyle, he sure could talk!

That was the last time I saw Kyle Olson.

I think of him often.

Milwaukee, Wisconsin, 2006

Eric took Kyle, along with one of Kyle's best buddies, to play golf for the first time. It was one of those beautifully crisp Wisconsin days when the air itself seems to sparkle like a dust made of diamonds.

Kyle shot a 77 on nine holes, and felt very good about it. Eric had shot only a slightly better score the first time he had played. Then Eric had gotten a full scholarship to play Big Ten golf, and then went on to play pro golf. Then fatherhood—and no golf.

Kyle knew all about his family's esteemed golf heritage: the glories of his grandmother, and his father, and now, possibly, him.

As he confidently lined up his last putt, Kyle looked up lovingly at his father and said, "Dad, I was born to play golf."

It was the first basketball game of the season. First minute. First possession.

Kyle Olson brought the ball up-court, checked for the open man, shook off a defender, faked right, went left. Looked for his shot. Up! And in!

Kyle made a fist, and pumped his elbow down to his side. He'd seen his dad do that. "*Yes!*" he said.

In a movie, Eric would have been in the stands, and Kyle would have locked eyes with him . . . fade to black.

But this was real life, and Eric wasn't there.

Eric was exactly where he should have been: at work in the shoe store, far away, sacrificing his day for his son, as he had most of the days of Kyle's life—with the glory days of his career now gone, and the glory days of fatherhood finally just ahead.

Elizabeth called right after the game and told Eric about The Shot.

Eric made a fist, and pumped his elbow down to his side.

"*Yes!*"

2. ADHD

CHAPTER SEVEN

BRAT GIRLS AND BAD BOYS

The Road to Rhinebeck

HERE ARE THE THINGS YOU THINK ABOUT AS YOU DRIVE A DAUGH-ter who hates doctors to yet *another* doctor, getting further by the minute from a husband to whom you'll never return: the early days, the days of love and health. But the good memories always dredge up the bad. If they didn't, you wouldn't be driving to Rhinebeck.

As little Alisa fidgeted against her car seat, Liza Winters remembered the days of love and ease that had blessed the early years of her marriage. She and Bill had both been making six figures, they owned a McMansion, and when they decided that it was time for Liza to get pregnant, the whole process had taken, like, ninety minutes. It had been so easy that Bill wouldn't even believe Liza was pregnant, so he called the doctor to check out her story—which was probably a bad sign, in retrospect. Bill was a little too controlling, Liza thought, and her sudden pregnancy was the first time he'd ever lost full command of Bill Universe.

The arrival of Alisa, though, made everything even better than before. She was gorgeous, for starters, with brown, round eyes shaded by little-puppy lashes, and a smile that warmed you from the inside out. Of course, the baby's beauty went well with the big house, the beautiful nursery, and the long maternity leave. Bill did play a lot of golf, but other than that: perfection. For ten months.

Liza's mother, a school psychologist, noticed it first: Alisa was suddenly different. She'd previously been so calm, so easy to cuddle and comfort, and so content to look at her books as she babbled happily to Liza. Then, at ten months, Alisa started to stay anxiously within the confines of a pattern on the carpet, as if it were a cage. She stopped looking at her books and started to chew on them. Her babbling ceased and she didn't seem to hear anyone. The formula she was drinking began to give her a mottled, scarlet rash, and when they switched her to soy, her reaction to it was so violent that even a drop of it on her skin made her blister and peel. Liza and her mother asked the doctor about the soy allergy, but he said that babies as young as Alisa couldn't get allergies, so obviously they didn't know what they were talking about.

Liza's mother, Beverly, remembers the next few months as the worst of her life, because: "I knew what was coming." She began to ease into the subject with her daughter, knowing Liza would be devastated.

Meanwhile, Alisa drifted away, into her own, lonely world.

At Alisa's eighteen-month check-up, Liza's mom took the doctor aside, to spare Liza's feelings, and told him that she feared Alisa was autistic. The doctor used the same phrase as before: "You don't know what you're talking about."

At twenty-seven months, though, Liza's world of contentment ended forever. Another doctor diagnosed Alisa with one of the vaguest and most common autism labels: Pervasive Development Disorder–Not Otherwise Specified. In plain English, it means Widespread Failure to Develop–Who Knows Why?

Parents tend to accept the diagnosis of PDD-NOS better than they do that of autism, but the prognosis is generally almost as grim: limited social and intellectual development, with probable adult institutionalization, or partial care.

Around this time, at the end of the 1990s, many parents were beginning to blame the childhood vaccinations for PDD-NOS, as well as the other types of regressive autism, but Liza had the feeling that something more complex had occurred. The vaccinations may have played a role, but Liza thought there may have also been problems in utero, possibly connected to her getting a flu shot while she was pregnant. Alisa also had gastrointestinal problems that seemed to somehow play a role in her condition.

Liza immediately sacrificed her lucrative career to work full-time with Alisa, and in Liza's opinion, "That was the beginning of the end of my marriage." She began to search feverishly for the most advanced care in the world, including biomedical treatment, but she felt that "the more involved I became, the more my husband backed off. He only went to a few doctors' appointments. He was still playing a lot of golf."

Liza couldn't bring herself to demonize Bill, though, because much of what they were going through was just unimaginable–like the plane trip to Colorado, for example.

They thought they could manage a short hop out to Denver to see Bill's parents, because Alisa seemed to be doing so much better by about age four. For over a year, Alisa had been on the gluten-free, casein-free diet, an anti-allergy diet, and an aggressive program of supplementation. She was also getting extensive–and expensive–occupational therapy, along with Floortime therapy, in which Liza spent an hour a day on the floor with Alisa, letting Alisa totally control the direction of their play. In addition, Alisa was in a speech therapy program. Her first coherent word had been, "Help!"

The therapies, all orchestrated by Liza, had lifted Alisa out of her silent, self-involved hiding place. It was no longer obvious to strangers that this little girl, now cuter than ever with dark curls, had been diagnosed as PDD-NOS. Now her primary diagnosis was ADHD with bipolar features. That was a huge improvement.

For a while, Alisa's treatment had also included a drug called Risperdal, an antipsychotic medication commonly given to kids with autism and PDD. It also seems to help some ADHD kids, even though it has the opposite action of most ADHD drugs. Most of them bump up the action of the attention neurotransmitter dopamine, but Risperdal drives it down. That didn't really make sense to Liza–or to her doctor, either–and it heightened Liza's distrust of drugs. She thought that ADHD drugs had too many side effects. Some of the kids who used them seemed to be zombies, and others bounced around like speed freaks. So, as Alisa had improved, Liza had weaned her off the Risperdal.

As they waited for the plane to take off, Liza and Bill let Alisa sit and color with a couple of other kids. Then Liza came to take Alisa to her seat, and Alisa started to tantrum. More precisely, in psychiatric jargon, Alisa began to cycle. Alisa's tantrums–similar to those of other kids with rapid cycling mood swings–extended far beyond normal meltdowns, into predictable cycles of mounting rage, followed by hysterical aggression, sometimes assault, and then exhaustion and remorse. The whole cycle could take almost an hour, and Liza, Bill, and the therapists had never found any way to shorten it with discipline, reason, or love.

Back in her seat, as the plane taxied, Alisa's protests escalated into screaming. As they lifted off, Alisa began to kick Liza and Bill, and her crying grew shrill and otherworldly, like the keening cackle of a witch. Liza and Bill tried to get Alisa to use her words, but there was no way.

Alisa, who still remembers the incident, felt as if she could no longer speak. Life, hateful and full of pain, seemed to be rushing in at her un-controllably, and forcing her to act as awful as she felt. It felt to her as if she were not even participating in her behavior, but was just reacting to the world's hurt in the only possible and appropriate way.

As Bill and Liza restrained Alisa, every pair of eyes on the plane seemed to be aimed at them.

"Let her *up!*" someone shouted.

"Give her some *candy!*"

As the screeching and struggling continued, Liza had to force Alisa to the floor, to keep her from hurting herself or the passengers in front of them.

When the flight attendant came by, Liza tried to explain, but the at-tendant just seemed disgusted with the whole family.

In about an hour, Alisa gradually cycled-out and grew still, and then suddenly fell asleep, as Liza stroked her face.

As the plane quieted, people were still buzzing about them, and seemed to want some of their words to be overheard, out of either anger, or genuine concern. Some of the words Liza still remembers were, "a good spanking," "overpower a child," "abuse," "crazy," "spoiled rotten," and "little brat."

Liza lifted Alisa's head to her lap. Humiliated, frightened, Liza began to cry, but wouldn't allow herself to make a sound.

She looked over at Bill, and tears were dropping off his face, too, as he stared straight ahead, lost in his own loneliness.

It was time to go back on Risperdal.

Those are the things you think about as you drive a daughter who hates doctors to yet another doctor. You see your husband's face, and feel some of what you once felt.

Detroit, Michigan

What Larry Smith couldn't understand was: Why do some of the people at Matthew's school seem to think that he's a *bad* boy–and why do they think that taking a drug will suddenly make him *good?*

To Larry, the whole thing seemed far simpler than that: "*Matthew hates school.*" Larry knew exactly how his son felt. He hadn't liked school either, and hadn't thrived in life until he'd escaped it. As nearly as Larry could tell, Matthew was a *great* kid–kindhearted, fun, and smart. He was a real boy's boy, hands-on, good at sports, and good at mechanical things. He was difficult sometimes, but he was *seven.*

That's not how the school saw it, though. The school counselor called in Larry and his wife, Kelly, for a special early-morning conference. She got right to the point. She told them that Matthew had the classic signs of ADHD. She thought Matthew should be evaluated by a doctor, who would, she believed, place him on the proper ADHD medication.

"But at home he's *good,*" Larry protested.

The counselor demurred. It was not a matter of Matthew being a "good boy," or a "bad boy." It was just that his *behavior* was bad: not conducive to a healthy educational environment for the school community.

The counselor looked over her glasses at them, and told them very patiently that ADHD was a complex neurological issue. There were two fundamental types of ADHD, she said. To simplify: the "AD" type, and the "HD" type. The AD children were the attention-deficit ones, who were categorized as being in the inattentive subtype, and the HD children were the hyper kids, in the hyperactive-impulsive subtype. Furthermore, there was a mixed subtype of children, who had characteristics of both disorders.

Each of the two major types had nine features, and to be diagnosed, a child had to have at least six of them. They were:

Inattentive Subtype

1. Is not good at details.
2. Has difficulty sustaining attention.
3. Frequently fails to listen carefully.
4. Doesn't follow through on tasks well.
5. Is not good at organizing.
6. Dislikes sustained mental effort.

7. Often loses things.

8. Is easily distracted.

9. Is often forgetful.

Hyperactive-Impulsive Subtype

1. Fidgets when seated.

2. Often leaves his or her seat in the classroom.

3. Is restless, and runs around excessively.

4. Doesn't like quiet activities.

5. Is often active, and on the go.

6. Talks excessively.

7. Blurts out answers before questions are complete.

8. Has difficulty awaiting turn.

9. Interrupts conversations and games.

As the counselor listed the characteristics, one at a time, Larry was thinking, "Me. Me. Not me. Me. Not me. Me. . . ." *Lots* of me's. In fact, he thought, almost *everybody* had lots of those traits—and in most adults, they were just considered quirky, or even signs of being a go-getter. Larry thought of saying something to the effect of, "You just described about one-fourth of the population, including me." But then she'd probably say, "Yes, it's an epidemic. And it's genetic."

He also thought of telling her that Matthew didn't get bored at home, and didn't act up at home—so maybe the *school* was boring and rigid. But that was a battle that would never be won.

Besides, maybe she was right. Larry and his wife were young parents, and all this was new to them. Nonetheless, neither of them liked the idea of giving their seven-year-old drugs for his brain. To Kelly, it seemed to invade her territory as a mother.

The counselor gave them the name of a doctor, and a week later they were in his office. The doctor talked to them for a few minutes, then talked to Matthew, who seemed confused by the whole thing. He just wanted to go play.

At the end of the exam, the doctor told them that Matthew didn't need drugs. Larry let out a quiet sigh of relief. Then Larry and Kelly went home and tried to forget about it. Matthew watched one of his favorite shows, *Full House,* and went outside to play. He was an outdoorsy kid, not a couch potato or a Nintendo Nerd.

Almost immediately, they got a letter from the school counselor. It said, "We had hoped you would have started Matthew on a trial of medication by now." She wanted another meeting.

This time she was much harsher. She said that Matthew needed to go on Ritalin *now*. She assured them that it was a very mild medication that would stimulate his brain stem and help him focus.

Larry didn't know much about the brain stem, but he wasn't sold. After all, the *doctor* hadn't prescribed Ritalin.

Then the counselor told them that if they didn't put Matthew on the medication, the state's Children's Services Division could charge them with neglecting his educational and emotional needs. If that happened, both Matthew and his older brother could be removed from the home.

Larry and Kelly were shocked, and frightened. They agreed to go back to the doctor.

The doctor was angry. He told them, "Remind the school that I am not a pharmacy." Larry assumed that this meant the school had sent other kids to him. However, the doctor wrote the prescription—10 milligrams of Ritalin, three times a day.

When they told Matthew he had to start taking it, he was dismayed, and seemed to feel that he'd let them down.

After he started taking it, his behavior changed. He often acted dopey and stoned. He didn't like it. "This stuff is gonna kill me," he said.

Rhinebeck, New York

Liza and Alisa pulled into Rhinebeck late in the afternoon, and were pleasantly surprised by the little town, as many people are. It's a quaint, woodsy place with lots of good restaurants, and Victorian and Federal homes, one of which houses the clinic that I operate with my brother, Steven Bock, M.D., and our associate, Michael Compain, M.D. Rhinebeck is overshadowed, however, by its more famous sister-hamlet of Woodstock, where I've lived for many years. Woodstock has been a magnet for diverse and creative people ever since it was put on the map by the 1969 rock concert, and also by Bob Dylan living there, and by the temporary residency of The Band, who'd recorded *Music from Big Pink* around here. In fact, I live in the house they were renting then, and the view from my bedroom window is on the back cover of the album. Woodstock is a great environment for innovation.

Liza drove straight to their hotel, and got a shock. She'd reserved a room with a refrigerator in it, because Alisa needed special foods, as do many kids with problems like hers. The desk clerk, though, said that Bill had called and that there'd been some confusion about paying extra for a refrigerator. Long story short, the reservation had been canceled. Liza shifted into overdrive and found another room with a refrigerator, but by then some of the food had spoiled. They had to eat at a restaurant, and that was always dicey. Restaurant food could trigger a cycle, and Liza wanted Alisa to be at her best for the appointment.

This wasn't the first time Bill had frustrated Liza by trying to econ-omize. He seemed to be appalled at how much Liza was spending on Alisa's treatment, some of which wasn't even effective. Supplements alone often cost hundreds of dollars every month, and their insurance wouldn't cover many of Alisa's biomedical treatments. Bill had recently implored Liza to return to work. She was working full-time for a non-profit organization she had founded—which focused on early interven-tion for autistic kids—but it wasn't making much money. Bill had told her that if her nonprofit couldn't become more economically feasible, she would have to give it up and find something else. It was easy enough to see his side of things, because they'd spent over $100,000 chasing down viable therapies, and were hurting financially for the first time. Even so, Liza thought her nonprofit was vitally important. Families needed to know that early intervention with behavioral and biomedical therapies *worked*—and the earlier, the better. Nobody else was telling them that—certainly not the vast majority of pediatricians, who still seemed collectively stunned by the new tidal waves of autism, ADHD, asthma, and allergies that were swamping their offices.

As Liza and Alisa sat down in my office for their first appointment, I could tell right away that Liza was one of the most medically sophis-ticated parents that I had yet met. Nonetheless, she was still struggling with Alisa's treatment. Liza began to go over the grab-bag of labels that had been applied to Alisa: PDD-NOS; mixed ADHD with features of both inattentive subtype and hyperactive-impulsive subtype; bipolar mood disorder; signs of oppositional defiance disorder; and attendant colitis, allergic rhinitis, and hypoglycemia.

Most of those behavioral labels explained very little about causa-tion. In my opinion, they were descriptions of behaviors, rather than di-agnoses. As always, I needed to uncover the root causes, as a good medical detective must.

As we talked, I looked carefully at Alisa, with her sniffly nose and other telltale signs of allergy, and my heart melted. She was one of the kids who could just look into your face and make you love them. She was a beautiful child, with friendly eyes and dark, shoulder-length hair. But her real charm came from the inside—she was just a good kid, and it shined right through.

Liza said that the only drug Alisa was on at this time was Risperdal, which seemed to be helping. They had tried several of the other standard ADHD meds—Ritalin, Concerta, and Tenex—but those three were disasters, she said. That made sense to me. Conventional treatment of ADHD usually revolves around using the Ritalin-type drugs to push up the activity of the stimulating neurotransmitter dopamine, which is associated with attention and energy. That approach works adequately for a number of kids, but it's a catastrophe for the significant percentage of ADHD kids who have been on the autism spectrum, whether it's been diagnosed or not. The autism kids tend to already have a relative excess of dopamine, and an excess of dopamine hurts their brains just as much as a deficit does. As the drugs push dopamine up even higher, it makes these kids anxious, agitated, and aggressive.

Many doctors still don't seem to fully realize this, and that's why these types of medications often fail in autistic kids. However, when I explained it to Liza, it clicked with everything she'd observed over the past few years and she got it right away. As I've said, *moms know.*

As Liza and I reviewed Alisa's history, Alisa became increasingly fidgety, then bolted up, as if her chair were electrified. She started to pick up things on my desk, examining each item for about a second and a half, then grabbing something else. Liza tried to settle her down. Then I said something, and Alisa shot a look at me out of a whole different pair of eyes. Gone were the friendly eyes. They were replaced by eyes that were just plain scary. She began to cycle, and suddenly I was seeing the full force of what I was up against.

Tears blurred Liza's eyes as she tried to penetrate Alisa's rage. For all practical purposes, the appointment was over.

Later on, I reviewed every aspect of Alisa's lab tests and treatment program, and here's the short version of the elements that caught my eye: low cysteine, low glutathione, low selenium, numerous IGE food allergies, low zinc, low vitamin A, and the presence of antibodies to neural antigens. Does some of that ring a bell, my fellow medical detective? As you probably noticed, many of these are the same essential biological issues that are involved in autism.

Alisa, of course, had a history of being on the autism spectrum, but that had been several years prior to this. According to conventional wisdom, her autism markers should have been gone.

They were not: Because autism and ADHD are both different faces of several similar, diverse root problems.

These shared root problems are centered around dysfunction of:

- **The immune system.**
- **The gastrointestinal system.**
- **The nervous system.**

Here is *my* perspective on ADHD: **ADHD is a catchall diagnosis, into which the medical system too often tosses children who suffer from complex, metabolic disorders.**

ADHD has many diverse causes.

ADHD has many diverse remedies.

Knowing this, I believed I could help this girl, and help this mother who had sacrificed her career, the security of her marriage—and most of the days and nights of her daughter's life—to save the little girl she loved.

The Myth of ADHD

The myth is *not* that our children are free from suffering. They *are* suffering. The myth is that they are all suffering from the same thing. *ADHD is not a single, monolithic disorder.*

There is currently an unprecedented epidemic of children with symptoms associated with ADHD.

- 3 percent to 10 percent of all American children have symptoms that result in a diagnosis of ADHD.

- 3.5 million children are on ADHD medications.

- 1.5 million adults are on ADHD medications.

- Two times as many adults are on ADHD medications now than in the year 2000, and the number keeps rising, as the Ritalin Generation reaches adulthood.

• $3.1 billion was spent on ADHD drugs in 2005, almost four times as much as the amount spent in 2000.

• 90 percent of all the ADHD drugs in the world are consumed in America.

The rise in the incidence of ADHD symptoms closely tracks the rise in the incidence of autism. Both conditions were relatively rare until approximately the late 1980s, then rocketed upward. Some researchers and clinicians, believe that this twin spike occurred primarily because of toxic factors in modern life—possibly including toxins from childhood vaccinations—coupled with the current widespread failure to *detoxify*, due mostly to heavy metal overload and nutritional deficits.

The net result has been an explosion of not just autism and ADHD, but also allergies and asthma.

The symptoms associated with ADHD that these children suffer are painfully real, but the catchall label of ADHD is frequently arbitrary, and misapplied. For example, some of the traits that are used to define ADHD are often just personality quirks or normal differences. These traits might include restlessness, an inability to work well in groups, impatience, verbosity, or a lack of interest in quiet activities. The fact is, many children labeled with ADHD do quite well when they are in unrestricted, unstructured environments, in which they are rewarded for their energy, independence, creativity, and individuality. Partly because ADHD is often just a normal variance in personality, at least half the children diagnosed with ADHD don't become adults who are diagnosed with ADHD, even though their personalities generally do not change very much. These people are simply more comfortable and effective in adult environments that are of their own choosing, as they work on tasks that interest them.

Furthermore, many people with ADHD, just like many people with autism, have very special gifts, which frequently exist in direct proportion to their deficits. It's wonderful to be well-rounded, but many of the greatest people in history were not at all well-rounded. They were single-minded, inspired, individualistic, quirky people who were highly focused in some areas and scattered in others. Realistically, many of them probably would never have been blessed with their notable mental surpluses *without* corresponding degrees of mental or emotional deficits. That is a fact of not only neurology, but also lifestyle. *You can't have it all.* A great example of the surplus/deficit phenomenon is Albert Einstein, the quintessential absentminded professor, who had many ADHD and Asperger's symptoms and couldn't even speak until he was three. As a matter of fact, Hans Asperger often referred to his young patients as "little professors." Consider this list of people who had numerous personality traits that are now closely associated with ADHD:

The ADHD Hall of Fame

Benjamin Franklin	Isaac Newton
Albert Einstein	Galileo
Thomas Edison	Wilbur Wright
Leonardo da Vinci	Walt Disney
Louis Pasteur	Winston Churchill
Henry Ford	Alexander Graham Bell
Beethoven	Pablo Picasso
William Randolph Hearst	Robert Frost
Frank Lloyd Wright	Nikola Tessla

This list illustrates the pointlessness of pathologizing people, particularly children, by applying arbitrary labels of illness to them, just because they're different. In psychiatry, pathology sometimes exists only in the eye of the beholder. For example, homosexuality was officially considered to be a mental illness until the 1970s. Another example of this is the mental illness once known as drapetomania, a disease characterized by an unnatural desire to flee, or escape. It was applied in the 1850s–to runaway slaves. A medical authority noted at the time that, "With the proper medical care, this troublesome practice that many Negroes have of running away can be almost entirely prevented."

This same pathologizing can apply to many ADHD kids, who would have once merely been labeled as daydreamers, bundles of energy, class clowns, characters, fireballs, absentminded eggheads ... or just plain *boys.*

This doesn't mean, though, that most ADHD symptoms are generally something to celebrate. More often than not, in most kids, the negative symptoms cause alienation, confusion, distress, and a failure to achieve. Our goal as parents and doctors should be to leave our children's unique personalities and mental powers intact, but to help them overcome the particular symptoms that cause them pain. We should do this by using individualized, noninvasive therapies that do not simply mask symptoms, but correct their root causes.

Unfortunately, conventional ADHD treatment—from its beginnings right up to our own current era—has not taken this individualistic and naturalistic approach. The general tendency has been to ignore subtleties and variances in each child, and to bombard children's brains and behavior with crude and occasionally cruel treatments.

The cruelest were those used in the earliest days of ADHD therapy. When ADHD symptoms were first recognized as a disorder, in 1902, they were classified as "a defect in moral control," and all the therapies applied against them were basically just clumsy and hurtful punishments.

Around World War I, though, there was a widespread American epidemic of brain infection, or encephalitis, and many doctors noticed that children who had this disease shared many traits with the kids who had symptoms of the so-called moral defect disorder. These symptoms included hyperactivity, a short attention span, impaired memory, and irritability. This helped doctors to realize that the problem was not a moral disorder, but a biological one. Shortly after this, doctors introduced the first psychoactive drug that seemed to help control the disorder: Benzedrine, a powerful stimulant—a form of speed—which is now a controlled substance.

By the early 1950s, symptoms of ADHD were referred to as "minimal brain damage," even though there wasn't any real physical evidence of brain damage. In the 1960s, the disorder was once again renamed. It became "hyperkinetic reaction of childhood," and doctors started to occasionally use a less addicting stimulant, methylphenidate, or Ritalin.

Ritalin seemed to work by enhancing the activity of dopamine, one of the brain's primary neurotransmitters, which is associated with attention, a positive mood, and physical grace. Most doctors had come to believe that almost all kids with ADHD had a deficiency of dopamine activity, and that when it was boosted, the children would feel happier, would be better able to control themselves, and would have longer attention spans. It seemed paradoxical that a stimulant could not only help calm down hyperactive children, but also wake up inattentive children, but that's how the drug seemed to work—most of the time.

In about 30 percent of all kids, though, Ritalin did not seem to work well at all.

- It made some hyperactive kids even more hyper.
- It made some hyperactive kids too lethargic.
- It made some inattentive kids even more inattentive.
- It made some inattentive kids too hyper.

Furthermore, most of the children experienced at least mild side effects, such as jitteriness, insomnia, or fatigue. Many experienced very serious side effects, such as impaired growth. Ritalin was, at best, a flawed pharmaceutical tool.

Ritalin was considered highly suspect by many doctors when I first began to treat ADHD symptoms myself, around 1983, partly because of widespread street use by kids who were taking it to get high. By '83, the name applied to ADHD symptoms had morphed once more, to Attention Deficit Disorder, even though hyperactivity was lumped in as a symptom. To me, at that time, using Ritalin was too much like trying to nail in a tack with a sledgehammer. You could pound down symptoms in a relatively adequate percentage of kids, but were you really helping them as much as possible? What about root causes? What about the high percentage of kids who weren't helped at all? What about side effects?

I was more interested in natural, innovative approaches that seemed to solve the underlying problems. The premiere natural approach back then was the Feingold Diet, which is still extremely popular. It was aimed mainly at restricting food additives, along with the natural food chemical called salicylate, which is found in a number of seemingly healthy foods, such as green peppers and mushrooms, which cause reactions in some people. The science behind this diet seemed a little fuzzy to me at the time, but parents and kids said it worked, and I couldn't ignore that. I've often thought that there are two basic types of doctors: those who listen to their patients, and those who don't. I've always said, if you don't listen, you won't hear, and if you don't look, you won't see. So I tried the Feingold Diet, and got relatively good results in some children.

Now, all these years later, I think I've figured out why restricting salicylates has been so helpful for many ADHD kids. It's not just because of the old theory that salicylates are frequently allergenic, but also because they are closely related to another natural food chemical called phenol. Phenols can cause physical, cognitive, and behavioral problems in people who have impairment of the natural detoxifying process of sulfation. Sulfation is closely related to methylation, and is often impaired in kids with autism and ADHD.

Now here's where this whole thing gets even more interesting: Methylation doesn't just help break down toxins. *It also helps break down neurotransmitters.* Therefore, it helps break down dopamine. And therefore, *it helps ADHD kids with autistic features get rid of their excess dopamine,* which is a terrible problem for so many of them, as it was for Alisa.

This more highly individualized, dietary way of treating ADHD is still not the standard approach that's taught in most medical schools. It's something doctors generally have to learn on their own. I would never have learned it if I hadn't simply listened to my patients.

In a larger sense, I was also learning at this time to listen to the wisdom of the body. I was finding that if I gave patients the full spectrum of metabolic resources that their bodies needed, their bodies' own phenomenal forces of self-correction and detoxification would remedy most of their root problems, and empower their healing processes.

Over the years, I have helped a great many children recover from ADHD by healing the root causes that result in symptoms of this omnibus, catchall diagnosis. Among the most frequent underlying causes of ADHD are:

THE ROOT CAUSES OF ADHD

1.   Toxification of the brain and body with heavy metals, particularly mercury and lead.

2.   Toxification from childhood vaccinations containing thimerosal, especially when given to a child who is sick, or on antibiotics.

3.   Toxification from various environmental pollutants.

4.   Nutritional deficits that impede detoxification and that impair neurotransmitter function.

5. Food allergies, sensitivities, and intolerances that harm brain chemistry.

6. Inflammation of the brain, particularly from autoimmunity that is related to streptococcal bacteria. This results in a disorder known as PANDAS.

7. In utero stressors, including environmental toxins, inoculations, bacteria, viruses, nutritional deficiencies, and emotional stress.

8. Thyroid disorders—most commonly low thyroid activity, resulting in impaired energy and cognitive function. A similar problem is autoimmune thyroid disorder.

9. Presence of testosterone in males, which exacerbates toxification.

10. Genetic factors that contribute to all of these various assaults upon the nervous system, immune system, and gastrointestinal system.

If you're learning to be a good medical detective, you're probably looking at that list and saying, "Those are the *same basic factors* that contribute to autism." You're right. The root causes of both disorders are similar. That is why I consider ADHD to be, in effect, part of the autism spectrum. It's why many kids have features of both autism and ADHD. It is also why many kids, such as Alisa, move from a diagnosis of autism to a diagnosis of ADHD, as their symptoms improve.

Now you may be thinking, "Gee, Dr. Bock, you're against pathologizing my son by saddling him with the ADHD label, but now you're saying he's on the *autism spectrum*. Thanks a *lot!*" Keep in mind, though, that in the prior chapters I also punctured the various, often arbitrary labels of the autism spectrum, because I believe those labels are also generally just descriptions of behaviors, rather than meaningful medical diagnoses of root causes. Even so, we must often use these words, accurate or not, to navigate in the medical milieu, and to communicate effectively with other medical professionals.

The key is: Keep reducing things down to root causes. That is what makes sense. That is what heals children.

When we fail to do this, the results can be tragic.

Detroit, Michigan

Matthew did everything he could to get out of taking his Ritalin. He spit the pills out, threw them away, and got mad when his mom and dad forced him to take them. He kept saying that the Ritalin was hurting him—making him feel like a zombie—but Larry and Kelly thought he was just making excuses. Kids hated *lots* of the things that were good for them, and it was a parent's job to fight through that resistance and make them do what was best.

Larry, though, was still not convinced that Matthew really needed Ritalin. Larry was almost certain that it was causing Matthew to have mood swings. However, he thought, maybe the mood swings were inherent in Matthew's personality, and the Ritalin was helping control them. The only way to find out would be to discontinue the Ritalin for a few weeks and see what happened. If they did that, though, the school might intervene again, and maybe even threaten once more to take Matthew away. After all, school authorities regularly checked on Matthew's medication status, and it seemed as if every time there was any little problem at school, they would tell Larry and Kelly that they should increase Matthew's dosage.

Therefore, over a period of seven years, as Matthew progressed from first grade to eighth, his daily dosage doubled from 10 milligrams to 20 milligrams, three times per day.

One of the worst problems with the Ritalin Matthew was taking was that it wore off about every four hours, often causing a slump of distress, lethargy, distractibility, and discomfort. The constant need for more medication had forced Matthew into a life that was somewhat like that of a drug addict, living from dose to dose. There were similar drugs that lasted longer, but they caused problems, too. Many of the kids on those drugs would lie in bed all night fidgeting and fussing with insomnia. Then, of course, they would be tired the next day, and run the risk of displaying inattentive behavior to the teacher, which could result in even higher dosages.

Larry tried hard to cooperate with the school authorities, but he could never get over his suspicion that medicating his son was actually more for the school's benefit than Matthew's. Matthew, with sandy hair and a sweet smile, continued to be a good kid at home. The only times he ever got into trouble were at school. Dealing with Matthew's school brought back bad memories for Larry. So much of what he'd learned as a child now seemed totally irrelevant. His memories of school often ran along the lines of: "Children, can you tell me something about Betsy Ross? She sewed the what? The flag? Class? Anyone?" Those old memories flared into consciousness whenever Matthew got into trouble.

Larry was also suspicious about the fact that Matthew's school, like most others, received extra federal and state aid for every ADHD child who was diagnosed and medicated. He had also learned that parents on welfare got more money when their kids were diagnosed and drugged. This was reasonable on one level, but it didn't offer any economic incentive for recovery—only for illness. Larry was also disturbed to know that Matthew, as someone who was older than twelve and currently on Ritalin, would be ineligible for military service (along with over 80 percent of his generation, which was riddled with the disqualifying disorders of learning disabilities, obesity, asthma, severe allergies, ADHD, and autism). The military obviously considered Ritalin use to be a stigma—who else would?

Despite all this, Matthew seemed to be making his way in the world. He had good friends, was a star on the school baseball team, and tried out for football but didn't like it. At fourteen, he was developing more sophisticated tastes in entertainment. He loved *The Shawshank Redemption* and *Saturday Night Live.*

Luckily, the end of all of this finally seemed near. Larry knew that about half of all ADHD kids didn't carry the condition into adulthood, for some reason (such as, possibly, that it *hadn't really existed* in the first place).

So he felt as if he could at last see the light at the end of the tunnel.

Also, he and Kelly were becoming interested in other approaches, such as dietary change, special ADHD supplements, and chelation.

Matthew's eighth-grade, midyear report card was the best of his life. He was *so* close. Still, he needed something *else*—something to put him over the top. He couldn't stay on Ritalin forever.

Matthew was in his aunt's basement, playing with his skateboard.

At age fourteen, Matthew Smith had a heart attack and died almost immediately. Larry and Kelly had no opportunity to speak to Matthew, or to hold him, before he died.

An autopsy by the county's chief pathologist showed that Matthew's heart was grossly enlarged, and was pocked with small vessel damage, consistent with extended use of stimulants. The chief medical examiner ruled that, "Death was caused by Long-Term use of Methylphenidate (Ritalin)."

Larry still wishes, among the many things he wishes, that he'd at least had a moment with Matthew at the end, to tell him that he was sorry.

Liza called me, sobbing. It was hard to understand her. Something terrible had happened to Alisa. I took a breath, and steeled myself.

CHAPTER EIGHT

EXECUTIVE FUNCTION

LIZA'S VOICE WAS HOLLOW AND CONVULSIVE, TREMBLING WITH emotion, tormented. "This is bad," she said. I could hear her take deep breaths that brought no calm.

"Alisa's locked in her room...out of control," Liza said. "I don't know what to do...." Deep breaths. "I think she broke my finger."

Alisa was cycling in intermittent waves of rage that blasted right through the phone lines.

"Just let her cycle out," I said. "She'll be okay."

Liza later told me that I sounded confident and reassuring, but listening to Alisa was alarming.

Suddenly there was the sound of something shattering.

"What was that?"

"Her lamp," said Liza. "That's the only thing left in the room. Everything else, I took out, so she couldn't break it. We were having a good *time*. She was *happy*. Then, *BOOM!*"

Now what? Have Liza go in after her? Risk confronting Alisa amid broken glass? "Just let her cycle out," I said.

As Liza fought to control her fear, I made myself slow down and think like a good medical detective. Rage was a classic symptom of heavy metal poisoning, but this kind of wild-animal, zero-to-sixty outburst was even more closely associated with the streptococcal disorder that I mentioned previously: PANDAS (Pediatric Autoimmune Neuropsychiatric Disorder Associated with Streptococcal Infection). PAN-

DAS, which usually strikes kids who've had several bouts of strep throat, causes brain inflammation. This inflammation occasionally reaches such a high threshold that it overwhelms the rational areas of the frontal lobes, and allows the tyranny of the lower brain to erupt in manic fear and anger.

Not many people in the medical community had, at this time, in the early 2000s, heard of PANDAS. However, I'd noticed a blurb about it, had done some research, and had gotten in touch with the physician who had discovered the condition, Susan Swedo, M.D., the Director of Child Psychiatry at the National Institutes of Mental Health. I learned that about half the kids with PANDAS had ADHD, that about half also had depressive disorders, and that about one-third had coexisting anxiety disorders. Apparently, PANDAS just cooked the brains of these poor kids. These children also often had facial tics and obsessive-compulsive problems—*as did Alisa.*

"I want you to check Alisa's antistrep antibodies," I told Liza. I told her which ones to check. *"Tomorrow."*

Liza said that Alisa had never had strep throat in her life, but I still insisted.

The racket from Alisa's rage gradually subsided as I discussed PANDAS with Liza. What a mom! Even in this hour of doubt and dread, she was keeping her mind lasered in on this one, new, narrow avenue that held some hope of saving her daughter.

When twenty minutes had passed without a sound from the room—the requisite time to ensure the end of a cycle—Liza said, "I'll let you go now."

"Call me tomorrow."

When Liza entered the room, stepping around the shattered glass, Alisa's whole face was bloated, and was the color of blood, as if she'd been beaten.

Even now, years later, Alisa can remember the primary emotion she was feeling as Liza came to her with open arms: *shame,* as a hot, sick sensation that seemed to flood her whole body.

Alisa still recalls that as the rage had advanced upon her, she had tried to use her words, and had tried to think things through, but it had swept over her like a blinding storm.

Alisa reached out. "I'm *sorry."*

"I know. I love you."

"I'm just. . . ." Her chest heaved. "A bad person."

Alisa began to cry. Her shoulders shook.

"You're a wonderful person."

Liza held her daughter very closely.

I stayed up late, thinking about the terrible mysteries of the mind.

When Sue Swedo had first started exploring PANDAS, many people in the psychiatric community had still believed that facial tics in children were caused by punitive toilet training.

We'd come a long way—and we had a long way yet to go.

The Terrible Mysteries of the Mind

Dr. Swedo discovered that one of the most damaging things that PANDAS does is to attack a part of the brain, called the basal ganglia, that is one of the primary links between the brain's calming, advanced areas and its more primitive, animalistic areas. The attack upon this important link can cause serious malfunctions of thought and behavior, including a tendency to fly into sudden, uncontrollable rages.

PANDAS isn't the only thing that can impair this link, though. It can also be harmed by a variety of other factors—everything from nutrient deficiencies, to toxins, to viruses, to inflammation from other causes. When this happens, drugs such as Ritalin can rev up the basal ganglia, and help compensate for the damage, but the problem still exists, because the root causes are still there.

The damage to the basal ganglia caused by PANDAS and other factors can wreak complete havoc upon the entire brain, because it is vitally important for the advanced areas of the brain to be in control of the lower areas.

The advanced areas consist essentially of the rational, inhibitory, logical regions of the upper brain, or neocortex—particularly the frontal lobes, which are located in the area of the forehead. These are incredibly powerful areas, dense with gray matter, that make humans more intelligent than any other creature on earth.

The more primitive areas of the brain—the ones that really aren't much different from those found in most animals—are located lower in the brain, near the brain stem, closer to the spine. These lower areas are governed by the highly emotional limbic system, which includes the brain's fear center, the amygdala.

The lower brain is the first stop for most of the information that comes in from the outside world, through senses such as sight and hearing. This information is sorted out by the thalamus—which is where problems often start for ADHD kids. Like autistic kids, ADHD kids often have weak function of the thalamus, and aren't very good at sorting out the information from the senses. ADHD kids often perceive the world as a chaotic jumble of sights and sounds. These kids can be overwhelmed by a busy environment, such as a shopping mall, or even a crowded classroom. Noisy, distracting environments can cloud their thoughts and judgments, and knock out their inhibitions.

Fear generally plays a big role in our brain's sorting process, simply because fear is our greatest single survival mechanism. Fear, unfortunately, plays *too* big of a role in the brains of many autistic children, as you may recall. Autistic kids tend to have overactive, enlarged amygdalas, and that's partly why they often feel so much anxiety. This same overactivation of the amygdala can occur among kids with ADHD, although it usually occurs to a lesser degree.

However, the biggest, single neurological problem that most ADHD kids have is that their brains are frequently not very good at sending messages from the lower brain to the upper brain, via the basal ganglia and a few other neural links. Their thoughts too often stay down in the lower, limbic area of the brain, which is governed more by emotion, fear, and instinct than it is by logic.

Furthermore, the path between the lower brain and the upper brain is a two-way street, capable of bouncing information back and forth, so that emotional and fear-based evaluation can work in partnership with rational and logical evaluation. Unfortunately, this process, too, is often impaired in people with ADHD. Thoughts and feelings tend to just get stuck. Sometimes they get stuck in the upper brain, creating a tendency for people to be overly rational, and too unemotional. In the jargon of psychology, these people live in their heads. Much more often, though, thoughts and feelings get bogged down in the lower brain, prompting behavior that's based far too much in fear, and in the emotion that's most closely associated with fear: anger.

When ADHD kids suffer from this difficulty in moving their thoughts and feelings up to the higher regions of their frontal lobes, they are at a terrible disadvantage. The frontal lobes are what enable people to pay attention, stay focused, figure things out, make good decisions, plan ahead, be considerate of others, defer immediate gratification, and remember things.

The frontal lobes are also the ground-zero home of inhibition. When people drink too much alcohol, part of its effect is to cut off the communication paths to their frontal lobes. When this happens, people sometimes lose their inhibitions, and do things they later regret. This condition of impaired inhibition can be practically permanent, though, among some people with ADHD. They just don't have a good neural highway between the lower brain and the upper brain, so when temptations and impulses arise, they aren't very good at evaluating them rationally. They tend to be too impulsive, and too quick to go for pleasure. They can't overcome the tyrannical dictatorship of fear, anger, and desire that resides in the lower brain. Feelings sweep over them like a whirlwind, and they get carried away.

It's been said that 70 percent of the brain is there to inhibit the other 30 percent. In some ADHD kids, however, this ratio seems to get reversed, and it's very difficult for these kids to control themselves. A person with this neurological makeup can go through his or her entire life feeling as overwhelmed by temptation as the proverbial kid in a candy store. This is part of the reason why so many kids with ADHD grow up to become adults who overindulge in alcohol, drugs, food, and other avenues of immediate gratification. Conventional wisdom says that these people are just masking their emotional pain with indulgences, but it's more complicated than that. They are also often simply incapable of knowing when to say when, because their frontal lobes don't get much of an opportunity to vote in the decision.

With the advent of modern brain imaging, we are now able to actually see physical signs of poor frontal lobe function. One sign is an excess of slow brain wave activity in the frontal lobes, as seen on the EEGs of people with ADHD. Another sign is a measurable deficit among ADHD people of brain cells in the frontal lobes, and also in the basal ganglia. Unfortunately, as time goes on, these deficits of brain cells can become more pronounced, and even self-perpetuating, because the brain, similarly to other parts of the body, is governed by the principle of use it or lose it.

Another important part of the brain that is often relatively dysfunctional in ADHD kids is the primary attention system of the brain, which is linked intricately to the frontal lobes. This attention system, known as the reticular activating system, is a network of connections that sends information all around the neocortex, trying to excite various clusters of brain cells into processing this information. If the reticular activating system is functioning sluggishly, the brain can have problems staying on task. This can result in the classic signs of the inattentive subtype of ADHD: lack of focus, easy distractibility, a short attention span, and difficulty in learning. If this system is overly aroused, though, it can create the opposite type of symptoms, those associated with the hyperactive subtype of ADHD: restlessness, impulsivity, a tendency to pick up and quickly discard random objects, talking too much, and becoming easily obsessed with things.

The reticular activating system is particularly sensitive to any excesses or deficits of neurotransmitters. Too much stimulating norepinephrine or dopamine can make it overly aroused, and too little can make it drowsy. Too much calming serotonin can also drive it down.

Neurotransmitters, of course, also play major roles in every other part of the brain, and various problems with neurotransmitters throughout the brain often result in symptoms of ADHD. It's very common for people with ADHD to have low levels of serotonin, and this almost always triggers agitation, restlessness, and anxiety. It's also common for ADHD people to have low levels of the thought-transporter acetylcholine. Without enough acetylcholine to carry thoughts from one neuron to another, thoughts can get lost in a thick, impenetrable brain fog.

The neurotransmitter that most frequently causes ADHD symptoms, though, is dopamine. A lack of dopamine is the main reason that Ritalin exists. Ritalin is, in many ways, the pharmaceutical Band-Aid for people who have a deficit of dopamine. Ritalin shares many characteristics with dopamine–primarily, the ability to trigger arousal. Dopamine wakes up the brain and perks up the mood, just as Ritalin often does. As I've mentioned, however, Ritalin is often the worst possible medication for ADHD kids who have autistic features, because these kids usually have too *much* dopamine. Dopamine, like all the other neurotransmitters, works well only within a narrow range–too much is as disastrous as too little.

One reason so many ADHD kids have a dopamine deficit is because their brain cells can't adequately accept entry of this neurotransmitter, even when it's present in sufficient quantities. Neurotransmitters need to enter brain cells through receptors, and if these receptors aren't working properly, the neurotransmitters can't get in.

There are twelve different types of receptors for dopamine on each brain cell, and one receptor, called D-4, is notorious for malfunctioning. A big reason it malfunctions is because this receptor needs to be methylated to function well. When the detoxification process of methylation breaks down, it allows too much dopamine to pile up in the receptor, just as it also allows too many toxins to pile up in the cells. This pile-up causes the D-4 receptor to shut down, and suddenly there's a shortage of dopamine activity. Once more, we see it: *the miracle of methylation.*

In fact, one reason that ADHD is so heritable—with genetic connections in almost 80 percent of all cases—is because malfunction of the D-4 dopamine receptor is commonly passed on genetically.

Too often, the medical community views genetic traits such as this as sadly inevitable, and impossible to overcome. However, simply methylating the D-4 receptor, using methyl-B-12, can often resolve the problem. Again, we see why it's so important to dig all the way down to root causes.

The net effect of all of these classic contributing factors to ADHD is a brain that just can't take good care of itself. In particular, it can't have a good talk with itself, in the same way that you might have a talk with yourself when you're trying to make a difficult decision. The higher brain simply can't engage in a smart dialogue with the lower brain. The lower brain hogs the conversation, and thoughts and feelings get bogged in a mire of fear, anger, and selfish desire. Negativity builds upon negativity, until bad behavior finally bursts forth like an uncontrollable fire.

When this unfortunate process occurs, people lose what neurologists call executive function. Losing executive function means that the frontal lobes aren't in charge anymore. The Boss is out of the office. Chaos reigns, and the lower instincts prevail. When people lose strong executive function, they can have the best of intentions, but just don't have the biological means to harness those intentions, and do the right thing.

The conventional remedy for lack of executive function is Ritalin, and similar drugs. These drugs usually stimulate the problematic parts of the brain, wake up the basal ganglia, and help people control themselves.

But Ritalin doesn't solve anything. The brain's problems are still there four hours later, when the drug wears off.

Building Executive Function

The Healing Program, however, can solve the root problems that impair executive function. It can help the body and brain to:

- Balance neurotransmitters.
- Methylate receptors.
- Regulate the reticular activating system.
- Provide the nutrients that become neurotransmitters.
- Restore the physical integrity of the basal ganglia.
- Activate and modulate neurons.
- Evacuate neural toxins.
- Improve blood flow to the brain, to get nutrients in and toxins out.

The Healing Program can trigger wonderful cascades of regeneration in brains that had previously been trapped in destructive spirals of degeneration.

As always, though, in the final analysis, it's not the Healing Program that ultimately creates the recoveries. It's the parents, and the kids. The Healing Program is a tool. It's the parents, with their limitless love–and their children, who are trying *so hard*–who do the work.

Executive Function

My medical detective's hunch was right: Alisa did have PANDAS. I recommended a course of antibiotics, which quickly quieted Alisa's chronic, subclinical streptococcal infection. When that happened, her immune system stopped producing its barrage of antibodies to the strep, and that had a powerful impact upon her brain, for an indirect reason. Strep bacteria, unfortunately, mimic a partial-protein that's found in the brain's basal ganglia. This mimicry confuses the immune system, and it begins to bombard the basal ganglia with strep antibodies, igniting a firestorm of inflammation. The inflammation then knocks down the proper function of the basal ganglia, impairing this vital link between the lower brain and the advanced brain. When this link is down, the fearful, angry, animalistic urges of the lower brain gain periodic dominance, no matter how hard people try to resist.

This ugly biological cascade had probably been harming Alisa's brain for years, but no one had been able to see it. All they'd been able to see was the horrible behavior it had caused.

Alisa had recently been having an average of four meltdown cycles every day, as her PANDAS had raged to new heights. When she started taking antibiotics, though, an entire day went by without a cycle. To Liza, even one day was an oasis of peace.

Another day came, with no rages. Then, a third.

On the fourth day, some of Alisa's friends were playing outside, and somebody told somebody else to shut up, and then it escalated, and Alisa got involved.

"Shut up, *psycho,*" one of Alisa's friends hissed at her.

Alisa thought it over. She thought that a reasonable response would be to see how much her *friend* liked being called a psycho. So Alisa said, "Yeah, *you're* a psycho." Then she hopped on her bike and rode away, feeling good, in full control.

Her executive function had returned! The Boss was back!

Well, at least midmanagement was back. The Boss would have said something even more frontal-lobe, like: "You don't define me when you insult me–you define *yourself*!" The Boss in each of us is always capable of saying those smart things that we later *wish* we'd said, but hadn't, in the heat of the moment. Executive function, in fact, is all about taking the heat *out* of the moment.

One more day went by without a blazing rage. Then, another.

The *real* Alisa was finally, once again emerging–the Alisa who had babbled happily in her crib, and had loved the world.

As a young child, Alisa had, with her mother's help, escaped the dark cage of autism. Now she was at last beginning to also free herself from the symptoms of ADHD. It was all part of her continuum of healing.

This exceptional degree of recovery could occur more frequently among children who have symptoms of both autism and ADHD, if only the medical community were more attuned to the similarities of cause and recovery between the two disorders. The conventional perception is that autism and ADHD are not related, other than that they are both developmental disorders.

I disagree.

The Autism-ADHD Connection

I am convinced that autism and ADHD are intimately related. I think ADHD is basically just the mildest form of symptomatology that is found on the autism spectrum.

More precisely, I believe that *both* disorders are merely similar neurological manifestations of a wide variety of related problems. These problems include:

- Toxicity.
- Nutritional deficits.
- Bowel dysbiosis.
- Inflammation.
- Immune dysregulation.
- Autoimmune disorders.
- Allergic reactions.
- Genetic vulnerability.

For the most part, when these problems are extreme, combined, and omnipresent, the result is frank autism. When they are less extreme, fewer in number, and exist only occasionally, the result is Asperger's or PDD-NOS. When they are relatively moderate, very limited in number, and occur only infrequently, the result is ADHD. When they are mild, isolated, and occur very rarely, the result is borderline ADHD, or neurological disorders as common and treatable as learning disabilities and speech pathologies.

Similarly, the degree of strength, variety, and frequency of these problems also has an influence on the intensity of a child's asthma, and upon the proneness of a child to allergy. Because of this, these two other 4-A disorders often co-exist with autism and ADHD.

One reason autism is generally viewed as being separate from ADHD is simply because of a quirky rule in the psychiatric diagnostic system. The rule says that when people have both a major disorder and a minor disorder, their basic diagnosis is only that of the major disorder. Therefore, when patients show simultaneous signs of both autism and ADHD, they are assigned a diagnosis of only the more severe disorder: autism. Because of this rule, even though autistic children may have a number of ADHD traits, their diagnosis of autism tends to focus their treatment on autism therapies.

This rule helps to obscure the many links between the two disorders. These links, which have been carefully documented by author and autism expert Diane Kennedy, include the following:

THE ADHD-AUTISM LINKS

Autism-Spectrum Traits	ADHD Traits
• Poor social skills; verbosity, inability to be empathetic.	• Disruptive, argumentative, verbose, and unempathetic behavior.
• Low awareness of physical danger.	• Frequent risk-taking behavior, with little regard for consequences.
• Tantrums, outbursts.	• Tantrums, outbursts.
• Overactivity in some people, lethargy in others.	• Overactivity and hyperactivity in some people, lethargy in others.
• Poor eye contact.	• Often avoid eye contact.
• Work can be careless and sloppy.	• Work is often careless, with poor attention to detail.
• Tendency to have poor gross and fine motor skills, including messy handwriting, awkward gait, and a lack of coordination.	• Tendency to have poor gross and fine motor skills, including messy handwriting, an awkward gait, and poor coordination.
• Resistance to change, and clinging to routine.	• Fear of new places and people; comfortable with habits.
• Tendency to have involuntary facial tics and body movements.	• Tendency to have involuntary facial tics and body movements.
• Poor memory among most people, but highly developed memory among some.	• Poor memory among most people, but highly developed memory among some.
• Speech pathologies.	• Speech pathologies.
• Tendency to be compulsively perfectionistic.	• Tendency to perfectionism.
• Frequent presence of notable mental gifts and skills.	• Frequent presence of notable mental gifts and skills.
• Tendency to focus very myopically on specific matters of interest.	• Common ability to focus intensely on matters of interest.

These links are closest between very high functioning autistic people, and people who have relatively extreme ADHD. In fact, people from these two groups often act so similarly that it can be hard to tell them apart. Among these people, making the distinction between autism and ADHD is often arbitrary.

Another revealing link between autism and ADHD is the fact that people with both disorders tend to share other specific mental and behavioral problems. Following are the co-morbid neurological and psychological conditions that frequently accompany both autism and ADHD.

AUTISM/ADHD

Disorders Associated with Both

1. Depression.
2. Anxiety and mood disorders.
3. Bipolar disorder.
4. Obsessive-Compulsive Disorder.
5. Learning disabilities.
6. Speech pathologies.
7. Oppositional Defiance Disorder.
8. Insomnia and sleep disorders.
9. Communication disorders.

From a conventional psychiatric perspective, Alisa had more than half of these co-morbid disorders, and could have been simultaneously treated for each of them, if Liza had not been such an astute mother. Alisa might have ended up taking a daily smorgasbord of drugs, each targeting a separate problem. These medications might have included antidepressants, anti-anxiety medications, bipolar meds, antipsychotics, OCD meds, insomnia medications, and, of course, Ritalin.

My approach to the broad scope of Alisa's problems was quite different. From my perspective, all these problems were interrelated, synergistic, and due largely to complex, metabolic root causes that required biomedical treatment. I believed that Alisa's wide web of problems indicated that her brain, *as a whole,* was metabolically impaired, and that the only effective treatment would be to nurture her entire brain, and her whole body.

This meant more than just reversing the PANDAS. It meant putting her on a full-scale Healing Program, which included the following:

- Anti-inflammatories, for lingering gastrointestinal problems.
- An anti-hypoglycemia diet.
- Restriction of several allergenic foods.
- Detoxification of heavy metals, with DMSA and methyl-B-12.
- Supplementation with a number of nutrients, including essential fatty acids.
- Antibiotics, used prophylactically, to control the chronic strep infection.

Even a multifaceted approach, however, held no guarantee of full recovery. Not all children achieve complete healing. The forces against them are fierce. Therefore, it's important to celebrate even moderate improvement.

There was one thing, though, of which I was certain: Without a comprehensive assault upon Alisa's entire constellation of interconnected issues, she would end up being just one more kid on the road to Ritalin. And that's a road that can lead to tragedy.

CHAPTER NINE

THE ROAD TO RITALIN

"I DON'T WANT TEIA ON DRUGS," LISA O'CONNOR TOLD HER DAUGH-ter's doctor.

"Then we've got to get you more *educated* about drugs," the doctor responded cheerfully.

"She's *six*. She's in *first grade*."

The doctor didn't respond, but continued to smile. Lisa felt trapped. "I'm not going to do this," she said.

The doctor became markedly less cheerful and insisted that Lisa at least take home a questionnaire. The doctor said that Lisa should fill it out, and then Teia's first-grade teacher would fill it out. After that, they would all decide together what was best for Teia.

Lisa took the questionnaire home, but as she filled it out, she began to feel as if the questionnaire had been constructed to steer parents toward describing their kids as having symptoms of ADHD. Teia *was* tired too often–there was no doubt about that–and she didn't focus well, but the questionnaire made it sound as if these traits had to be symptoms of a mental disorder, and couldn't possibly indicate anything else.

Lisa studied the questionnaire after she finished it. "They've got her on the road to Ritalin," she murmured to herself. She threw the questionnaire away. She thought that was the end of it.

A year later, though, Teia's second-grade teacher called Lisa in to the school. Lisa thought she knew what was coming–Ritalin–so she brought her husband with her, and also her sister, who was a grade-school principal.

The teacher told them Lisa needed to repeat second grade. Further-more, she needed to repeat it on Ritalin.

"We need to get Teia to concentrate," the teacher said. "She's just *not* going to be able to get better without the medication."

To help drive home her point, the teacher called Teia into the room, along with the school's math teacher. The math teacher showed Teia some geometric shapes, and Teia began to identify them. He showed her a cylinder.

"It's an oval," Teia said.

The second-grade teacher shook her head, and drilled a look into Lisa.

"If you look at it from Teia's perspective," said Lisa's sister, turning the illustration around, "it *is* an oval."

Teia, confused and nervous, thought the whole thing was a little crazy. Here were all these grown-ups, arguing about giving her a medi-cine that would make her tiredness—her goopy feeling—get better. But she didn't want to take a medicine that would make her feel less goopy. She wanted actual *energy*—a bunch of it—like the other kids had.

Lisa put her foot down: no Ritalin, no way.

The teacher let them go, but didn't seem too concerned about her defeat. The decision about holding Teia back was hers to make. Time was on her side.

RITALIN

The Most Common Side Effects

1. **Insomnia.** Some children require sleeping pills at night to counteract Ritalin's stimulation.
2. **Addiction.** Dependency sometimes occurs, occasionally even after relatively short courses of the medication.
3. **Decreased appetite.** Ritalin often has the same basic effect upon appetite as pharmaceutical diet pills.
4. **Growth delay.** The drug can interfere with growth hormones, and can also delay growth by interfering with a child's appetite.
5. **Weight loss.** Ritalin triggers weight loss by interfering with eating, and by increasing the metabolic rate.

6. **Heart palpitations.** The stimulating effect of the drug can cause not only palpitations, but also increased heart rate. In rare cases, it causes heart enlargement and vessel damage, which can, uncommonly, result in death.

7. **Nervousness.** Ritalin can trigger anxiety in some people, and often causes restlessness.

8. **Tics.** This occurs in about 1 percent of the patients who had not previously had involuntary motor tics. It includes facial twitches and excessive blinking.

9. **Headaches.** They are most common early in treatment, and may be accompanied by stomach pains.

10. **Crying.** Some patients have less control over emotional outbursts than they did prior to drug administration.

11. **Rebound effect.** When the drug wears off every few hours, some patients experience elevated anxiety, depression, or restlessness.

12. **Blood sugar destabilization.** Patients with diabetes or hypoglycemia may experience rapid shifts in blood sugar levels.

Rhinebeck, New York

Teia slumped down in one of my office chairs as if she had melted into it. She was sniffly and stuffy, inattentive, sluggish, and withdrawn. One-word answers. Poor eye contact. Moderately dilated pupils. She also had little white bumps on her arms, known as keratosis pilaris, which could indicate a deficiency of essential fatty acids and vitamin A. Teia was small for her age, and had a long history of bladder infections, which had been treated with antibiotics. She also had a history of cold intolerance, hypoglycemia, and constipation.

In retrospect, I realize that she was a very beautiful child, with gorgeous hair and a sweet little face, but she wasn't projecting it, so I didn't see it. Her eyes were dull, almost dead, and seemed to somehow be drawing light in, instead of reflecting it.

Her lab work showed low glutathione, low cysteine, low plasma sulfate, and normal thyroid levels in her blood.

So, Detective, what do you think?

Low thyroid? You're right. So many clues pointed at low thyroid: cold intolerance, small stature, constipation, and, of course, lethargy and impaired cognitive function.

Although Teia did have normal levels of thyroid hormones in her blood, it didn't necessarily mean that enough thyroid hormones were getting into her cells. In that regard, thyroid hormones are somewhat like the hormone insulin: You can have plenty of insulin in your bloodstream, but if it's not moving glucose into your cells, due to a condition such as insulin resistance, you've got a problem. Too often, however, when doctors look for thyroid problems, the only thing they do is check the blood level of thyroid hormones. With this limited testing, they can accurately diagnose laboratory-proven hypothyroidism, but they often miss the signs and symptoms of a milder form of the disorder, that I refer to as functional hypothyroidism. When their lab results come back within the normal range, or even the low normal range, they frequently overlook the abnormalities of daily, physical function that are caused by moderately low thyroid.

As I looked deeper into the root causes of Teia's functional hypothyroidism, I found that she had elevated thyroid antibodies, indicating that she was suffering from a relatively common but often overlooked autoimmune problem known as Hashimoto's disease. Hashimoto's disease is by far the most common of all the autoimmune diseases, but it often has relatively subtle symptoms that are mistaken for other problems, such as, in Teia's case, inattentive subtype ADHD. Unfortunately, most doctors generally don't test for Hashimoto's, and as I've said, if you don't look, you won't see.

Similarly, some doctors also disregard moderate *excesses* of thyroid hormones, which can cause symptoms resembling those of hyperactive subtype ADHD.

In addition to Hashimoto's disease, Teia had another subtle thyroid problem, which is also relatively common: a deficit of the enzyme that is involved in the metabolism of thyroid hormones. Activity of this enzyme, called deiodinase, can be impaired by a deficiency of selenium, and also by mercury overload. So, once again, we see that mercury, from vaccinations and other sources, can create symptoms of a behavioral disorder in a very indirect way.

In addition, mercury toxification also appeared to be having another, very *direct* impact upon Teia. She had low glutathione, low plasma cysteine, and low plasma sulfate, all indicating impaired detoxification, through the processes of sulfation and methylation. Mercury was, in all likelihood, the primary root cause of Teia's impaired ability to detoxify.

Teia also had a secondary heavy metal problem: toxification from lead. Lead is a classic contributor to ADHD. It's not only neurotoxic, but also drives down two minerals the body and brain desperately need–iron and zinc. A high percentage of ADHD kids are low in iron–which is needed to make dopamine–and this saps their mental and physical energy. One study showed that 80 percent of ADHD kids were low in iron. Unfortunately, many doctors don't pay attention to iron deficiency until it hits rock bottom, resulting in frank anemia. This same lack of regard for subtle deficiencies is also true of zinc, which is a critically important nutrient for cognitive function, because it protects neurotransmitters. In fact, one of the aphorisms of neurological nutrition is, "No zinc, no think." Zinc, however, is typically depleted in ADHD children–by an average of two-thirds, according to a recent study.

Teia's toxicity, according to other lab tests, was also creating dysfunction in the internal power centers in each of her cells, which are known as the mitochondria. It's very common for people to have mitochondrial problems. That's why practically every supermarket in America carries a supplement that boosts the function of the mitochondria: co-enzyme Q-10. Many people find that when they start taking this supplement, their energy levels soar.

This supplement can also indirectly help many people to overcome hypoglycemia, since people sometimes start eating too many sweets, triggering hypoglycemia, when mitochondrial problems pound down their energy. Therefore, I was hoping that as the function of Teia's mitochondria improved–through detoxification and supplementation with Co-Q-10–her hypoglycemia would go away.

Hopefully, Teia's toxicity would be easier to resolve than a similar level of toxicity in a boy, since testosterone tends to exacerbate heavy metal poisoning. *This negative effect of testosterone may be a reason why boys have 400 percent more autism than girls, 400–800 percent more Asperger's, and 400–600 percent more ADHD.*

Teia's hypoglycemia–a condition that can absolutely destroy energy–was probably also being aggravated by several food allergies, including an allergy to dairy. Teia's mom had been giving her a lot of yogurt, during her many courses of antibiotics, to help restore Teia's healthy bowel bacteria, which are often killed by antibiotics. The antibiotics had definitely triggered candida overgrowth, which was hammering Teia's energy, but the strategy of giving Teia yogurt was backfiring, due to her dairy allergy. Many people, I've noticed, eat large quantities of yogurt when they take antibiotics, but it's often unwise, since so many people are reactive to dairy products. A better strategy is to take probiotic supplements, which contain acidophilus and other healthy digestive bacteria, but no dairy.

Teia was also allergic to chocolate, which she loved to eat, and that was probably another part of her energy problem. Food allergies wreak havoc on stable levels of blood sugar, and can even cause psychiatric symptoms, such as spaciness and depression. Symptoms of food allergy, in fact, often closely mimic symptoms of ADHD, and this frequently results in a misdiagnosis of ADHD.

Another reason that Teia may have craved chocolate is because it contains a potent chemical that boosts dopamine production, phenylethylamine. This chemical is probably the main reason that some people actually seem to get high from eating chocolate.

Teia was still having chronic bladder infections, and was put on a low, prophylactic dosage of antibiotics to stop the infections before they became established. I was concerned that antibiotics might disrupt her detoxification, but I thought the probiotics might help with that.

I talked with Teia's mom about adjusting her diet and supplement program. The centerpiece of Teia's treatment, though, was restoring her thyroid hormones to their proper levels. I was certain that her functional thyroid deficiency was her worst problem, simply because low energy was her strongest complaint. I gave Teia a relatively high dosage of vitamin D, to regulate her immune system, and to help stop its autoimmune attack upon her thyroid. I also put her on a treatment for low thyroid: Armour thyroid, a prescription medication that contains actual thyroid hormones. Armour thyroid can restore thyroid hormone levels quickly and dramatically.

I was confident that the Healing Program could help Teia, because it addressed her entire, interwoven web of problems: low thyroid, heavy metal toxification, nutritional deficiencies, impaired detoxification, candida overgrowth, allergies, chronic bladder infections, and hypoglycemia.

It *could* help her. But would it? That depended mostly on Teia's mom, Lisa. It's easy enough for me to spot problems. It's hard for parents to solve them. It takes all the energy and all the love they've got. It can stress marriages, overwhelm entire extended families, and decimate finances. But that rarely stops families from doing what's best for their children.

It certainly didn't stop the family of another of my ADHD patients, nicknamed the Million Dollar Kid. But it almost destroyed it.

The Million Dollar Kid

Brian Dunn's parents spent everything they had on him, more than a million dollars, before they gave him that nickname. They mortgaged their home three times, burned through their life savings, and asked every member of their extended family to contribute to the Save Brian Fund. Brian's grandfather donated a small fortune to it. They spent most of the money on behavioral therapies, but a lot went to private schools, which were more accepting of quirky, difficult, ADHD kids, like Brian. The whole ordeal was shattering to the family. It made Brian's parents afraid to risk the chance of having another child, and hurt the intimacy of their marriage. Brian's dad knew that if they had another child with problems like Brian's, they'd soon be bankrupt, and everybody in both their families would be bankrupt. But they never gave up on him. It didn't even enter their minds.

Brian's mom, Mary, now thinks that Brian had problems from the very beginning, possibly because of his vaccinations, and possibly because she ate tuna practically every day during her pregnancy. Even as an infant, his eye contact just wasn't right. His speech started to develop normally, then shut down. He had so much trouble learning to crawl that Mary had to get down on the floor with him and teach him to move his arms and legs in sequence. When he was a baby, he always seemed to have diarrhea, and he threw up his formula so frequently that Mary was afraid he was starving.

As a toddler, Brian had a hard time playing with other kids. Mary tried to boost his social skills by putting him in a Montessori preschool when he was two. She hoped that would help hook him into the real world. But one day she was watching him through a window at school, as he sat by himself, alone, anxious, and disconnected, and she began to cry. Something was terribly wrong.

They took him to the Eden Institute, in Princeton, New Jersey–a famous autism treatment center–and he was diagnosed with PDD-NOS.

Mary, a nurse, began interviewing doctor after doctor, trying to find someone who could offer more than just the behavioral therapies. Finally, she met a dynamic autism support group leader, Maureen McDonnell–a registered nurse who's now a prominent conference coordinator with Defeat Autism Now–and Maureen put Mary in touch with some doctors who really helped. They put Brian on a careful diet and a supplement program, and gradually, with great effort, he emerged from his isolation and limitation.

But not enough. He tried to fit in at public school, but almost every day he came home crying, because the work and the environment overwhelmed him. He would try to focus, but his mind would fly away, and soon he'd be in trouble. He sometimes had panic attacks so severe that his teacher wanted to rush him to the emergency room. Mary knew that wouldn't solve anything, though, and would just drive up their stack of bills even higher, so she would take him home, and calm him down.

Sometimes in school he was dreamy and lost, and sometimes he was loud and selfish. He had no friends. When he didn't get his way, he would tantrum, and the tantrums would often blaze into cycles of rage and assault that frightened everyone around him. Mary and her husband frequently had fights about how to deal with him. How could they *not* disagree, since nothing either of them did really seemed to work?

Brian's grade school years crawled painfully past. He grew older in a life dark with loneliness, anger, and alienation.

Mary, though, could see the sweetness beneath his surface. Brian wanted so *badly* to be good. He was dying to please his parents. He wanted to be able to somehow thank them for making him the Million Dollar Kid. But it wasn't happening. His level of executive function was extremely low, and he was a slave to his own anger and urges.

High school was approaching. Mary would lie in bed dreading what was just ahead: a world in which she could no longer protect her son.

What *happens* to a kid with this degree of pain and dysfunction? How does life treat a young man who knows only how to fail? What would he get involved with? *Alcohol.* That would probably make him feel good–for a few hours. Drugs, maybe. Cigarettes to tone down the anxiety. Angry, alienated friends. Fights. Stupid stunts to show off. Dangerous driving. Careless sexual behavior. He'd end up with some crummy job–or none at all–living alone in a dingy apartment, or in one of their back bedrooms.

Those are the things that moms of ADHD kids think about. With good reason.

Putting Out Fires with Gasoline

An alarming 30 percent to 50 percent of all adults with ADHD, it is now estimated, self-medicate their conditions with excessive amounts of alcohol and street drugs. This futile attempt by ADHD adults to feel better has been likened to trying to put out fires with gasoline. It just makes the situation worse.

Many ADHD adults and adolescents turn to stimulating drugs, such as cocaine, crack, amphetamines, and methamphetamines. These dopamine-enhancing drugs can temporarily soothe not only the symptoms of the inattentive subtype of ADHD, but also those of the hyperactive-impulsive subtype. Ritalin, of course, can also be abused, and is often the abusive drug of choice among many adults and adolescents with ADHD. Ritalin is a popular street drug, and in some cities it's sold for a price that is approximately equivalent to that of heroin.

Depressive drugs can also be alluring to people with ADHD, particularly those who chronically feel hyperactive and overstimulated. Alcohol is by far the most commonly abused depressant in America, accounting for 18 million alcoholics. Many of these alcoholics have severe deficits of dopamine, as do many people with ADHD. Other depressants that are often abused by people with ADHD are heroin, pharmaceutical painkillers such as Vicodin, and anti-anxiety drugs such as Valium and Xanax.

Self-medication by ADHD adults appears to be increasing in incidence of late, because controlled pharmaceutical substances are now easier than ever to acquire, due to their availability on the Internet.

In addition, adults with ADHD are more vulnerable than most people to the overuse of less acutely harmful substances, such as nicotine, caffeine, and even sugary foods. Because of this, there is a higher rate of smoking among people with ADHD, and a higher rate of obesity, despite the fact that hyperactive symptoms burn calories.

The main reason people with ADHD are overindulgent with alcohol, drugs, and food is to mask physical and emotional malaise. Another reason is increased impulsiveness, due to impaired executive function.

Partly because of increased incidence of substance abuse, and partly because of chronic oppositional and impulsive behavior, adults and older adolescents with ADHD are more likely than others to commit antisocial acts. One study indicated that they are approximately twice as likely as others to be involved in property crime, domestic violence, and assault. They are also twice as likely as others to have their driver's licenses suspended.

ADHD symptoms also make it much harder for people to make good livings. People with ADHD symptoms are less likely than others to complete high school, less likely to attend college, and are less likely than others to hold full-time jobs. In one study, ADHD adults with high school diplomas were found to earn an average of $10,800 per year less than other high school graduates, and ADHD adults with college degrees earned $4,300 less than other college grads. This study, conducted at Harvard, estimated that ADHD costs Americans approximately $77 billion each year in lost wages. Employers tend to be very wary of people with ADHD symptoms, and those symptoms are more frequently recognized now, as awareness of ADHD grows.

Furthermore, divorce rates are also higher among adults with ADHD symptoms, approaching approximately 65 percent.

Adults with ADHD are also significantly less likely than others to report satisfaction with their other relationships, including those with friends, family members, and coworkers. They tend to have significantly lower levels of satisfaction with life than others do, and are less likely to have positive self-images, and are less likely to be optimistic.

Due to all of these factors, as well as to the intrinsic emotional pain of ADHD, there is a significantly increased risk of suicide among adults, adolescents, and children with ADHD. Furthermore, unlike most other neurological disorders, ADHD has high rates of suicide that are associated not only with the disorder itself, but also with the drugs most commonly used to treat it, including Ritalin. Many suicides among children, attributed to Ritalin use, occur every year.

This was the possible future that Mary had to face. If she and her husband refused to face it, and did not struggle to help Brian recover, this future of pain and failure would be even *more* likely to occur.

This was also the reality that Lisa faced with Teia.
It was the reality Liza faced with Alisa.

What happens to these kids, when they must finally face the world without the protection of their parents?

The answer to that is easy: Not all of them make it. Life doesn't always have a happy ending, no matter how hard you try.

Brian, 2006

It was the famous Disney World Parade of Lights, coming closer, the music rising, fireworks overhead. Mary was in the crowd, surrounded by kids, thinking about her own son, and wondering where he was.

At this moment, she was remembering Brian's early years, when he couldn't even look at her, couldn't talk, and couldn't play. She remembered her fears back then—of him remaining in diapers as a young man, and living in one of their back bedrooms, as he stayed a child forever. Then later, even when he'd improved, there had been the constant dread that he would live a life of loneliness and defeat, dulling his pain by getting drunk or high on drugs, just to get through each day. But Brian had worked *hard*. They all had, even her father, who'd contributed so much to the Save Brian Fund, only to die just before Brian had finally begun to recover.

It had taken almost three years to solve all of Brian's root problems: the toxification, the allergies, the candida overgrowth, the immune deficiencies, the nutrient deficits, the lingering PANDAS, and the neurological inflammation.

They had fought each battle as a family, hoping each battle would be the last, then had to fight again, and again, until finally: the gradual emergence of Brian Dunn as a fine young man.

What a *winner* he was! He had a million dollar smile and a steel-trap mind. These days, Brian could almost effortlessly soak up facts, and he kept them forever. As Mary put it, "He still has that fabulous autistic memory." It was a happy irony, and one Brian deserved. One they *all* deserved.

Brian was in honors classes in math and language. Straight A's in Spanish. Lots of buddies. He was a great lacrosse player. A guitarist. He had a girlfriend. College loomed, a beacon.

The music—louder now. The Million Dollar Kid! His band was leading the parade!

The Million Dollar Kid: Looking for his mother's face in the crowd. Finding it.

"Brian!"

The million dollar smile.

Teia, 2006

Teia's mom Lisa brought me her report card as if it were a Nobel Prize.

Teia was doing *great*. She was energetic, outgoing, and athletic. "This is a *fantastic* report card," I told Teia.

"Thank you," she said simply. But she was *so* proud, this little girl who only a few years before had been in special-ed classes, and had been threatened with having to repeat second grade. Her eyes, once dim, now danced with light. Now her face, in every moment, reflected all the beauty around her, and she was luminous. She was one of the most beautiful little kids I've ever seen.

"Tell me something, Teia," I said to her. I really wanted her opinion. "Tell me what I should say to kids who feel sick. So they don't feel so scared."

"Oh, that's eeee-zy, Dr. Bock." Her eyes were gleaming. "Just tell them their *mommies* will take care of them."

I looked over at Lisa, but her eyes were lost in her daughter's face. They stayed that way for quite some time. We all sat there quietly, just enjoying life.

Alisa, 2006

Alisa was skating in the Rockefeller Center ice rink, as television cameras filmed her. They were shooting a documentary about kids who'd made remarkable recoveries from autism and ADHD. Alisa's movements were fluid and beautiful–full of rhythm and power–and when she executed a perfect waltz-jump, Liza clapped spontaneously.

Alisa's recovery had finally hit high gear when we'd knocked out her PANDAS. The PANDAS had been the driving force behind her ADHD symptoms. It had intensified her neural inflammation, and had amplified the neurological damage that was being done by allergies, nutritional deficits, toxification, and hypoglycemia. When at last we got all those interrelated problems under control, Alisa's executive function had suddenly blossomed, and now she had powers of self-control and judgment that Liza had barely dared to dream possible. Alisa still had every bit of her charm, though, and all of her electric charisma. She had more friends than she could accommodate. The violent little tyrant that had once been part of her was gone, just as surely as her baby teeth were gone.

Liza called Alisa over. There had been a change in plans. They had to leave immediately. Liza knew this would be a huge disappointment for Alisa, who loved skating, particularly here, in the mecca of America's ice rinks. As recently as a year ago, telling Alisa to grab her skates and go would have meant *war*: a scene, a cycle, one more ugly humiliation for both of them.

Liza told her they had to leave. Alisa's face clouded. Reflexively, Liza began to apologize.

Alisa cut her off. "It's okay, Mom. I understand."

"Thanks, honey. I love you."

"Love you too."

So simple. After *everything*. Finally, *finally*–so simple–almost as if it had been inevitable.

Alisa took her skates off, and together they headed home–just the two of them now–where they would watch *ER* together before bedtime. It was Alisa's favorite show. Alisa, who had once hated doctors, liked them now, and was even thinking of becoming one.

They left holding hands, happy and laughing, content to live one more simple day.

Matthew, 2006

Approximately a year after Matthew Smith died, his parents, Larry and Kelly, created a website in Matthew's honor, and in his memory, focused on the dangers of Ritalin.

They also began to lobby the U.S. Congress to pass a bill that would make it much more difficult for school systems to insist that children take Ritalin, against their parents' wishes. The bill passed by a landslide vote and became a federal law in 2005.

At this point, more than 2 million people have visited their website, which is named ritalindeath.com.

Due to those high numbers of website visitors, and due to the passage of the law that they sponsored, Larry and Kelly Smith believe that their work, on behalf of Matthew, has probably helped to save the lives of many children.

Knowing this is enough to make them feel, from time to time, almost happy.

3. ASTHMA

CHAPTER TEN

A LITTLE ANGEL

ON THE DAY HER DAUGHTER WAS BORN, ANJU USMAN FELT AS IF she herself had been born once more, into a better world—one that was reconnected to her own childhood, and was linked for the first time to a future now infinite.

Priya was a little angel. She had luminous eyes that seemed to take up about half her face, and she was able, even as an infant, to look deeply into her mother's eyes and inspire in Anju a sense of peace that was greater than any she'd ever known. Anju, at that time, was treating AIDS patients and drug addicts at Chicago's Cook County Hospital, and that work brought her an intense sense of satisfaction—but compared to *Priya*? There *was* no comparison. The idea of living without Priya suddenly seemed not just pointless to Anju, but practically impossible.

On the other hand, life with Priya was pretty impossible, too. Cook County Hospital was a medical combat zone. Cook County is the place that the show *ER* is based on, and Anju still can't watch that program, because every melodramatic moment of it brings back memories of days careening into nights, as people screamed, cried, and died.

At the end of her shift, Anju would rush home to Priya, who would also be screaming—with colic—her face red and contorted, her belly as hard and big as a melon.

But Anju would work her mother's magic, and Priya's eyes would light with recognition as she grew quiet and calm. Anju would become hypnotized by her daughter's eyes and drift into mom-heaven, holding Priya to her heart, as they both plummeted into sleep.

Part of the colic problem seemed to be caused by Anju's schedule as a doctor. It prohibited her from breast-feeding Priya, and Priya could barely hold down conventional formula. Anju tried some soy formulas–even Alimentum, which was predigested–but most of it came back up. The Alimentum was supposed to be the easiest for newborns to handle, but it had corn oil in it, and Priya seemed to be sensitive to anything that contained corn oil or corn syrup.

As Priya got a little older and started to eat solid foods, Anju found that a number of foods made Priya gassy, bloated, and irritable. Priya was a sensitive baby. She seemed to cry a lot, and tossed and turned in her crib at night. She wasn't growing well. She was beautifully delicate, but too tiny.

Anju spoke to Priya's pediatrician often, but he wasn't concerned. He said that he saw babies every day who spit up their food and were fussy, but they all outgrew it. He thought Priya was generally healthy– no infections, no illnesses, and normal behavioral development.

When Priya was nine months old, Anju was eating an ice cream cone, and she thought, why not let the baby have a lick? Her first ice cream–one more happy little ritual! So Anju put a dab of it in Priya's mouth. Priya's lips started to swell. Then her throat began to constrict. Priya started to choke, and struggle for air. Anju ran to the medicine cabinet and grabbed a syringe filled with the stimulant epinephrine, which her husband kept around because he had a severe allergy to shrimp. Anju jabbed the needle into Priya's thigh. Priya's anaphylactic shock quickly subsided, and her face deflated. She began to cry. Anju held her closely, and massaged the site of the injection.

Anju, worried, took Priya to an allergist. Tests showed that Priya was allergic to milk, wheat, corn, and eggs. Anju began to restrict Priya's diet drastically. One problem that loomed, though, was Priya's vaccination for measles, mumps, and rubella, which was based in egg. Anju didn't want to miss that vaccination, because she believed vaccinations were critically important. Priya hadn't missed any of her shots yet, not even the hepatitis-B vaccination on the first day of her life. So Anju took Priya to the hospital, where doctors tried to desensitize her to eggs, by giving her an extremely small dosage of the vaccine. The moment it hit her system, though, Priya became violently ill.

Soon after that, Priya began to suffer from asthma. Almost every day, she would begin to wheeze and fight for air. As a toddler, and then as a preschooler, she was never very far from her inhaler.

Anju began to research methods of reversing asthma. She devoured issues of the publications she trusted most: *The New England Journal of Medicine, The Journal of Pediatrics, The Journal of the American Medical Association,* and *Lancet.* But she found virtually *nothing* about reversing the condition. The standard treatments for asthma were not aimed at reversal, but at just controlling symptoms.

Anju was dismayed. At Cook County Hospital, there seemed to be a sudden explosion of asthma cases, but no one seemed to know why it was happening, or what to do about it. The doctors mostly just gave the kids inhalers, sent them home, and told them not to feel too bad, because so many *other* kids had asthma. Asthma, in an insidious way, was beginning to be accepted as a frequently inevitable element of childhood. It was becoming a source of humor on television sitcoms, and a topic of cocktail chatter among moms. Anju felt that too many parents, and even doctors, were just shrugging their shoulders at the epidemic, and waiting for the pharmaceutical industry to come up with a magic bullet.

The best approach to asthma, Anju was starting to believe, would never consist of merely suppressing its symptoms with conventional pharmaceuticals. That was a classic example of too little, too late. And too dangerous—kids died from asthma in every state, every day.

Anju began searching outside the realm of conventional medicine. And in so doing, Anju Usman, M.D., became a member of a growing group of physicians who were trying to save their *own* children from the new childhood epidemics, by exploring natural types of treatments. Frustrated by the failure of conventional techniques, and frightened by the threats to their own families, they were searching for the root causes of the new epidemics.

The majority of these doctors had children or grandchildren who were suffering from autism. These doctors—including Jaquelyn McCandless, M.D.; Jeff Bradstreet, M.D.; Jane El-Dahr, M.D.; and Amy Holmes, M.D.—were coalescing regularly in conferences sponsored by groups such as Defeat Autism Now. They were being joined by researchers, writers, and other medical professionals who also had children with autism and other 4-A disorders: Bernard Rimland, Ph.D.; Jon Pangborn, Ph.D.; Karyn Seroussi; Nancy Wiseman; Stan Kurtz; Lauren

Underwood, Ph.D.; Jim Adams, Ph.D.; Lyn Redwood, R.N.; Sallie Bernard; and a number of others. Their individual concerns, born of love for their own children, were becoming a major medical movement.

It was hard for some of these physicians and researchers to look beyond their traditional training, but they had discovered that when their own children had begun to suffer, it had forced them past philosophical attachments into pure pragmatism.

It was at one of these conferences that I met Dr. Usman. After I finished a lecture, she approached me, accompanied by six-year-old Priya, and by her two younger daughters, who also had serious problems.

Anju was fascinated by the fact that I thought asthma could sometimes be reversed—except for rare, mild symptoms—by modulating the immune system. As an AIDS doctor, she was aware of the incredible power of the immune system—and also of its frightening vulnerability.

Anju had by this time vaulted far past conventional medical wisdom, and was working with autistic and other chronically ill children at the Pfeiffer Institute in Chicago, which specializes in treating biochemical imbalances and heavy metal toxification.

Anju, I learned, had been on an arduous intellectual journey. Born in India, she'd grown up since the age of two in the prairie town of Fort Wayne, Indiana, and had graduated from the excellent Indiana University School of Medicine. She described herself to me as "a normal Hoosier, nothing special," but her work at Pfeiffer was cutting-edge. She had already done a superb job of correcting some of the root causes of Priya's asthma, with nutritional therapy and supplementation. Priya had never required hospitalization, nor even a trip to the emergency room, as do so many children with asthma. Priya didn't even seem to be particularly preoccupied with her asthma, in contrast to many asthmatic children, who become perpetually anxious about their painful asthma episodes, and allow asthma to dictate their activities. Even so, Anju was struggling to find something that could accelerate Priya's healing, and get her over the asthma, once and for all.

As Anju and I spoke, Priya held Anju's hand, and the love the little girl felt for her mom radiated from her warm eyes. Priya had a fragile, vulnerable beauty, and was soft-spoken and very intelligent, like her mother.

I wanted to help Priya—as I invariably do when I meet a child who has a serious problem—but I knew that she was in good hands. Anju was a fine doctor, and an extraordinarily caring and loving mother.

Nonetheless, the dark forces Priya was up against–the forces that so *many* of our children are now up against–were terrible and strong. Asthma and allergies, even during Priya's short lifetime, had become ever more deadly.

The Asthma Epidemic

Incidence of asthma has rocketed wildly upward over the past twenty-five years, in tandem with the other new childhood epidemics of autism, ADHD, and allergies.

The combined increase of these four disorders is not a coincidence.

Asthma is part of a larger pattern. The pattern consists of four primary childhood epidemics that are triggered by the following root causes:

- **Increased** exposure to toxins, from the environment, and from childhood vaccinations.
- **Decreased** ability to detoxify, due to heavy metal overload and nutritional deficits.
- **Genetic** predispositions that impair the ability to detoxify, and thus create vulnerability to negative lifestyle and environmental factors.
- **Dysfunction** of the immune, gastrointestinal, and nervous systems.

These root causes have resulted in a wide array of childhood illnesses and problems, most of which generally appear unrelated. However, as a rule, only the most obvious *symptoms* of these disorders are unrelated. Asthma, for example, has symptoms that are quite different from those of autism, ADHD, and most food allergies. Nonetheless, asthma, autism, ADHD, and allergies are all often caused by the same forces, which have varying effects upon the body.

Furthermore, all four of these disorders can even be present in the same child. This combination of combined disorders is not at all unusual.

Making the Connections Among Asthma and the Other 4-A Disorders

• Children on the autism spectrum commonly have ADHD traits, typically have allergies, and have a higher incidence of asthma.

• Presence of asthma or allergies during a mother's pregnancy doubles her chances of having an autistic child.

• Children with asthma, according to a recent, large study, had significantly higher rates of ADHD behaviors, including poor concentration and conflicts with other children.

• 77 percent of asthmatics have chronic gastroesophageal reflux, a common symptom of food allergies.

• People with asthma are approximately 300 percent more likely than others to be obese, even when they exercise as much as others, partly because inflammation contributes to both disorders.

• Asthma, hypothyroidism, and allergies are the three most common co-morbid physical disorders among people with autism.

• 90 percent of all children who have asthma also have allergies.

Allergies, in fact, are now known to be *the single most common trigger of asthma.* When people with asthma have an allergic reaction, it often tends to localize in their airways. This allergic reaction is generally most severe in the bronchial tubes that supply the lungs with air. It causes these bronchial tubes to become clogged with mucus, and it makes the muscles around them go into spasm, creating a powerful constriction. This squeezing and clogging results in such drastic narrowing of the bronchial tubes that it often makes people who are enduring an asthma episode feel as if they are trying to breathe through a straw. During a severe episode, they frequently feel as if they are being slowly strangled. They can become dizzy, disoriented, and so sick at their stomachs that they vomit. They can begin to turn blue–first in the extremities of their fingertips and lips–as their bodies run out of oxygen and congest with carbon dioxide. They often panic, and this heightens their sense of strangulation. As they fight for air, they often become drenched with sweat, to the point of dehydration. Unable to drink, their throats become parched, and this makes breathing even harder. Their chests heave and struggle against the oppressive lack of oxygen, as their muscles begin to burn and weaken. After hours of this, they can become utterly exhausted. Exhaustion itself, leading to suffocation, is generally the cause of death among the approximately 5,500 Americans who die of asthma every year.

Fatalities from asthma are now twice as common as they were in 1980, despite advances in hospital crisis care. The main reason for this is simply that during this period the incidence of asthma tripled. In addition, more people have very serious cases of asthma.

Without question, we are in the depths of history's worst epidemic of asthma, even though the condition has been recognized since the time of the ancient Greeks. The Greeks coined the term "asthma," which also meant "oppression."

Tracking the Epidemic

• From 1980 to 2000, the number of doctor visits for asthma increased almost 300 percent, from 6 million annually to 17.3 million.

• Twenty million people in America have asthma.

• Nine million Americans eighteen or younger have asthma.

• In high-incidence zones, such as the Bronx, or Central Harlem in New York City, up to 25 percent of all children now have asthma.

• Forty thousand people worldwide die from asthma each year, mostly in advanced, industrialized nations.

• In very large regions of high incidence—including New Jersey, New England, and New York—12 percent to 15 percent of all children have asthma.

• Each year, there are approximately 2 million emergency room visits for asthma.

• Children who take antibiotics before age four have 400 percent more asthma than others.

• During spikes of air pollution, asthma hospitalizations generally increase by 20 percent to 30 percent.

• Approximately 40 percent of asthmatic adults have asthmatic children.

• Asthma now costs $11.5 billion annually in medical care.

• Workplaces with indoor air pollution are a leading trigger of asthma.

• Asthma causes 14 million missed school days each year, and 12 million missed work days.

• Almost 6 percent of all Americans have asthma.

These statistics strongly suggest that the new epidemic of asthma is closely tied to the recent increased toxification of America. Episodes of asthma are clearly linked to air that is polluted from smog, industrial chemicals, particulates, and pollen.

Many doctors, though, don't realize that toxins do not have to be in the air to contribute to asthma. Toxins in food and water, and even in home furnishings, can trigger asthma episodes. Furthermore, heavy metals, including those that are included in vaccinations, can also be an indirect but powerful cause of asthma. The link between toxins and asthma exists because of two primary reasons:

1. **Toxins**–from any source–increase inflammation in the body, including inflammation in the airways.
2. **Toxins**–including those that we eat, breathe, drink, inject, and touch–destabilize the immune system, which is intimately linked with asthma.

Understanding the immune system is the key to understanding asthma. However, many people with asthma do not fully appreciate the causative role that the immune system plays in asthma. This role is enormous. Dysfunction of the immune system is the ultimate root cause of most cases of asthma.

The immune system is the root source of most asthma simply because it is the root source of allergy:

- **The immune system creates all allergies.**
- **And allergies create most asthma.**

The immune system creates allergies when it becomes confused. It mistakenly believes that a harmless substance–such as gluten, milk, or pollen–is an invading pathogen, such as a germ, or poison. It goes to war against this presumed invader by triggering inflammation. The immune system triggers this inflammation to get rid of the invader with extra heat, extra blood flow, and extra mucus and fluids. But if this inflammation hits the airways, as it often does, it can cause asthma. The inflammation produces the mucus that clogs the bronchial tubes, and it also contributes to the tightening and spasm of the muscles that girdle the bronchial tubes.

Uncontrolled inflammation is one of the body's worst enemies. Sometimes, when the immune system becomes extraordinarily confused, it can cause inflammation that results in systemic swelling throughout the body. When this swelling occurs in the joints of the skeletal system, it creates the painful and crippling symptoms of rheumatoid arthritis. Rheumatoid arthritis hurts as much as ordinary, age-associated osteoarthritis, but it can endanger the whole body. More often than not, this condition strikes adults. But not always. On frequent occasions–more commonly these days than ever before–it strikes children. When it does, it becomes one more terrible, auto-immune element of the new childhood epidemics. It can twist the bodies of children into sad, crippled caricatures of the very elderly.

It began to cripple little Priya.

CHAPTER ELEVEN

THE ROOT CAUSE

WHEN PRIYA HAD REACHED AGE TEN, SHE HAD CAUGHT A VIRUS.
That wasn't unusual for her. She seemed to catch every bug that came
around. Her immune system just didn't seem to function well. In fact, all
three of Anju's daughters had problems with immunity.

Priya's virus had begun to gradually subside. As it did, though, a
new catastrophe struck. Priya's joints began to swell with fluids. She
could no longer hold a pencil–her hands were too sore, and were suddenly fat with fluids. The swelling moved into her knees and hips. She
couldn't walk.

Priya was good about it, as usual, despite the pain and disablement.
But it broke Anju's heart to see her suffer.

Anju took Priya to a local rheumatologist in whom she had faith.
She'd heard he was a good doctor. He said that Priya was having an unusual reaction to the virus, and that the pain and swelling would soon
go away. They waited. For two months. Priya still couldn't walk. The
pain was eating away at her.

The rheumatologist wanted Priya to start taking steroids, to bring
down her joint inflammation.

Anju didn't want to do it. She thought Priya was too young to go on
oral steroids, possibly for the rest of her life. Her system was too sensitive, and the side effects were potentially horrendous: severe mood
swings, systemic swelling, and uncontrollable fat deposits in the ab-
domen, face, and neck. Some of the side effects were, in fact, quite sim-

ilar to those of rheumatoid arthritis itself, and that made Anju worry that Priya's regular use of a steroid inhaler might have initially triggered many of the symptoms, and might still be perpetuating them.

Anju began to search frantically for alternatives. By this time, the spring of 2000, Anju was doing highly sophisticated metabolic rebalancing at Pfeiffer, and she knew that sometimes yeast, or candida overgrowth, caused serious joint pain and swelling. She tested Priya for candida overgrowth, and found that Priya had very high levels of yeast. Anju put Priya on an herbal antifungal medication. She felt that the herbal medicine would be safer for sensitive little Priya than a pharmaceutical antifungal, such as Diflucan.

Simultaneously, Anju became much more strict about Priya's diet. For years, Anju had restricted gluten and dairy products from Priya's diet, but as Priya's asthma had begun to improve, Anju had loosened the restrictions, and had allowed Priya to occasionally eat dairy products and wheat. After all, it was hard for Priya to constantly pass up the cookies, ice cream, macaroni, pancakes, and sandwiches that all her friends were eating.

Priya responded fantastically to Anju's therapies. Two weeks after the dietary change and herbal medication, Priya's symptoms of rheumatoid arthritis completely vanished. She could walk. She could run. Her hands felt fine. She went back to her normal routine.

When I heard about Priya's response, I was impressed with Anju's clinical acumen. Anju had eliminated the root cause of the problem. Many doctors, by the year 2000, were dabbling with natural types of modalities, but too many were just using them for the old-fashioned purpose of knocking down symptoms, instead of employing them as part of a comprehensive program that reversed root causes.

However, the DAN doctors—as we'd begun to call ourselves—were becoming ever more ambitious about reversing root causes. We had to be. As a group, we were treating some of the most intractable conditions that existed. They were hard to treat mostly just because they were so complex. For example, many serious diseases occur merely because the immune system becomes weak, and gives illness an opportunity to flourish. The 4-A disorders, though, have a much more complex relationship with immunity. Allergies and asthma, in particular, are generally caused by *overactivity* of the immune system, rather than underactivity. To overcome them, the immune system must be made to function at just the right level.

The particular part of the immune system that can become overactive, resulting in allergies and asthma, consists of white blood cells known as T-cells. Unfortunately, many people with asthma and allergies have never even heard of T-cells, because the standard treatments for asthma and allergies generally don't address these root causes. That's why these treatments typically fail to achieve a full reversal. *Reversal, however, is possible.*

It is possible when the T-cells are directly addressed.

T-cells are named after the thymus, the hormone-producing gland located behind the breastbone that helps direct the activity of the immune system. There are several types of T-cells, including some that kill cancer cells, some that help stimulate the immune response, and some that help turn off the immune response, after a health crisis has passed. One type of T-cell that helps activate the immune response is called a helper T-cell. There are two different kinds of helper T-cells: Th-1 (or thymus-helper 1), and Th-2 cells. They work in concert with one another, but have very different functions.

- **Th-1 cells.** These immune system cells are involved in immunity that is performed by the cells themselves, known as cell-mediated immunity. They attack pathogens directly, or send messages to encourage other immune cells to attack. They do this even when the pathogens are already lodged inside infected cells.

- **Th-2 cells.** These immune system cells also attack pathogens, but in a different way. They do it by producing different messages that encourage other immune cells to produce antibodies. These antibodies then attack foreign substances, including bacteria, viruses–and also allergens. Th-2 cells do not enter infected cells.

Because these Th-1 and Th-2 cells work together, it's important that they stay in balance. *But this doesn't always happen.*

Quite often, in many people, there is a skewing of this balance, with an increase of Th-2 antibody production, and a decrease in the activity of Th-1 cells. This skewing can be caused by a variety of factors–including, for example, stress, and yeast overgrowth–but the primary factor that now appears to cause this skewing toward Th-2 dominance is the presence of toxins. Mercury in the body promotes excessive activity of Th-2 cells. So does lead. So does aluminum. These heavy metals aggravate and overexcite the immune system, resulting in allergy, impaired immunity, and in autoimmunity, in which the immune system inadvertently attacks healthy tissues and organs.

This skewing of immunity to Th-2 dominance makes it harder for people to fight off the viral, bacterial, and fungal infections that lie within their cells. It makes them prone to many common illnesses. The excess activity of Th-2 cells also triggers an overactive immune response, which can result in allergy and autoimmunity. Priya, for example, almost certainly had Th-2 overactivity and Th-1 underactivity, and that's probably why she was sick so often, and had so many allergies.

Overactive Th-2 immunity results in too many attacks on substances that don't need to be attacked, including pollen, and common foods, such as milk and wheat. The final result, of course, is allergy.

Allergy then triggers inflammation, as the body fights to free itself from presumed invaders. When the inflammation strikes the airways, asthma can occur.

This imbalance in the immune system, combined with widespread inflammation, is the main reason that there is now an epidemic of asthma and allergies. *We are a Th-2 skewed society.* It's just one more result of too much toxicity.

Kids with autism and ADHD usually tend to be Th-2 skewed. That's why they often have more colds and flu than other kids, and it's why they so frequently have allergies. These allergies can contribute to these kids' negative neurobehavioral traits, including spaciness, obsessiveness, lethargy, poor cognitive function, and irritability.

Unfortunately, kids with asthma tend to be even *more* Th-2 skewed than kids with autism. Asthma is an absolutely classic consequence of Th-2 skewing—there's no doubt about it.

Correcting this Th-2 skewing can be tough. It can require a full-scale program of detoxification, combined with a rebalancing of the immune system. Generally, a child must adhere to the Healing Program for an extended period of time to overcome Th-2 skewing, since this skewing is so deeply embedded. Another smart tactic that helps children who are Th-2 skewed is simply to protect them from the toxins, irritants, and allergens that overexcite their Th-2 cells. In almost all cases, both of these strategies must be applied.

However, all children must be treated individually, because some autistic children, in contrast to kids with asthma, are actually Th-1 skewed, instead of Th-2 skewed. This, too, can cause inflammation. The key is *balance*. Another type of T-cell, regulatory T-cells, help balance Th-1 and Th-2–but not always sufficiently.

There are no easy ways to achieve this balance, and solve these problems.

But it *can* be done.

In many children, it *must* be done. Achieving this balance is the only way to fully ensure these children's health, and to spare them and their families from the suffering that asthma, allergies, autism, and ADHD so commonly inflict.

Anju's Suffering

Right after Priya was born, Anju had felt so electrified with the new feeling of maternal love that she couldn't wait to have another child. Even ministering to Priya's terrible problems had given Anju a sense of primal satisfaction. She liked taking care of people. When Anju had been a child herself, she had left Fort Wayne once to visit India, and had come back home saddened by the suffering she'd seen, and certain that her mission in life was to help those who were most helpless. In the AIDS and addiction wards of Cook County Hospital, she had fulfilled some of that mission. But then she'd become a mother, and had begun working with autistic children at Pfeiffer, and had found the true center of her life.

Anju's second daughter, Aniyka, had been born only a couple of years after Priya, and Anju had prayed that Aniyka would have an easier time in life than had little Priya. For a time, Anju's prayers seemed to be answered. Aniyka was a happy baby. Easy. *Healthy.*

At four months, though, Aniyka–who'd missed her day-of-birth vaccination because of a logistical problem–got her first vaccination. The next week, she began wheezing. The week after that, she got an ear infection. Anju took Aniyka to the pediatrician, and he gave the baby antibiotics for her ears and steroids for her wheezing. The treatments seemed drastic to Anju, but she trusted her doctor, and didn't know what else to do.

The ear infection persisted for almost a year, though, despite course after course of antibiotics, which triggered several yeast infections. Finally, Aniyka's ear, nose, and throat specialist implanted tubes in her ears, to drain the fluids, and Aniyka began at last to feel better.

Two years after Aniyka was born, Anju had another baby. Vaniya, like her two older sisters, was delicate, beautiful, and easy to love. Vaniya, similarly to Priya, got her first vaccination on the day she was born, and almost immediately began to have problems. The inside corners of her eyes, where her tear ducts drained into her nose, became intermittently red and swollen. Anju suspected allergy, but she couldn't determine the source. Then one day Anju put Vaniya's head on her shoulder–without first putting a cotton diaper over her shoulder to protect her clothing, as she normally did–and Vaniya's eyes got red and puffy. That was the clue: Vaniya was allergic to synthetic fibers. Anju found that whenever she dressed Aniyka in anything other than cotton, her eyes would swell. Avoiding all synthetic fibers was practically impossible, though, and over the next two years Aniyka contracted ten inflammatory eye infections, and was hospitalized four times. The condition, called periorbital cellulitis, can transport bacterial infection straight to the brain. In the hospital, they had to give Vaniya intravenous antibiotics to protect her brain from infection.

When Anju began to attend DAN meetings, and to later speak at them, I would talk to her about her kids' problems. Priya, Aniyka, and Vaniya seemed to be classic examples of Th-2 skewed kids. Their bodies were good at fighting harmless substances, such as polyester and milk, but bad at fighting real foes, including viruses, bacteria, and fungi.

Anju was doing everything that could possibly be done–as a physician and as a mother–but these allergic, infectious, and asthmatic conditions can be dreadfully persistent. In retrospect, it appears as if detoxification might have helped Anju's children during these difficult times, but back then, we simply didn't realize its tremendous potential.

These days, when those of us in the battle against the new childhood epidemics look back at those recent years, we realize how far we have come in such a short time. But it's sad to think about how many more children we might have been able to help, if we'd known then what we know now.

Even so, despite all these difficulties, Priya's asthma was getting *better*. When she would start to wheeze, Anju would just remind her to use her inhaler, and that would be the end of it.

Priya's most stubborn problem, though, was allergy. Right after Priya overcame her rheumatoid arthritis, she began to be reactive to a wider variety of things. Sometimes Anju couldn't even determine what Priya was reacting to. Priya would just get a tight feeling in her throat, from something as seemingly inconsequential as walking into the lunchroom at school, and then it would go away, for no apparent reason.

The uncertainty that surrounded Priya's allergies was not unusual, because allergies can be maddeningly mysterious. They can morph from one symptom to another–from wheezing, to hives, to indigestion–and their source can keep changing, from milk, to pollen, to polyester. That is why it's so important to try to repair their root cause: an overactive immune system. As long as the immune system is too touchy from being Th-2 skewed, anything can happen.

Aniyka's allergies, similar to Priya's, were also persisting, despite everyone's best efforts to help.

Then another crisis hit. Aniyka developed an infection, and Anju had Aniyka's blood sugar checked. It was four times too high. Aniyka had juvenile-onset diabetes, at age eight.

Anju was shocked. As she researched diabetes, though, her shock congealed into anger. Several studies that had just been completed strongly implicated the HIB vaccination as one cause of juvenile-onset, or Type 1, diabetes. That is the type of the disease that is not triggered by obesity, but by a failure of the pancreas to produce enough insulin. Anju found, in fact, that the risk of children developing diabetes after receiving the HIB vaccination was even higher than the risk of their developing the disease itself, which can usually be effectively treated with a course of antibiotics. Studies indicated that the HIB vaccination may cause approximately two thousand to four thousand new cases of Type 1 diabetes every year. Advocates of the HIB vaccination dispute this perspective. However, doubts about the HIB vaccination may account for the fact that approximately one in every twenty pediatricians now refuses to give the vaccination to his or her own children.

Around the time Aniyka was diagnosed with diabetes, Anju had her fourth and final child, Rajan. She refused to allow him to be vaccinated.

In a bittersweet irony, Rajan has remained abundantly healthy, and is notably larger and stronger than his older sisters.

In September 2001, Priya walked into the lunchroom at school and her chest began to tighten. Her throat felt thick and clogged. She began to wheeze.

The school administrators immediately called Anju, and she hurried over. She took Priya home, and began to give Priya the standard treatments for an asthma episode, including the use of an inhaler to open her bronchial tubes. For the first time ever, nothing seemed to help. Priya was wheezing desperately. She was flushed and tired. Anju was frightened.

She rushed Priya to the nearest emergency room. As the E.R. doctors began to treat Priya, no one acted particularly alarmed. By 2001, these doctors were dealing with asthma emergencies almost every day. But Priya didn't respond. The mood in the E.R. started to shift. The doctors began to shout and bustle about in quick, urgent bursts of activity. They couldn't help her. Priya was gasping. Turning blue.

The head of the E.R. grabbed a phone, and in a matter of minutes a helicopter swooped down outside. The doctors ran Priya's stretcher cart out to the helicopter, a Lifestar Flying Emergency Room. There wasn't enough space for Anju. The 'copter shot into the air and was gone, headed for Chicago's best treatment center for acute asthma crisis, the Loyola University Hospital, thirty miles away.

Anju jumped into her car. She drove as fast as possible. She hit clumps of traffic that seemed to last forever. She felt dazed, dreamlike. She said out loud, "She's too young to die. I'll die without her." Over and over, as she drove, she kept repeating, "I'll die without her," as if saying this, somehow, would keep it from happening.

At the hospital, doctors inserted IVs into Priya's veins. They pushed huge amounts of steroids into her system. They forced pure oxygen into her lungs. Priya struggled and gasped, and then grew still.

Anju finally got there. She slammed her car door and ran inside. She found Priya's room.

Priya was alive.

When some of Priya's strength came back, four or five hours later, Priya held her mother's hand and gazed warmly into Anju's eyes, bringing Anju the pure, unconditional child's love that Anju now felt she needed as much as she needed air itself.

"Mom," Priya said, "I had this dream. I dreamed that I went to heaven, and that God was there, and angels were there, and that people I didn't know were there. And some people were telling me to stay in heaven, because it's a really nice place. And some people were telling me to go back home, because my mom really needed me. And then God asked me, 'Priya, what do you want to do? Do you want to stay, or go back home?' And I said, 'Well, I'd better go back home, because my mom will die without me.' "

As tears formed on Anju's face, she felt blessed, and beyond happy, because she was suddenly certain that God had purposefully let Priya come back, and that her little girl would never go, and that they would be happy together forever.

CHAPTER TWELVE

HAPPY ENDINGS

ANJU DISCOVERED, BY DOING SOME DIFFICULT MEDICAL AND parental detective work, that Priya's asthma episode at school had been triggered by her just *smelling* some peanut butter sandwiches that kids were eating in the lunchroom.

Anju went to the school and talked to the administrators about restricting peanuts from the school grounds. They sympathized with her, but wouldn't do it.

These days, only several years later, it's not uncommon for schools to ban peanuts, due to the recent sharp increase in deaths among children from peanut allergies. Now, approximately two hundred people, most of them children, die each year from reactions to foods—primarily to peanuts—often because their reactions cause fatal asthma attacks.

Not only do peanuts now cause more deaths than any other allergen, but many people with severe peanut allergies can have reactions from just smelling or touching peanuts. No one is certain why peanuts are so uniquely lethal. They do contain complex proteins, which can confuse the immune system, and they may be harder than other high-protein foods for the body to recognize, because of the fact that they were one of the last staples to enter our food supply. But the reasons for their unmatched capacity to kill remain largely mysterious.

Anju and her husband, therefore, had to take Priya out of school. They couldn't possibly take the risk of her being exposed to peanuts again.

The family's range of activities began to shrivel, out of fear of contact with peanuts. They could no longer travel on airplanes, because the airlines often passed out bags of peanuts. They couldn't go to restaurants, because someone near them might be eating a dish with peanuts, or because they might inadvertently order a dish containing peanuts or peanut oil. Priya couldn't even go into grocery stores. Anytime she came near an aisle that contained a peanut product, she would begin to react, and would have to rush out.

At one point the family checked into a hotel room, and Priya said, "Mommy, there's a peanut in here."

Anju couldn't spot any. "Are you sure?"

"I can feel it."

They began to pull apart the whole room. When they lifted the couch, they found a Reese's Peanut Butter Cup.

Another time, Aniyka wanted to sell Girl Scout cookies, but Anju was worried about it, because one variety, Tagalongs, contained peanuts. "You can sell the cookies," Anju told Aniyka, "but they're not allowed in the house."

After Aniyka took her cookie orders from the neighbors, though, the scout troop sent her home with a big box of cookies to distribute. Anju was frightened by the presence of the cookies. She was beginning to feel frightened all the time. "'Niyka," she said, "you weren't supposed to bring them home. Priya could react."

"I'll pass all of them out tomorrow," Aniyka said. "I promise."

To be on the safe side, Anju wrapped the cookies in a plastic bag, and took the bag down to the basement. For good measure, she put it in the crawl space.

Later, Priya went down to the basement. "Mom," she called up, "there's peanuts down here." Her throat started to tighten. She ran upstairs.

When fall came, and it was time for Priya to register for school, Anju went to Priya's pediatrician and asked her to write a letter to the principal, requesting permission for Priya to be tutored at home, due to severe allergies. The pediatrician refused to do it, even as a professional courtesy. She said she couldn't believe that a child could have a severe reaction from just *smelling* a food. It wasn't consistent with her training.

Anju was sickened by the refusal. For so long, she had thought that almost all doctors shared her mission of wanting, above all, to help the most helpless. Now she was beginning to doubt it. Some doctors seemed to care more about staying safely within the confines of the mainstream than about expanding their horizons to help desperate patients. Anju began to go through what she later described as "a grieving period." She felt betrayed, not only by her own profession, but also by the federal government. Government officials were still denying that any harm had come from thimerosal–even after they had removed it from the childhood vaccinations. Federal officials were also maddeningly steadfast in their assertion that no harm had come from any other element of America's expanded vaccination program, such as the accelerated shot schedule. There wasn't even any official recognition that the new childhood epidemics *existed*.

This perspective, though, didn't fit with the reality that Anju was seeing every day. Each new day now, she was treating members of a generation of children who were suffering from horrendous new onslaughts of autism, ADHD, asthma, allergies, juvenile rheumatoid arthritis, childhood cancers, Type 1 and Type 2 diabetes, and obesity. Every day she was trying to repair the bodies of kids who suffered from toxicity, brain inflammation, skewed immunity, depleted neurotransmitters, nutrient deficiencies, and inflamed bowels. Why was all of this happening? Why wasn't anyone in a position of power rising up to defend America's children?

Anju herself, however, was making tremendous clinical progress against the new epidemics, as were so many of the DAN doctors. She was achieving recoveries and remarkable improvements among autistic kids and other chronically ill children who had basically been abandoned by their own doctors.

Anju had, in particular, made a stunning clinical breakthrough in linking the aluminum in vaccinations to immune dysfunction. Aluminum, she believed, was causing as much damage as mercury, but mostly to the immune system, instead of the brain. For example, her own children were suffering from terrible immune problems, but no neurological problems–they were extremely bright, and emotionally mature. Therefore, Anju was becoming convinced that many children, including hers, were not suffering primarily from mercury toxicity, which tends to do most of its damage to the brain, but instead were suffering from aluminum toxicity, which is generally more destructive to the immune system.

It was a brilliant connection. It appeared to be one more piece of the baffling puzzle of the new childhood epidemics.

Despite the promise of this important insight, though, Anju was re-ceiving no government grants to pursue it, nor was she being offered any special support from Chicago's community of mainstream medi-cine.

Anju, myself, and the other DAN doctors were, to a painful degree, engaged in this struggle by ourselves. We stood alone on a new frontier of medicine.

As a parent, Anju was even more alone. Her isolation existed for a simple reason: There is no one in the world who feels more alone than the parent of a seriously ill child.

Failure to Thrive

"He's not *responding*," the doctor told Peggy Renieres. "That's not *good*. He should be admitted. *Immediately*."

Peggy suddenly went weak. She had brought her moderately ill baby to the doctor's office only as a precaution. Now the doctor was saying that Loukas, who'd suddenly begun to wheeze, had to check into the hospital–*now*.

"Breathing problems in babies are like chest pains in adults," the doctor said. "You can't wait around."

With her fear mounting by the moment, Peggy looked down at Loukas, just ten months old, as he struggled to push away the nebulizer mask that the doctor had placed on his face. It wasn't helping him. He was still wheezing, and his chest was retracting spasmodically, as he fought to force air into his inflamed lungs.

Loukas had woken up that morning with an upper respiratory in-fection, a common occurrence for him, and that was the only reason Peggy had brought him here. But when they'd arrived, he'd suddenly started wheezing. He'd *never* wheezed before–just coughed a lot. Since birth, he'd barely been able to fight off any infectious illnesses, and the illnesses had always seemed to lodge in his lungs. When the infections would begin to burn in his chest, he would whimper for days with pain, until the antibiotics would kick in and kill the bacteria. Right after one infection would end, though, another would begin.

The frequent illnesses seemed to be taking a toll on his weight and physical development–or maybe it was the other way around. In either case, he was in the lowest tenth percentile of weight, and appeared to be getting thinner every week, instead of heavier. One problem was simply that he hated to eat. He could say only three things: "Yes," "No," and–whenever they offered him food–"No more."

Peggy hurried over to the hospital with Loukas, hoping for the best, but things got worse. One doctor listened to Loukas' lungs and said he might have the frequently fatal illness of cystic fibrosis. Another examined Loukas' spindly body and said it looked as if he were suffering from failure to thrive, a vague but ominous diagnosis that could open the door to unlimited catastrophe. When Peggy heard that, she lost it, and broke down in front of everyone. Loukas was her first and only child, and it felt to her as if he'd suddenly been ripped from her maternal protection, and was out in the cold world on his own.

For two days and two nights, Loukas squirmed and wheezed in an oxygen-infused tent that was draped over him to help him breathe, as Peggy and her husband, Nikolaos, sat in his room and waited. Doctors came in periodically to insert IVs into Loukas, to give him shots, and to tap his sore chest. After a while, every time anyone in a white coat entered the room, Loukas would moan, "No more," and his big green eyes would float in tears.

Toward the end of it, an allergist came in and did the standard test for allergy, scratching holes in Loukas's skin, as Loukas wailed and fought. Then the doctor wiped the scratches with potential allergens, and looked for the telltale red wheals of inflammation.

When the allergist finished, he pronounced Loukas free of any allergies, except for a mild reaction to cats.

They sent him home with an inhaler, and some drugs to help hold down the inflammation in his airways, a symptom that is present in almost all asthma patients. They told Peggy to cram as much food into Loukas as possible. They said ice cream would be a good choice. Kids *love* ice cream! It will fatten him up!

Peggy nodded dutifully and got out of there as fast as she could. *Ice cream?* Were they out of their *minds*! Peggy didn't know much about asthma, but her sister had suffered from it, and Peggy's mom hadn't let her sister eat any dairy products at all. Peggy's mom had been taught by her own mother, Loukas's great-grandmother, that milk often makes a child with lung problems even more phlegmy and croupy. It was folk wisdom. And it is true. *Moms know.*

Peggy took Loukas off dairy products right away, and his lung problems improved.

Not long afterward, the family visited Peggy's parents in Hong Kong, where her father worked as an international businessman, and Peggy's mother–a health buff who looked about half her age–insisted that they take Loukas to a local doctor that she really liked. The Hong Kong doctor did some allergy tests that were different from the standard scratch test, and his tests indicated that Loukas was sensitive not only to milk, but also to gluten.

Peggy quickly found out that it is extremely common for the standard scratch test to be contradicted, because it checks only for the allergic antibody IgE, and not for other allergic antibodies, such as IgG. When Peggy got home, she mentioned this discrepancy to her growing cadre of regular doctors, but they were all dismissive. Virtually all of them gave Peggy the Crazy Mom treatment–as in, "*Hong Kong?* Hmmm...." After that, she learned to keep most of her doubts to herself.

Of course, she kept Loukas off dairy and gluten. She also began an aggressive program of supplementation. It helped. But not nearly enough. Loukas, by age two, was still too small. His muscles were flaccid, and his lungs were still touchy and twitchy from chronic inflammation. At least once a day, Peggy had to give Loukas a lengthy anti-inflammatory nebulizer treatment, and it appeared as if this treatment schedule would stretch into the distant future.

Loukas was also often irritable and spacey, and could only stay focused for moments at a time. Peggy thought that these mental traits were tied to his physical problems, but she was afraid that if these characteristics persisted into his grade school years, his teachers and his doctors would start pushing Ritalin at him.

Loukas's doctors were already pressuring Peggy to put Loukas on a continual, high-level dosage of oral steroidal medication, to reduce the inflammation in his lungs. She wouldn't do it. One of Loukas's cousins was on steroids for asthma, and it appeared to be stunting his growth, as it often does.

At night, Peggy would find herself hovering over Loukas as he slept–listening, listening–in case he stopped breathing.

Sometimes the whole treatment routine seemed crazy. There must, she thought, be a way to get to the bottom of the problem.

The Root Cause of Asthma

When I first began to treat asthma, in the early 1980s, most doctors still thought that the fundamental root cause of asthma was bronchospasm, or sudden contraction of the bronchial tubes that bring air to the lungs. Therefore, their basic treatments revolved around the relatively new procedure of dilating the bronchial tubes when they went into spasm.

Many doctors, though, were not content to merely treat asthma when it flared up, but wanted to prevent it, by determining the underlying causes of the bronchospasms. They found that most bronchospasms were touched off by several classic triggers, including mold, pollen, pollution, infection, and pet hair. Therefore, they told their patients to try to avoid these triggers. They believed that this was the best possible solution to the problem.

However, other practitioners continued to dig even more deeply into asthma's root causes. Some of us who were treating asthma almost every day came to believe that there was an even more basic root cause than that of the classic asthma triggers. This more fundamental root cause appeared to be inflammation. It seemed as if the bronchial tubes went into spasm from the classic asthma triggers only when they were already aggravated by inflamed muscles that had become overly sensitive, and by inflamed tissues that poured out too much mucus.

Over the next decade, the medical mainstream began to agree that inflammation was the root cause of asthma, so doctors added a new treatment. In addition to the existing treatment of dilating bronchial tubes when asthma episodes struck, doctors began to also put patients on continuing courses of steroidal, anti-inflammatory drugs, to help prevent asthma episodes from being triggered.

These days, most doctors still use these two standard approaches: (1) dilating bronchial tubes during asthma episodes, and (2) prescribing steroidal anti-inflammatories to help prevent episodes.

Even this approach, however, fails to reach the real root cause of asthma. The root cause of asthma is: *the original source of the inflammation.*

Therefore, to defeat asthma, we must dig all the way down to the basic sources of airway inflammation, and eliminate them.

This can be hard to do. It's much easier to just give patients steroids to decrease their inflammation. Doing that can make them less reactive to asthma triggers—as long as they stay on the steroids. In contrast, it can take months of medical detective work to identify the original sources of inflammation, and to remove them. When this is achieved, though, the patient can become free from any serious asthma symptoms.

One confusing factor in the quest to eliminate the original sources of inflammation is that these sources can also be the direct *triggers* of asthma. This can make it harder to identify them as the culprits that kicked off the whole chain of events in the first place. Fungus, for example, can cause infectious inflammation, and then later fungus can act as the direct irritant that triggers an asthma episode. When this happens, patients sometimes remove themselves from the mold that triggered the episode, but they still might have a low-grade fungal infection simmering away, just waiting for another trigger to transform it into an asthma episode.

Another confusing factor in eliminating the sources of inflammation is that there's usually more than one source, and these sources can all combine to create inflammation that's very resistant to treatment. In fact, there are three primary sources of inflammation, and each of the three has several subcategories.

THE THREE MAIN SOURCES OF ASTHMATIC INFLAMMATION

1. **Infections.** They are a notorious source of inflammation. Infections can also be a common trigger of asthma episodes, after inflammation has already taken hold. These infections can be caused by a virus, a bacterium, or a fungus. The infections can originate in the airways, or they can start somewhere else, such as in the gut, and then migrate to the airways.

Furthermore, the infections might even stay in a location distant from the airways, but create inflammatory chemicals that travel to the airways. For example, a chronic infection in the gut can create so many inflammatory agents that some travel to the airways.

Therefore, asthma can be caused by an infection that may seem totally unrelated to asthma, such as a chronic yeast infection, or perhaps chlamydia, or even a lingering measles infection in the gut.

Infections can also indirectly contribute to asthma by skewing immunity and increasing the activity of Th-2 cells. This not only heightens inflammation, but also makes people more prone to allergic reactions.

Asthma can therefore sometimes be reversed by helping patients overcome their infections. This is why diverse treatments—such as administration of antibiotics, or antivirals, or antifungals—can result in dramatic improvements in asthma symptoms.

2. Allergens. Like infections, allergens not only trigger asthma episodes, but can also cause inflammation. Even eating the wrong type of diet can contribute to inflammation.

The conventional treatment of asthma, unfortunately, fails to place enough emphasis on food allergies and good nutrition. Many doctors ignore this aspect entirely.

Food allergies not only trigger inflammation, but also cause other symptoms that contribute to asthma, such as allergic overproduction of mucus, and excessive sensitivity of the nervous system, which can contribute to bronchial muscle spasms.

Milk products are the most common food factor in the causative cascade of asthma, and wheat is second. Many children get profound relief just by switching from cow's milk to soy or rice milk, and by staying away from wheat. The gluten-free, casein-free diet can work wonders.

Asthmatics can also benefit from probiotics, because these digestive aids not only reduce the incidence of food reactions, but also help to regulate the immune system, and overcome Th-2 skewing.

Another dietary measure that can be hugely helpful is taking supplements of essential fatty acids, such as fish oil, borage oil, evening primrose oil, or flaxseed oil. EFAs are potent anti-inflammatories, and several studies indicate that they can help reduce the frequency, intensity, and duration of asthma episodes.

Similarly, it's important to avoid the common foods that directly increase inflammation. The most important foods to avoid are those that are high in saturated fats—especially the *trans*-fatty acids found in many processed foods. Also, too much salt can have a pro-inflammatory effect.

3. Toxins. Virtually any toxin can create inflammation, as the body struggles to eliminate the toxin. However, heavy metals, even more than other toxins, appear to most frequently create the high level of toxicity that can result in widespread inflammation.

In my own practice, the toxins that seem to be most commonly found in asthmatic children are mercury, lead, aluminum, cadmium, tin, and arsenic. The high incidence of toxicity from mercury and aluminum, of course, makes me suspect that part of the current asthma epidemic was caused by the childhood vaccinations that contained mercury and aluminum. The vaccinations may have caused not only systemic inflammation from heavy metals, but also may have contributed to immune skewing, and to the creation of low-level chronic infections.

Several clinical studies support the link between the vaccinations and asthma. For example, in a study in England, 10.7 percent of children who received a pertussis vaccination developed asthma, compared to 2 percent of children who didn't receive it. In America, a large epidemiological study showed that children vaccinated with DTP were twice as likely to develop asthma as those who weren't.

The vaccinations, though, are not the only source of toxicity among kids with asthma, just as they are not the only source of toxicity among children with autism and ADHD. Environmental toxins also play a huge role.

Outdoor air pollution contributes to asthma, not only as a trigger, but also as a cause of inflammation. About 20 million American children live in areas that do not meet federal standards for clean air, and when air pollution spikes in these areas, hospitalizations for asthma typically increase by about 20 percent to 30 percent. Even indoor air pollution is a terrible problem. Air is often excessively recycled within homes, and frequently contains not only chemical gas emitted by home furnishings, but also dust, mold, mildew, dust mites, and insect waste products.

All of these various toxins add up, and reach a cumulative toxic level that is often underestimated. For example, if air is moderately high in lead, and also moderately high in carbon monoxide, it can escape the attention of federal regulators, but still create such a high cumulative toxic burden that some people can get sick from it.

Because toxins are a major cause of asthma, kids with asthma often respond dramatically to programs of detoxification. As their bodies gradually become cleansed of toxins, their inflammation decreases, and they suffer markedly less from asthma.

These are the three most important root sources of the inflammation that leads to asthma. Sometimes all three are present at once. The damage done by these sources cannot be permanently eliminated by just taking a drug. As a rule, a patient must adhere to the comprehensive Healing Program for weeks, months, or even years to eliminate the inflammation caused by these root sources, and to be free from significant symptoms of asthma. This takes time, but it works. On the Healing Program, most asthma patients improve considerably, and many achieve reversal of the condition.

A multifaceted program is the kind of help patients need. Unfortunately, though, it's not the kind of help they usually get.

Chicago, Illinois

Priya, in fifth grade now, had to stay away from school, and was tutored at home, as Anju searched laboriously for treatments that could help her.

At one point, Anju went to a doctor who recommended a special nutritional formula designed to promote growth and development. The formula, though, had soybean oil in it, and Anju told the doctor that Priya was very reactive to soybean oil.

"That's not possible," said the doctor. "People are allergic to proteins, not fats and oils. There's *nothing* in the literature about allergies to oils."

"I don't care what the literature says," Anju replied. "She reacts to soybean oil."

The doctor sighed, and began to give Anju the condescending Crazy Mom treatment. Because Anju was a physician herself, she was generally spared from that attitude, but she knew all about it, because the mothers of her autistic patients often mentioned it. Their hometown doctors rarely tried to hide the scorn that they felt for the mothers who questioned their conventional approaches.

Shortly after that, Anju took Priya to an allergist. During the visit, Priya began to wheeze, and Anju told the allergist how worried she was about Priya's asthma.

"Oh, that's not wheezing," said the allergist. "She's just making a noise with her larynx."

Anju was shocked. "Of course it's wheezing."

"No. She just needs to do some throat exercises. That will make it go away."

Anju was beginning to believe that the only person who could save Priya was herself. It was a terrible feeling.

Rhinebeck, 2002

Loukas sat sullenly in my office, fidgeting and fitful, obviously miserable, as I began his first appointment.

Peggy was polite, but I later learned that she didn't have a lot of optimism about my program. She'd already been to too many doctors, and was fed up with their treatments, and even their egos. At her most recent appointment with a new doctor, she'd mistaken the female physician for a nurse, and the doctor had just gone *off* on her. Peggy had managed to keep her mouth shut, but she was sick of the system.

She'd come to me because she had seen my second book, *Natural Relief for Your Child's Asthma,* in her Hong Kong doctor's office, of all places. She knew, therefore, that I tried to do more than just suppress symptoms. But she wouldn't let herself get her hopes up.

As the appointment went on, though, she became more animated and enthusiastic. Years later, she told me that this was simply because I was listening to what she had to say.

The first thing I realized, as she described her family's health history, was that Loukas was definitely a member of what I call an atopic family. An atopic family is one in which there is widespread allergy. Atopic means prone to allergy–particularly to allergy that shows its symptoms in a part of the body that's distant from the site where the allergen entered the body. For example, if someone eats strawberries and gets hives on their skin, that's an atopic reaction. Another common atopic reaction is asthma. Asthma is not always caused by direct contact between an allergen and the airways. Sometimes it's caused by foods and chemicals that are nowhere near the airways.

The condition of being atopic often runs in families. That's why asthma tends to run in families. It's not necessarily the asthma that is directly inherited, but the atopy. Thus, once again, we see that the reality of a disorder is easier to understand when root causes are revealed.

Just looking at Loukas, I could tell that he was an atopic kid. He had dark circles under his eyes, which is almost always a sure sign of allergy—usually food allergy. He was sniffly, pale, tired, and irritable, all of which can indicate allergy. For Loukas, poor digestion was almost certainly a primary cause of his allergy, as it generally is, and it was probably also a major factor in his small size. At age six, he only weighed 48 pounds. I also suspected that he had an underlying immune imbalance, with Th-2 skewing. This skewing was probably feeding into his allergies, and also making him prone to infection. The immune skewing, the allergies, and the infection then contributed to his asthma, in his terrible downward spiral of illness.

Even though he was just six, Loukas had all the classic features of the inattentive subtype of ADHD. At this time, he was probably on the road to Ritalin. If that happened, though, it would be a disaster. The last thing in the world that he needed was a stimulant that would mask the physical exhaustion that was destroying him. There was nothing wrong with this kid's brain that couldn't be remedied by restoring the health of his body.

After I reviewed all of his lab work, I put him on a Healing Program that was individualized for his own particular needs.

LOUKAS' HEALING PROGRAM

- **Restriction** of several allergenic foods.
- **Continuation** of a strict gluten-free, casein-free diet.
- **Supplementation** with cod liver oil, probiotics, essential fatty acids, and vitamins A, C, and E. These supplements would reduce his inflammation and boost his immunity.
- **Administration of transfer factor,** to reduce his Th-2 skewing, by promoting the activity of his Th-1 cells.
- **The anti-candida diet,** to help control his chronic fungal infection, and improve his bowel dysbiosis.
- **Echinacea and other herbal anti-microbials,** to help him overcome other lingering infections.
- **Calcium and magnesium,** to help reduce the oversensitivity

of the muscles around his airways, and to replace the calcium from his nondairy diet.

- **Supplemention with DMAE,** to improve his mental energy, focus, and attention.
- **Co-enzyme Q-10,** to boost his physical energy and increase his antioxidant levels.
- **Melatonin,** to help him sleep better, and decrease his chronic inflammation.
- **The anti-hypoglycemia diet,** to help build his strength and energy, and to restore his metabolic balance. This diet would complement his gluten-free, casein-free diet, and the anti-candida diet.

That was it. Nothing dramatic. Even so, I was hoping for dramatic improvement. When you give the body what it needs, great things can happen.

Chicago, 2002

Thank God—Priya was getting better! Anju had embarked on a cautious but ambitious program to build up Priya's body, so that she wouldn't be so overreactive to allergens, and so vulnerable to asthma triggers.

I talked with Anju from time to time, and for the most part, she was employing therapies that were extremely similar to those that I was applying to my own young patients with asthma, allergies, autism, and ADHD. In her own practice, Anju was continuing to have success with the autistic children she was treating, and this helped to fuel her growing sense of confidence that she could improve the health of her daughter, whose immune system was as oversensitized and as damaged as that of any child I'd ever heard about.

Anju was bringing down Priya's inflammation, modulating her skewed immunity, desensitizing her to potential allergens, reducing her level of toxicity, and building her strength and vitality.

Priya, as usual, was great about doing all the treatments, and that gave Anju hope, too. After all, it's the kids themselves who bear the brunt of their own healing, and when they embrace it, instead of resist it—as some children do—it gives them a tremendous advantage.

Priya went back to school! It was such a happy day when that happened. She'd missed a whole year, and now she was back to socializing with her friends, feeling like a normal kid, and having some fun.

They kept her away from the lunchroom, though. Each day, she ate lunch with the principal in his office, and was allowed to invite one of her friends for the special private lunch. She became good friends with the principal.

She could even cheat on her diet. Every so often, she'd have a cookie or even some ice cream. No problem. To her, these ordinary things brought great joy. Through her suffering, Priya had become a very mature, spiritual child, who'd learned to appreciate the little things in life that most kids just couldn't.

Anju, for the first time in years, was beginning to savor optimism. The many sacrifices she had made to help the most helpless were finally coming full circle, and bringing peace to her own life. Life, she was starting to believe, really could have a happy ending.

Rhinebeck, 2003

"*Loukas!*" I said, "you look *terrific!*"

What a tremendous leap this tough little kid had made! In just a year, he'd gained almost 50 percent more weight. His asthma had virtually vanished. His muscles were strong, and his cheeks were pink, and wrinkled with a perpetual smile. The dark circles under his eyes were gone, and he was calm, focused, and attentive. This was the kind of child you'd look at and think, "Nice healthy kid–big for his age."

Peggy looked ecstatic. "For the first few months," she told me, "every time he coughed, I held my breath, waiting for the other shoe to drop. But it never happened. He doesn't *get* sick anymore. He hasn't used his inhaler since I don't know when."

"I know when," said Loukas. "The last time I used it was the first time I was here."

For the rest of that day, I felt like I was walking on air. Sometimes I think that I've got the best job in the world.

Chicago, 2003

For Priya, January 2003 was good. February was great. March was perfect.

It was spring break, and Anju and her husband were going out to dinner with friends. Their friends brought over their own children to play with Anju's kids, and to eat some Chinese take-out.

Priya no longer had to be extraordinarily careful about what she ate, but she did need to avoid peanuts entirely. Because of that, they ordered take-out only from a particular Chinese restaurant, where the chef knew about Priya's allergy, and never gave them anything with peanuts. The chef always made a special egg roll, just for Priya.

As the four parents were leaving, Priya said, "Mom, I can eat this egg roll, right?"

"Sure."

Right after they left, Anju got a call on her cell phone. It was Priya.

"Mom, there might have been peanuts or something in my egg roll. My tongue's real itchy."

"Take some Benadryl. If it doesn't go away immediately, call me back. Right away, okay? *Right away.*"

A minute later Anju's phone rang again. It was Aniyka. "She's still having problems."

"Give Priya an epi!" Aniyka knew how to give epinephrine injections, because she was diabetic. "Call 911! I'll be home in a second!"

The local fire station was only a few blocks from their house. The paramedics arrived in a matter of moments.

Anju and her husband burst into the house just after the paramedics arrived. The paramedics were bent over Priya, trying frantically to revive her. She wasn't responding. They rushed her to the hospital. Doctors there tried to revive her, but they could not. Priya was dead.

Loukas, 2006

Loukas was in his tae kwon do class, in his little white uniform, sparring with another child. Peggy watched from outside, in her car, through a large, plate-glass window. Suddenly Loukas made a wrong move, and split open his finger. Blood began to drop from it. Loukas grabbed his hand. He ran outside.

Peggy opened the car door, and ushered him in. She put a Band-Aid on his hand, and gave it a kiss. Loukas began to run back to his class. Peggy called him back, for no real reason—mother's instincts—and held him tightly, dearly, until he squirmed away and went back to play.

4. ALLERGIES

CHAPTER THIRTEEN

LIFE
AND DEATH

Washington, D.C.

"I HAVE ALWAYS BEEN THE TYPE OF PERSON THAT FOLLOWS RULES. I obeyed my parents and teachers. I completed high school and my undergraduate work without getting into any trouble.

"I respected authority, and rarely questioned the teachings of my medical school professors. I did everything by the book.

"Even when our first child, Priya, was born, I took my vitamins, drank four glasses of milk per day, and had her immunized on day one.

"She cried almost constantly, she wouldn't nurse, and she seemed to be in distress. But we took her to the finest doctors, who assured us she would outgrow it."

Anju, still shocked and raw from Priya's recent death, looked out at the faces in the large DAN Conference auditorium, and she seemed to notice me and the people with whom I was sitting. Most of Anju's closest colleagues were in the audience. We were there to honor Anju's courage, and to try to learn something new that we could all use to help save our kids.

Most of us DAN doctors, by this time, usually referred to the children we were treating as "our kids," because of our close bonds with them. There's something about children who are suffering–perhaps their combination of innocence and bravery–that makes you adopt them into your heart. Around me were people who'd dedicated their lives to these kids, and who ached for Anju's loss: Sid Baker, Jill James, Stephanie Cave, Tim Buie, Jackie McCandless, Jeff Bradstreet, Andrew Wakefield, Jane El-Dahr, Lauren Underwood, Liz Birt, Dick Deth, Karyn Seroussi, Jon Pangborn, Jim Neubrander, and many others. Some had sons and daughters of their own who'd been hit by the new epidemics, and I knew that these people felt Anju's pain on a gut level.

The title of Anju's speech was "Courage in the Midst of Chaos." With steely control but terrible sadness, she said, "At six months, Priya had an anaphylactic reaction to some eggs that she accidentally ate. Tests revealed that she had allergies to gluten, casein, soy, eggs, and peanuts. Priya never received her MMR, due to her egg allergies, but otherwise she was fully immunized.

"After putting her on an elimination diet, she improved greatly. She started to grow, and to sleep better. She was happier and more alert. The dietary changes helped her, but her immune system remained hyperactive and hypersensitive, and never fully recovered."

Anju took a breath. "Priya died of an anaphylactic reaction to a trace amount of peanut in an egg roll.

"I wish I could turn back time. I wish I knew then what I know now, about the effects of vaccines and heavy metals on a developing immune system. I sought out the people I thought would help, but I was sent down a path that led to tragedy.

"I applaud your efforts for being here. It takes courage to go against the establishment, and to speak out for what you know is true. In my talk, I will discuss treating the autism spectrum disorders using nutrient therapy, and a biomedical model. I hope this helps you down a path that leads *away* from tragedy—toward recovery."

Then she began her detailed PowerPoint presentation.

I was moved—we all were moved that day—by the greatness of Anju's heart. She had many things on her mind at that time, other than helping us, and our kids. I knew, as did most of my other friends in the auditorium, that Anju's daughter Aniyka was beginning to have severe allergic reactions, similar to those that had killed little Priya.

Aniyka would eventually overcome the problems, but there was no way to know that at this time. Uncertainty hovered like a black cloud.

The Universal Threat

Allergies are among the most powerful and destructive of all the interwoven forces that compose the new childhood epidemics.

• *Allergies contribute immeasurably to the epidemics of autism, ADHD, and asthma.*

• *Allergies are an epidemic in their own right. Food allergies have increased by approximately 700 percent in just the last ten years, and fatal allergies are far more common than ever before.*

Only the crippling force of toxins matches the damage that is done every day by allergies.

Many people, however, vastly underestimate the harm that allergies do. They don't perceive allergies as a life-or-death issue, but only as a minor annoyance that causes sniffling and hives. Part of the reason most people generally associate allergies with only their mildest, most common symptoms is because allergies themselves are so common, and their symptoms are so evident in everyday life. About 75 million Americans, or one-fourth of the population, have allergies.

Another reason that the threat of allergies is underestimated is because allergies are usually not the only element that contributes to various disorders. Allergies get lost in the crowd of combined factors that cause disease.

Therefore, most people simply don't realize that allergies are a dark, deadly force that can kill children, destroy their brains, and cripple them with symptoms. *The vast majority of all children with autism, ADHD, and asthma have serious allergies.* As a general rule, these three disorders can *not* be overcome without alleviating the damage done by allergies.

Take a look at the following table, which shows the percentage of autistic children who improved when they avoided certain foods. As you can see, the rate of improvement was remarkably high. All of the following foods, except for sugar and yeast, are notoriously allergenic. Although sugar is generally not a cause of classic allergy, many children are still intolerant to it, because it destabilizes their blood sugar levels, and feeds yeast and pathogenic bacteria in the gut.

DIETARY FACTORS IN AUTISM THERAPY

FACTOR	% of Patients Who IMPROVED	% of Patients Who DETERIORATED	% of Patients Who Experienced NO EFFECT
Gluten-Free, Casein-Free	65	3	32
Anti-Yeast (candida)	54	3	43
Additive-Free	54	2	44
Chocolate-Free	49	2	49
Dairy-Free	50	2	48
Sugar-Free	48	2	50
Wheat-Free	49	2	49
Egg-Free	40	2	58

Chart extrapolated from Defeat Autism Now Syllabus, Spring 2006, from information compiled by the Autism Research Institute.

Following is another table that also shows how important it is to restrict allergenic foods from autistic children. This table rates the order of importance of various autism therapies, according to the opinions of parents. The parents rated the restrictions of several highly allergenic foods as being among the best possible therapies for autism. The only therapy that was considered more important was detoxification.

This table shows that the worst foods for autistic kids generally are: (1) dairy products, (2) chocolate, (3) yeast-proliferating foods, and (4) the combination of gluten and casein. All these foods are common allergens, except for the yeast-proliferating foods—such as sugar, vinegar, and yeast—which do their damage not through allergy, but by exacerbating intestinal candidiasis.

EFFECTIVENESS OF THERAPEUTIC
MEASURES FOR AUTISM
Rated from Best to Least Effective

THERAPY	% of Patients Who IMPROVED	% of Patients Who DETERIORATED	% of Patients Who Experienced NO EFFECT
Detoxification	75	3	22
Dairy product restriction*	50	2	48
Chocolate restriction*	49	2	49
Vitamin A	40	2	58
Yeast-proliferating foods restriction*	54	3	43
Zinc	48	3	49
Gluten-casein restriction*	65	3	32
Vitamin C	56	2	42
EFAs	54	2	44
Calcium	62	3	35
Digestive enzymes	58	3	39
Folic Acid	42	4	54
Vitamin B-6	51	13	36
Nystatin	49	5	46
Diflucan	52	5	43
Depakene	31	26	43
Risperdal	55	18	27
Prozac	37	33	30
Adderall	34	26	40

*Allergy or food reaction-related therapy

Chart extrapolated from Defeat Autism Now Syllabus, Spring 2006, from information compiled by the Autism Research Institute.

The incidence of allergies is every bit as high among ADHD kids as it is among autistic children. In fact, it's extremely rare for me to treat an ADHD child without finding evidence of a reaction to at least one allergen. In addition, practically all asthmatic kids react to certain foods or airborne allergens.

Sometimes kids who are misdiagnosed with ADHD don't have the classic features of that disorder at all, but instead have allergic symptoms that mimic ADHD symptoms. These allergic symptoms can include restlessness, insomnia, poor cognitive function, depression, and hyperactivity. These mental and emotional reactions to allergens are sometimes referred to as cerebral allergies, because their most obvious symptoms are neurological.

Allergies also often mimic other disorders, besides ADHD. For example, they can cause symptoms that are extremely similar to those of irritable bowel syndrome, even among people who don't have classic IBS. Because allergies so often mimic symptoms of other disorders, they are sometimes referred to as "the great pretenders."

Furthermore, allergies not only mimic the symptoms of various disorders, but also play an important role in the *causation* of a wide variety of disorders and diseases. Unfortunately, the role that they play in disease causation is frequently overlooked, since many doctors and patients tend to underestimate the power of allergy. When this oversight occurs, patients are often unsuccessfully treated with medications for many years, as their chronic conditions fester, and continue to be fueled by allergies.

Following are various problems that allergies often trigger, contribute to, or mimic.

DISORDERS ASSOCIATED WITH ALLERGIES

ADHD symptoms are commonly made more severe by allergy, and sometimes allergy is the primary underlying disorder among people who are misdiagnosed with ADHD.

Arthritis is often made far more painful by the swelling caused by allergic inflammation. In addition to exacerbating osteoarthritis, allergic symptoms also often mimic the symptoms of rheumatoid arthritis.

Asthma is inextricably linked with allergy. Almost all people with asthma have allergies, and allergies are the most common trigger of asthma episodes.

Candida problems are exacerbated by food allergy, and food allergy is exacerbated by candida overgrowth, in a self-perpetuating cycle.

Chronic ear infections are frequently triggered by allergic congestion. When these infections require repeated courses of antibiotics, it can harm the immune system and gut.

Chronic fatigue syndrome is closely associated with allergy. Allergic symptoms mimic and trigger the symptoms of this syndrome, including those of malaise, fatigue, poor cognitive function, depression, swollen glands, and night sweats.

Chronic pain is often amplified by the inflammation of allergic reactions, and by the decreased activity of serotonin that allergies can precipitate.

Cognitive and mood disorders are commonly linked with allergies. This includes depression, anxiety, impaired cognitive function, and hyperactivity. Allergies can initiate these conditions, or contribute to existing conditions.

Diabetes can be made much worse by allergy. Food reactions disrupt insulin metabolism, destabilize blood sugar levels, and contribute to inflammation of the pancreas.

Digestive disorders go hand in hand with food allergy. Food reactions commonly cause symptoms of indigestion, including heartburn, gas, and bloating. Autistic children with bowel dysbiosis can be particularly sensitive to problems with digestion and elimination.

Eating disorders often occur among people with food allergies. Food reactions typically trigger craving, which then causes people to binge on favorite foods. Allergies also contribute to bulimia and anorexia, by lowering serotonin levels.

Eczema, acne, and hives are extremely common reactions to food allergies and sensitivities. In one study, 100 percent of patients with hives, and 66 percent of patients with eczema responded positively to restriction of various allergenic foods.

Fibromyalgia, or widespread chronic muscle pain, has been linked to low levels of serotonin. Low serotonin is often caused by food reactions.

Hay fever is typically caused by airborne allergens, and when food reactions occur simultaneously, they can make hay fever much worse.

Headaches are a common symptom of food reactions. Migraines are frequently triggered by various foods. In one study, 93 percent of young migraine patients stopped having headaches when they eliminated all of their reactive foods.

Hypoglycemia commonly results from food reactions. The food reactions spike blood sugar, which then plummets.

Insomnia can occur when food reactions disrupt the normal balance of hormones and neurotransmitters, including serotonin and melatonin.

Irritable bowel syndrome, which accounts for about one-third of all visits to gastroenterologists, is often triggered by dairy products, animal fat, sugar, citrus, and cruciferous vegetables, such as cauliflower and broccoli. Symptoms of food reactions also often mimic symptoms of IBS.

Obesity is much more common among people with chronic food reactions. Weight gain is often triggered by allergic inflammation, which disrupts the metabolism. Food reactions also cause food cravings. In addition, food reactions typically create a false fat of tissue swelling, abdominal bloating, and water weight.

Sinusitis is very common among people with airborne allergies, and also among those with food allergies. Both types of allergies cause swelling of nasal tissues, as well as inflammation, and production of excess mucus.

- **Allergies** make many existing problems worse.
- **Allergies** initiate or trigger a variety of serious disorders.
- **Allergies** create symptoms that mimic those of many other disorders.

Sometimes the dreadful damage that allergies can do begins subtly, and almost innocently—as a runny nose, or a cough, or heartburn. But the damage can escalate, step by step, until tragedy is suddenly just one step away.

The Spinal Tap

Hugo Frank, barely two years old, needed a spinal tap. His doctors had to determine if his brain was inflamed with the often deadly infection of meningitis. When the doctors told Hugo's dad, Ron Frank, that they needed to do a spinal tap, they referred to the procedure with its modern name–lumbar puncture–but Ron knew what was coming, and felt jittery with dread. As the moment for the procedure approached, Ron sat with Hugo in his hospital room, read him books, held him, and hid his own fear.

Hugo and Ron were exceptionally close. During the first few weeks after Hugo's birth, Ron played a large role in caring for him and immediately discovered that he liked everything about parenting–even the diapers and sleepless nights. His life had a new kind of love in it. A Woodstock transplant from New York City, Ron worked at home as an investor, and had plenty of time to be a hands-on dad, especially after he clicked off his computer screens when the stock markets closed. He didn't hire a nanny, but sometimes he took Hugo to day care in the morning for a few hours, if his wife wasn't feeling well, so that he could get some work done.

Ron began to worry that the day care might be a source of germs, though, when Hugo began to have problems. When Hugo was about a year old, he caught a cold that quickly infected his lungs. The doctor put him on a course of antibiotics. It went away, and everything seemed fine. Hugo was his usual self again, a fireball of energy. Even as an infant, Hugo was a fun, frisky little kid, the kind that dads are naturally drawn to.

Just a few days after the infection ended, though, Hugo again began to cry and cough, and they went back to the doctor for more antibiotics.

Ron was concerned that milk might be causing the congestion, so he switched Hugo to soy formula, during the times Hugo wasn't nursing. Hugo loved the stuff, and began to drink bottle after bottle of it. The doctor agreed that avoiding dairy was a wise course of action.

Then the colds and infections began to come in waves, forcing repeated courses of antibiotics. The infections inflamed Hugo's lungs, his sinuses, his throat, and sometimes his middle ears. At one point, he developed the oral yeast infection known as thrush, probably from all the antibiotics, but it eventually cleared. Hugo was in pain much of the time, and sometimes he would cough so violently that he vomited. He had a hard time sleeping through the night, due to his choking, congestion, and fevers. But he was an unusually tough little guy, resilient and cheerful, and his bravery and good nature made his parents adore him that much more.

Around the time he turned two, though, Hugo caught an infection that he just couldn't kick, even with his standard antibiotics. His breathing turned gurgly, and his chest and face stayed hot and wet with sweat night and day. At the same time, he developed a viral skin infection called parvovirus B-19, or Fifth Disease, that streaked his cheeks and chest with a red rash.

Ron and his wife, Adah, took Hugo to the doctor for more diagnostics. They got bad news. Hugo's white blood count, indicating his degree of infection, was an off-the-charts 37,000. Time for the hospital.

In the hospital—hacking with a deep, pertussal cough and reeling with fever—Hugo was diagnosed with pneumonia. They bombarded him with stronger antibiotics, but he didn't respond. He was alarmingly young to have such a persistent pneumonia.

That was when the doctors decided that Hugo needed to be tested for meningitis, with the lumbar puncture.

Hugo, barely old enough to talk, would need to lie motionless on his side in a fetal position, to open the spaces between his vertebrae, as the doctor slid a hollow needle into the membrane covering Hugo's spinal cord, to withdraw fluid. Ron would have to hold Hugo down, so that he wouldn't jerk away from the pain, and drive the needle into his spine.

So Ron waited with Hugo, stroking his hot face, and keeping him calm.

He wondered how all this had come so far, so fast.

How could he protect his little boy?

Chicago, Illinois

After Priya's death, Anju felt, as she later put it, "like one of the walking wounded." On the surface, she was functional, but her inner self was hollow with hurt. In that regard, she identified with her young patients who looked fine, but were suffering from autism, ADHD, allergies, and asthma. Their outward appearances were usually shockingly normal: cute faces, healthy-looking bodies, and no scars. But the young victims of the "invisible epidemics," as the 4-A disorders are sometimes called, were suffused with pain, as was Anju.

Even so, Anju and her husband had three other children to raise, and a life to continue. They persevered, boats against the current.

Aniyka's situation was particularly troubling. For most of her life,

Aniyka had been struggling against the destructive force of her own immune system. Only her first four months in life had been easy. She'd missed her day-one hepatitis-B vaccination, and that had seemed to help her avoid the colic that had tormented Priya.

However, almost immediately after Aniyka had gotten her initial immunizations, at four months, she'd begun to wheeze, and to develop ear infections. From age four months to twelve months, she'd suffered from recurrent ear infections, and had been given almost continual courses of antibiotics and steroids to treat them, and to help prevent them. The antibiotics, though, had allowed the yeast on her mucus membranes to proliferate, and she'd developed recurrent candida infections throughout her diaper area, as well as thrush on her tongue.

For many years, she continued to have trouble with yeast. Then at age eight, she'd been diagnosed with childhood diabetes, the autoimmune form of the disease. After that, she'd had to add sweets to the list of foods she couldn't eat, along with dairy, corn, and soy. That was hard for a little kid.

As her teen years approached, she wasn't overcoming any of her allergies, despite comprehensive and sophisticated treatments.

'Niyka was emotionally strong, though, as are so many of these kids who must deal with terrible distress so early in life. Each day, she endured the heartbreak of her sister's loss, and the uncertainty that shadowed her own future, with a bouyancy and grace that made her parents proud, and stronger themselves.

On Memorial Day weekend, when Aniyka was twelve, she went on a camping trip with her Girl Scout troop, and stayed in a camp that was very moldy. When she came home and mentioned the mold, Anju was concerned, because mold is a fungus that's similar to yeast. But Aniyka seemed to be okay.

A couple of days later, though, Aniyka began to wheeze, and huff for breath, which was unusual for her. She'd never had serious asthma symptoms before.

"Let me give you a nebulizer treatment," Anju said.

It didn't work. Anju gave her another one. It didn't work. Another. Another. Aniyka kept wheezing.

Anju rushed her to the closest hospital. From there, they immediately hurried Aniyka to the asthma crisis center at Loyola University Hospital, where Priya had gone.

When Anju arrived there, she felt sick that it all seemed so familiar.

CHAPTER FOURTEEN

THE HOSPITAL

ANIYKA KEPT DETERIORATING. HER BREATH FADED TO GASPS. SOON she couldn't breathe at all. The doctors at Loyola put her on a ventilator in the Intensive Care Unit, and forced pure oxygen into her lungs.

They pumped her system full of drugs–steroids, albuterol, anything they could think of that might open up her lungs.

Days passed. Anju and her husband hovered over Aniyka, and prayed. A week crawled by. Aniyka was still on the ventilator.

After two weeks of almost constant crisis, Aniyka began to breathe on her own. She gradually began to look like herself again: delicate, beautiful, and more vulnerable than ever.

When she finally came home, she was the same as always, but only on the outside. Now Aniyka, too, was one of the walking wounded.

Fighting with Doctors

Hugo, still in the hospital after several days, seemed to be sinking. He actually appeared to be getting worse, if that were possible. In their efforts to quell the pneumonia, his doctors gave him a cephalosporin antibiotic, in an IV drip. Right after that, though, he developed bright red rings under his eyes, and his joints began to swell and ache. He could hardly speak.

Hugo began to fear the doctors. When any of them entered the room, he would croak, "I'm full," which was his two-year-old way of saying, "No more."

Finally, one of the doctors mentioned the possibility that Hugo might be having an allergic reaction to cephalosporin.

"Then let's use another drug," Ron said. Ron, who'd gained some expertise in antibiotics from all of Hugo's illnesses, wanted to try erythromycin, which tends to be less allergenic.

The doctor, however, wanted to administer another drug in the cephalosporin family, because erythromycin could not be delivered intravenously, which allowed for higher dosages.

"That would defeat the purpose," Ron said. The pivotal problem, he suggested, seemed to be the allergic reaction.

The doctor appeared to be offended by Ron's input. He reiterated his point.

Ron reiterated his.

The doctor's studied forbearance began to harden. He started to give Ron the sex-appropriate version of the Crazy Mom treatment: the Idiot Dad treatment.

Ron, unaccustomed to condescension, and fiercely protective of his son, let loose his frustration. The argument became heated. At the end of it, Ron said, "Give me twenty-four hours. If the white blood count doesn't go down, we'll stop."

Twenty-four hours later, the white count was down, and Hugo was beginning to brighten with color. His cough quieted.

Ron became convinced that he had to take an even more active role in overseeing Hugo's health care. Most of Hugo's short life had been straight downhill, and there wasn't much downside left. Hugo's decline had to *stop*. Now.

Rhinebeck

The first thing I noticed about Hugo was his allergic shiners. Dark circles under the eyes are more than just a clinical clue of allergy—they're a dead giveaway. You don't need to be much of a medical detective to determine atopy from allergic shiners—you just have to look for them. Another clue to look for is a horizontal crease under the lower eyelid, which is called a Dennie-Morgan fold. Both of these signs are simple reactions to nasal congestion, swelling, and increased blood flow to the ethmoid sinuses, which are near the tear ducts.

If the tear ducts become congested and obstructed, it can also give kids a watery, glassy-eyed look. If this congestion persists for years, it can even result in the appearance of a long face, and occasionally a warped palate, due to constant open-mouth breathing.

These signs of chronic allergy are so obvious that I'm always surprised when doctors and patients fail to recognize them. In Hugo's case, not one of his doctors had ordered any allergy testing.

Even if conventional allergists had tested Hugo, though, they might have missed some of his most virulent allergies. Allergies frequently remain undiagnosed, for several reasons. One reason they're missed is because the majority of allergists rely primarily, or even exclusively, on the skin scratch test, or prick test, in which they scratch open the surface of the skin and apply a potential allergen, to see if it causes inflammation. I consider this test to be relatively unreliable, because it doesn't place the allergen deeply enough into the body to achieve a consistently clear result. I much prefer the intradermal test, in which the allergen is placed significantly deeper into the skin. The intradermal test is a more sensitive tool, and helps eliminate false negatives, in which existing allergies go undetected.

The intradermal test hurts a little more than the prick test, though, so kids are often resistant to it. Therefore, when I'm testing children, I often use a variation of the RAST (or radioallergosorbent) blood test, known as the ELISA (Enzyme-Linked Immunosorbent Assay) test, which requires only one needle poke, to withdraw blood. In this test, a blood sample is checked for the presence of the specific immune antibodies that various allergens provoke. This is a good test, even though it's not 100 percent reliable, since it only looks for antibodies, instead of obvious physical signs of allergic reaction. Because of this, it sometimes provides false positives, indicating allergy when none actually exists.

Due to these occasional false positives, the ELISA test is not very popular among most allergists. In my opinion, though, it's still the most practical and revealing test, even though it's not perfect. The false positives aren't very common, and when they do occur, the only harm to patients is the unnecessary restriction of certain foods. These restrictions usually don't last very long, because most patients soon try the foods in a food-challenge test, and find that they don't cause problems.

The ELISA test, I believe, is sufficiently reliable, and it often uncovers many subtle and mild allergies that would otherwise go undetected.

Another reason food allergies are missed is because most allergists tend to focus primarily on inhalant allergens, instead of food allergens, especially when patients have nasal or pulmonary congestion. My approach is different. Whenever I am searching for the root causes of congestion, as well as other metabolic problems, food allergies are always high on my list of the Usual Suspects. As I'm performing a differential diagnosis, sorting out possible causative factors, I almost always screen for food reactions.

Furthermore, I usually screen for more kinds of food than do most allergists. I often screen for as many as twenty-four or more foods, instead of the standard ten to twelve.

The main reason I find more food reactions than most allergists, though, is because I screen for a broader spectrum of reactions. As the following material indicates, traditional allergists tend to screen only for IgE allergies, and therefore they miss two other important types of reactions.

FOOD AND INHALANT REACTIONS

The Three Primary Types

1. **IgE Allergies.** These are the reactions that most doctors do recognize. They are reactions to foods or inhalants that involve the immune system's IgE antibodies. They are the only type of classic, "true" allergy, according to the conventional definition of allergy. They are relatively uncommon, affecting only a small percentage of all people who have reactions to foods. They are generally the most severe type of reaction, and usually occur almost immediately upon contact with the allergen. They can remain troublesome throughout life.

2. **IgG Sensitivities.** Technically, these are not classic allergies, because they involve the immune system's IgG antibodies, instead of the IgE antibodies. Therefore, they are often ignored by allergists. These sensitivities are far more common than classic IgE allergies, although they usually have milder symptoms. Generally, symptoms don't become evident for several hours. Occasionally they take as much as a day or two, or even longer, to produce symptoms. They sometimes go away after a reactive food has been avoided for several months, or longer.

3. **Intolerances.** These are simple, chemical reactions, usually to foods, that do not involve the immune system. Because they don't involve the immune system, they are not considered to be classic allergies. Therefore, they are often completely overlooked by allergists. Even so, intolerances can cause severe

symptoms. For example, when some people eat the food substance known as tyramine, which is in wine and cheese, it triggers dilation of the blood vessels in their brains, and causes
migraines. Another well-known example of food intolerance is
lactose intolerance. People tend to think of lactose intolerance
as an allergy, but it's not, because it doesn't involve the immune
system. It's simply a chemical reaction to lactose, or milk sugar,
which occurs among people who don't have enough of the enzymes that are needed to break down lactose. Thus, many people can test negative for milk allergy, but still react strongly to
dairy products. This happens very frequently.

Ten to twenty years ago, most allergists were extraordinarily skeptical about the potential harm that could be done by sensitivities and intolerances. They often told patients that they were just imagining their
reactions. These days, the trend is gradually changing. There is generally
more recognition now of the importance of sensitivities and intolerances.

Unfortunately, though, the harm that is commonly caused by food
reactions—including classic allergies, sensitivities, and intolerances—is
still generally underestimated by most clinicians. This can be disastrous
for patients.

It was almost disastrous for little Hugo Frank.

At Hugo's first visit, I determined with ELISA testing that he had IgG
reactions to chocolate and wheat, and IgE reactions to dairy products,
oranges, eggs, soy, cat hair, dog hair, mold, dust, and dust mites. He was
a notably atopic child.

Each of his inhalant and food reactions, by itself, might not have
caused significant damage. Added together, though, they presented a
serious, cumulative threat. Each one added to Hugo's total immune
load, which had become far too heavy for a little child to bear. His immune system should have been focused on killing viruses, bacteria, and
fungi, but instead it was preoccupied with eliminating harmless things
like molecules of cat hair and oranges.

Hugo's immune system appeared to be dangerously skewed toward
Th-2 dominance. He needed to rebalance it, so that his Th-1 cells could
handle his infections, while his Th-2 cells decreased their activity, and
decreased his body's attack on harmless allergenic substances.

If he didn't achieve that rebalancing, it was possible that future bouts with pneumonia might be even worse. If that happened, it could be fatal. Pneumonia is the fifth-leading cause of death in the United States. It kills about 100,000 Americans every year, many of them very young, or elderly. It kills about 3.5 million children worldwide every year.

To help Hugo, I put him on the following Healing Program.

Hugo's Healing Program

• **Antifungal medication.** Drugs such as nystatin could help eliminate the candida overgrowth in Hugo's gut, which was exacerbating his allergies and contributing to the heavy load that was dragging down his immune system. The candida overgrowth had almost certainly been promoted by the many antibiotics he'd taken, and, unfortunately, he would probably need to keep taking them, on occasion. Therefore, he needed something to counteract the antibiotics' side effects.

• **Probiotic supplements.** Along with antifungal drugs, probiotics would help stop his yeast overgrowth, and overcome the yeast-proliferating side effects of the antibiotics. It would also promote Th-1 immunity, thus helping to balance his Th-2 skewed immune system.

• **Restriction of reactive foods.** He needed to completely avoid chocolate, eggs, soy, oranges, dairy, and wheat. These reactive foods were the root cause of his congestion, and his congestion was the root cause of his opportunistic infections.

• **Environmental controls.** He needed protection from the inhalant allergens in his immediate environment. This meant using a mattress cover and an air purifier, and getting rid of his stuffed animals. The inhalants were magnifying the damage done by Hugo's food reactions.

• **Supplementation.** He needed a good pediatric multivitamin with some extra vitamin C. This would help give his immune system the boost it needed.

Obviously, there was nothing very exotic about Hugo's treatment program. Once again, the emphasis was simply on (1) reducing the on-going insults against the body, (2) killing existing pathogens, and (3) providing optimal nutritional support. This would enable the innate wisdom of his body to rebalance his metabolism and his immune system. When these simple, fundamental elements are addressed, healing is often fast and dramatic.

Even just the act of restricting allergens, by itself, often works wonders. For example, consider the following three cases. In each of them, the mere restriction of a few troublesome foods was pivotal in overcoming disorders that could have destroyed these kids' lives.

John Peters, October 2005

When John first visited my office, at age two, he'd been diagnosed as being on the borderline of the autism spectrum. He suffered from delayed speech, poor social skills, and obsessive-compulsive behavior, with stimming. He was put on the gluten-free, casein-free diet, with concurrent restriction of soy. Almost immediately, he went into a state of severe withdrawal. His mother reported that his behavior became "bizarre." She said he acted "totally autistic, and had no eye contact." This lasted for forty-eight hours. However, just two weeks later, he began speaking coherently for the first time in his life. He also showed further behavioral and cognitive improvement from methyl-B-12, DMG, vitamin A, GLA, and Co-Q-10. Within less than a year, his mother noted that he was "doing great, with notable neurodevelopmental bursts." With additional dietary modification, he continued to develop even further. As a preschooler, he became very social, learned his ABCs, learned a number of songs, and continued to progress.

Patrick McCauliffe, May 2000

Patrick had a diagnosis of Asperger's when I met him, at age four and a half. He had poor language and social skills, was very withdrawn, was uncoordinated, was spacey and hyper, had poor eye contact, tended to blurt out profanities, was too thin, and exhibited obsessive-compulsive behaviors, such as singing numbers repeatedly. He was often sick, and had chronic rhinitis that was worse in fall and winter. ELISA testing revealed that Patrick had IgE allergies to mold and milk. He was also sensitive to the feathers in his pillow. He was low in magnesium and vitamin A. He went on the gluten-free, casein-free diet, and also on an anti-candida diet, and an anti-hypoglycemia diet. He took cod liver oil, probiotics, and some antioxidants. His improvement was fast and profound. In three months, his behavior was much better, and his OCD symptoms had decreased considerably. One year after his first appointment, Patrick's father reported that Patrick was "doing absolutely great." He was reading far above his age level, was funny and happy, and was socially adept. Four years after the first appointment, he was doing excellent academic work and was a very popular child, with no symptoms of any autism-spectrum disorders.

Christopher Bronson, September 2003

Christopher had been diagnosed as PDD-NOS at age two. He had suffered an autistic regression as a toddler, which had resulted in the loss of his acquired language, as well as in poor eye contact, hyperactivity, and poor social skills. He'd had nine ear infections between six and eighteen months, and suffered from chronic diarrhea. At his first visit, during which he could not hold a conversation, he tested positive for allergies to eggs, milk, peanuts, cat hair, and trees. His parents reported that his developmental symptoms were worse every spring, when the trees bloomed. He had low zinc, low vitamin A, low plasma cysteine, and low glutathione. Because he was very allergic to cat hair, I had to recommend that they find another home for their cat. When the cat was gone, and when Christopher began to avoid his allergenic foods, his neurological problems improved suddenly and dramatically. In less than three months, he had much better interactive language, improved eye contact, smoother coordination, and less bowel dysbiosis. Within one year of his first appointment, he was fully conversant, and had suddenly become very popular at school. Within two years, he had overcome his tree and egg allergies, and no longer regressed behaviorally in the spring, when the trees bloomed. He was no longer getting sick, was doing extremely well academically, and loved to ski and swim. The last time I saw him, three years after his initial visit, he told me that he'd recently read a book to his brother's class at school. He said that during the presentation, "I was stylin'."

Those are typical responses to the relatively simple action of restricting reactive foods and inhalants.

Of course, not every child achieves a full recovery. That's something I tell every parent. In this world, there are no guarantees of a happy ending. We live in the shifting sands of an uncertain time, surrounded by poisons that are new to the earth, and by toxins that are sometimes included in our medicines.

We are all vulnerable, and all fallible, with mortality our only certainty, and our love for our children, too often, the only shield against their suffering.

But that love can be so strong! Consider Ron and his wife Adah, and their love for Hugo. I sent them home, as I do most parents, with a dozen directives, but no foolproof way to enforce them. Hugo's success would depend almost completely on the degree of their devotion and daily care.

Just to get started, they had to wean Hugo away from his favorite foods, including soy milk and chocolate. The reason they were his favorites was because kids invariably crave the foods to which they're most allergic.

Even taking away Hugo's stuffed animals would be tough. Kids love their teddy bears. It's even harder for kids when I have to tell their parents that they need to give away their cats or dogs. When those moments happen, only the love of moms and dads can fill the void, and nurse the hurt.

They stuck it out, though, and within three weeks Hugo was vastly better. Most of his congestion had cleared, and the bacteria that had been festering in that congestion was mostly dead. His cough calmed down, and at last he could get a full night's sleep. His immunity was finally beginning to build, rather than wither.

Months passed, with no further colds, flu, or infections.

During this time, I got to know Ron and Adah, my fellow Woodstock residents, and we became friends. It was nice to have the family of a patient living in town, since so many of my kids come from all over the country, and even other countries. I looked forward to watching Hugo grow up.

The Hospital

For years, as my practice grew and I became ever more comfortable in Woodstock, I enjoyed watching Hugo become an extraordinary little kid. Children who've suffered very early in life are sometimes more mature than others, and more compassionate. They've seen more of life than most kids. A lot of the time, they're also stronger emotionally, and even physically. They know how to take a hit, bounce back, and keep playing. Hugo was like that. He became a special child, strong and kind–very well liked in the community–and it was my privilege to be at least a small part of his maturation.

He was exceptionally outgoing, a bundle of energy and cheer, and he and his parents stayed extremely close. When Hugo got a little older, Ron and his wife separated, but Adah stayed in town and they both made sure that Hugo felt secure. Hugo focused most of his energy on athletics, and became such a gifted dancer that he joined a local professional modern dance troupe. It was always exciting to see him perform, or play sports–this healthy, resilient kid who'd once been so frail.

Too often, children don't get the second chance in life that Hugo did, just because people don't realize that something as innocent as an orange or a kitten can make a child sick.

As a physician, I didn't see a lot of Hugo over the next few years, because he hardly ever got sick. I saw him for a sore throat once, a rash once, a headache, and a couple of routine physicals. In 2001, I treated him for amoebic colitis, in conjunction with an infectious disease specialist. Hugo had apparently contracted the disease while whitewater rafting in Costa Rica. From time to time, when I was traveling to conferences, he'd see other local doctors for his minor ailments.

In 2002, when he was ten, he came to me with a more serious problem. A doctor had diagnosed him with mononucleosis, and he was feeling really weak. He had a cough, a fever, swollen glands, a headache, and no energy.

I reviewed Hugo's lab work, and I didn't like how it looked. Maybe the lab reports were indicative of standard mono–but certain details made me uncomfortable. For one thing, there were too many atypical white blood cells. Almost 30 percent of Hugo's lymphocytes were atypical.

I wanted someone else to look at it. I gave the lab work to a pathologist. He also thought it could be mono. But maybe not.

I immediately sent the lab work to a pediatric hematologist.

I waited. I was very worried. There are no guarantees of happy endings. Our love for our children, too often, is their only shield against suffering, and sometimes even that love is not enough.

Hugo had acute leukemia. We needed to get him to the hospital right away.

CHAPTER FIFTEEN

LOVE
AND LOSS

HUGO HAD ACUTE MYELOID LEUKEMIA, ONE OF THE MOST DEADLY forms of childhood cancer.

Ron immediately arranged for him to be treated at the Memorial Sloan-Kettering Cancer Center in New York City. Sloan-Kettering uses a multidisciplinary approach and is generally considered to be among the best treatment centers in the world, particularly for childhood cancers.

All I could do was wait, keep my heart open, and hope.

THE OTHER CHILDHOOD EPIDEMICS

The 4-A epidemics have not occurred in isolation. They are part of a larger picture of increased incidence of illnesses and disorders among America's children. The other health issues that are most closely associated with the 4-A epidemics, and that are most threatening and disruptive, are: (1) childhood cancers, (2) diabetes, (3) obesity, and (4) learning disabilities. For the most part, these problems revolve around the same essential issues as the 4-A disorders: toxicity, nutritional deficiencies, immune dysfunction, metabolic imbalance, and failure to adequately detoxify.

Childhood Cancers

In 2006, the National Institutes of Health reported that America has recently experienced an "abrupt rise" in childhood cancers, which began in the early 1980s. From the early 1980s to the early 1990s, the incidence of cancer in American children under ten years of age rose 37 percent. In more recent years the increase in childhood cancers has continued to climb at approximately this same rate. Over a twenty-year period, ending in 1998, the incidence of all childhood cancers increased from 11.4 cases per 100,000 children, to 15.2 cases per 100,000 children.

The incidence of malignancies in children is rising most quickly among the types of cancer that are generally associated with exposure to toxins. These cancers include leukemia and brain cancer. Approximately one-third of all childhood cancers are now leukemia, and incidence of brain tumors in children rose from 2.3 per 100,000 children to 3 per 100,000 children from 1975 to 1998. Leukemia and brain cancer combined now account for approximately half of all childhood cancers.

Among the toxins most frequently linked to the rising incidence of these cancers are those found in pesticides and industrial chemicals.

Currently, one in every 330 American children gets cancer. Approximately 25 percent of all children who get cancer die from it. Some cancers, including acute myeloid leukemia, have significantly lower survival rates.

Diabetes

Both Type 1 and Type 2 diabetes are increasing in incidence among America's children.

Type I diabetes, the form of the disorder associated with an autoimmune attack upon the pancreas, which secretes insulin, appears to be increasing in children at a rate of approximately 30 percent per decade. About 13,000 American children are now annually diagnosed with the disease, which results in a decreased life expectancy of fifteen years.

The most alarming recent evidence concerning Type 1 diabetes is its apparent link to childhood vaccinations. In one study, conducted in New Zealand, researchers documented a 60 percent increase in Type 1 diabetes in children that began in 1998, when the country began vaccinating children for hepatitis B. A similar study in Finland showed a 64 percent increase in Type 1 diabetes that began when the HIB vaccination was introduced.

Researchers in America have linked the aluminum that is added to vaccinations to the rise in incidence of Type 1 diabetes that has occurred among American children.

Interestingly, supplementation with vitamin D, which is known for its ability to help modulate the immune system, has been shown to decrease incidence of Type 1 diabetes.

Type 2 diabetes in children is increasing even faster than Type 1. Until recently, Type 2 diabetes was very rare in people under thirty, but its incidence began to surge around 1990. Until 1990, only 4 percent of all children with diabetes had Type 2 diabetes, but that percentage has increased five-fold, and is currently 20 percent. In some high-risk groups, such as obese African American children, incidence of Type 2 diabetes is as high as 45 percent.

Obesity is the leading risk factor for Type 2 diabetes, but many researchers now believe that the condition known as insulin resistance is the root cause of both obesity and diabetes. Insulin resistance is characterized by poor ability of the cells to process insulin.

Furthermore, it now appears as if insulin resistance is often triggered by inflammation. Therefore, inflammation is now linked closely to both obesity and diabetes.

Inflammation has also been linked to many forms of cancer, and is intimately associated with autism, ADHD, and asthma.

Another common disorder that has been linked to inflammation is atherosclerosis, or plaque build-up in the arteries. Atherosclerosis is now often present in children, particularly obese children, although it was very rare in previous generations.

Approximately 6 percent of the American population, or 16 million people, now have Type 2 diabetes. It is the seventh leading cause of death in the country, and is one of the most frequent causes of limb amputations, blindness, and kidney disease. This rate of death and disablement seems certain to climb, as America's diabetic children reach adulthood.

Obesity

The obesity epidemic tracks the 4-A epidemics, as well as the diabetes epidemic, and is closely related to them. One link among all of these disorders is the presence of inflammation, which is now regarded as a significant trigger of obesity.

Obesity has doubled among children and adolescents during the past twenty years. Now, an estimated 20 percent of all American children are obese or overweight. Obesity is inextricably linked with Type 2 diabetes and atherosclerosis, and is closely associated with liver disease, orthopedic problems, insulin resistance, depression, hypertension, sleep apnea, and asthma. There is also evidence that obesity is significantly higher among children with ADHD symptoms. Obesity appears to be particularly linked to problems with the D-4 dopamine receptor, the receptor that's most closely associated with ADHD symptoms. It's theorized that problems with this receptor interfere with feelings of satiety, or satisfaction after eating.

Learning Disabilities

Learning disabilities are approximately 55 percent more common now than they were twenty years ago. They are now present in approximately 20 percent of all American children. The most common learning disabilities are dyslexia (language-based disability), dyscalculia (mathematical disability), and auditory and visual processing disorders. These disabilities are much more severe than the common intellectual deficits that many people have in certain areas. They are neurological problems that make various mental pursuits exceedingly difficult, and sometimes almost impossible.

Learning disabilities are closely linked to the symptoms of ADHD. Similarly to ADHD, learning disabilities are now believed by many researchers to often stem from exposure to environmental toxins. Some researchers believe that toxins from pollutant sources, as well as toxins from childhood vaccinations, contribute significantly to learning disabilities. It's been estimated that up to 50 percent of all children with learning disabilities suffer from high levels of heavy metals, including cadmium and lead.

Similarly, reduction of IQ has also been tied to exposure to heavy metals, particularly lead.

Pesticides also can affect intellectual function and the ability to learn. Some children appear to be more vulnerable to damage from pesticides than others, due to insufficient production of the enzymes that are needed to break down two of the most common pesticides, diazinon, and chlorpyritos. One study showed that a subset of children who were enzyme deficient were 50 to 65 times more likely than others to have high levels of these common pesticides in their bloodstreams.

One indicator of the important role that toxins play in learning disabilities is the link between learning disabilities and motor skills. Children with learning disabilities are significantly more likely than others to have problems with coordination and muscle control. The seemingly disparate problems of learning disabilities and poor motor skills have both been closely associated with toxification, particularly with heavy metals. In this regard, children with learning disabilities are similar to those with Asperger's syndrome, who also tend to have impaired motor skills.

There are no easy answers to this wide array of problems that now face our children. If there is a silver lining to this dark cloud, however, it is the recent discovery that so many of these seemingly unrelated problems have similar causative factors. If the causative factors are similar, then it may well be reasonable to assume that the remedial factors will also be similar.

Thus, to oppose the destruction of each of these terrible disorders, it appears prudent to apply similar, comprehensive programs of healing, in conjunction with behavioral programs, and appropriate medical protocols. The fundamental elements of these healing programs are relatively simple: good nutrition; detoxification; reduction of further exposure to toxins; supplementation with concentrated nutrients; exercise; stress management; avoidance of reactive foods and inhalants; and use of appropriate pharmaceutical and natural medications.

The simplicity of these comprehensive programs is their strength. There are many ways to become ill, but there are only a few fundamental paths that lead to healing.

MEMORIAL DAY

As Memorial Day weekend of 2005 approached, Anju felt an almost constant gnawing uneasiness, remembering the Memorial Day weekend of the prior year, when Aniyka had suddenly, for no apparent reason, begun to gasp for breath. The two weeks that Aniyka had spent in the Intensive Care Unit at Loyola Hospital had assaulted whatever small, uncertain sense of security that Anju still had left.

Even so, Anju still had her kids at home to raise, and her kids at the clinic to heal.

For strength, she often meditated and prayed. She used these moments of stillness to connect with the soul of the daughter that she would not see on this earth again. Priya, she believed, had become a messenger. Priya conveyed to her, from a source of greater wisdom, the direction that Anju needed to take, in order to learn from her pain, and to use it to help her heal the children of other mothers.

Aniyka, now a pretty young teen, was animated by less philosophical forces. She did not dwell upon the vagaries of fate, nor the threat of fatal allergies, but instead focused upon the more age-appropriate issues of boys, school, and fun.

But it happened again. On Memorial Day weekend Aniyka ran to Anju and said, "Mom, I feel short of breath."

"Okay, let me give you an inhaler."

It didn't work, they tried again, and again it didn't work. Anju rushed Aniyka to the hospital, but by then Aniyka was fighting so hard for air that they had to take her to Loyola, again.

Why?

WHY WE GET ALLERGIES

We get allergies because of three fundamental factors: (1) nutritional factors, (2) immune factors, and (3) inflammatory factors. Feeding into each of these three general factors is an array of harmful, interwoven forces. For example, the force of yeast overgrowth can stress the immune system, and contribute to immune factors that cause allergies and other food reactions. Similarly, the force of enzyme deficits can contribute to the nutritional factors that cause food reactions.

Even one isolated force can create an allergy. When many forces combine, they can create allergies that are so severe that they can last a lifetime, and even be fatal.

Nutritional Factors

Nutritional deficiencies are a singularly important force that triggers food reactions. These deficiencies are especially common among autistic children, who are notoriously picky eaters, and who frequently have digestive difficulties. The deficiencies often result in food not being properly broken down. When food is not completely broken down, it creates partial proteins and other molecules in the body that the immune system misidentifies as foreign invaders, and attacks with the allergic response. Improper breakdown also creates intolerances.

Probiotics are often deficient in 4-A children, and this can be extremely harmful. Probiotics are vitally important for complete digestion, and help provide important nutrients. They also promote Th-1 cellular immunity, which helps to overcome Th-2 skewing. In addition, they help correct yeast overgrowth in the gut.

Essential fatty acids are also often deficient, contributing to the inflammation that helps trigger allergies, sensitivities, and intolerances. To overcome this deficiency, EFAs should be taken as supplements, and should also be consumed in foods. Similarly, it's important to avoid foods that are pro-inflammatory, such as the *trans*-fatty acids found in margarine and other saturated fats.

Immune-modulating nutrients are also often insufficient. They are another immune-related factor that can influence the immune system's overreaction against allergens. It's important to have sufficient intake of vitamins A, D, and C, along with zinc. Many children with 4-A disorders are low in vitamins A and D, and some are low in vitamin C and zinc.

Intestinal hyperpermeability is also an extremely important nutritional problem. The walls of the intestines often become far too permeable, and allow the absorption of food molecules that have not been fully digested, thus triggering allergy. Many things contribute to intestinal hyperpermeability, but one of the most common contributors is intestinal candidiasis, or yeast overgrowth. Yeast can loosen the adhesion between cells in the gut, and allow partially digested food molecules to escape from the gut and enter the system.

Other important causes of intestinal hyperpermeability are: excessive intake of alcohol; taking too much aspirin or ibuprofen; presence of lingering viruses; bowel dysbiosis; drinking too much coffee with meals; and eating foods that are high in chemical additives.

A deficiency of stomach acid is also a common cause of food reactions. Many people are low in stomach acid, known as hydrochloric acid, and this deficiency tends to worsen with age. Stomach acid is essential for breaking down foods. Oddly enough, one telltale symptom of this insufficiency is heartburn, because when the stomach doesn't have enough hydrochloric acid, it often overreacts by secreting too much, causing discomfort in the esophagus.

Lack of the digestive enzymes that break down food is another common digestive deficiency. The most well known of these enzymes is lactase, which breaks down lactose, or milk sugar. When people don't have enough lactase, they can't adequately digest milk products, and are said to be lactose intolerant. These shortages of enzymes are often genetic. For example, African Americans are significantly more likely than Caucasians to suffer from lactose intolerance. Other common enzyme deficiencies among autistic children include an insufficiency of enzymes that digest carbohydrates and fats, such as isomaltase and lipase.

Refined, processed food contributes to food reactions. When fiber and other natural factors are removed from foods during processing, the foods can then congest the GI system and contribute to constipation, and also to food reactions. Furthermore, refined foods are far more likely than whole foods to contain artificial substances, which may cause adverse reactions.

Poor eating habits are the final nutritional force that can contribute to food reactions. One bad habit is eating too narrow a range of foods. Another is eating too quickly, because this can overwhelm the digestive processes. It's also important to chew foods completely, in order to initiate the digestive process in an effective way. In addition, it's wise to avoid excessive amounts of liquids with meals, because liquids can dilute digestive juices. Furthermore, it helps to avoid stress during mealtime, because the stress response shifts blood away from the organs of digestion, as part of the fight-or-flight reaction, and thus impairs digestion.

Immune Factors

Because all classic allergies are triggered by the immune system, anything that harms the immune system can contribute to allergies.

Immune overload is arguably the most important single force that causes allergies. Picture the immune system as a kettle that can hold only a certain amount of water. If you keep filling it, the kettle will eventually overflow. Similarly, if the immune kettle is filled to the brim with pathogens and foreign material—including viruses, bacteria, fungi, heavy metals, environmental toxins, artificial foods, and inhalant allergens—it will simply be unable to accommodate anything more. When this happens, a mildly innocent food allergen—such as corn or an egg—can give the immune system more than it can handle.

There's always a natural limit to how much the immune system can tolerate, and people often exceed this limit. During pollen season, for example, the immune system might be far less able to tolerate allergenic foods. Therefore, it is very important to reduce the immune load as much as possible, at all times, and especially during the pollen season. The most practical way to do this is by simply avoiding reactive foods and substances. Even avoiding stress can help, because emotional stress depresses the immune system. Stress can also contribute to Th-2 predominance.

Overactivity of Th-2 cells is, by itself, also a primary contributor to allergy. It can even create a cycle of almost perpetual allergy. This occurs when Th-2 skewing promotes immune hyperactivity, which then promotes further Th-2 skewing. This cycle can last indefinitely.

Antibiotic overuse, particularly during infancy, also contributes to Th-2 skewing, as well as to other important forces that promote allergy, sensitivity, and intolerance. Antibiotics, for example, commonly destroy healthy bacteria in the gut, and this can lead to yeast overgrowth. Yeast overgrowth then adds to the immune load, and also contributes to intestinal hyperpermeability.

The damage to the intestines that's done by yeast overgrowth can then extend beyond the gut, and become a factor in inhalant allergies. Many inhalant allergies, in fact, are more rooted in gut problems than in airway problems. This phenomenon was recently proven in an animal experiment, in which mice that had been given antibiotics became substantially more allergic to inhaled mold.

The hygiene hypothesis accounts for another probable cause of allergy. According to this theory, people are actually more vulnerable to allergy and intolerance if they live in very clean, hygienic environments. These ultraclean environments, it is believed, don't challenge the immune system to develop enough natural resistance. Theoretically, when people live in less clean, less hygienic environments, they are more likely to develop more balanced immunity, with more resistance and tolerance, and are less apt to overreact allergically to things like dust, mold, and animal hair.

Childhood vaccinations may also be one element that contributes to allergy, in a way that is similar to the mechanisms of the hygiene hypothesis. The vaccinations that prevent childhood illnesses may actually be making children more vulnerable to allergic disorders, by changing the natural function of their immune systems. Specifically, the vaccinations appear to make kids' immune systems too Th-2 skewed, with a relative deficit of Th-1 activity. For example, when children actually contract a virus, and the virus gets into their cells, they fight the illness primarily with Th-1 cells, which lead the attack on the intracellular viral material. On the other hand, if kids are vaccinated against a virus, and never develop the actual disease, they may never activate a robust Th-1 response against it. When this happens, they may develop too much Th-2 activity, creating too much allergic response.

Also, receiving vaccinations with thimerosal, prior to receiving the measles-mumps-rubella vaccination, can lead to further Th-2 skewing. This skewing can then contribute to an improper immune response to the MMR vaccination. This improper response can result in a chronic, low-grade measles infection. It can also sometimes result in autoimmunity.

Thus, the body gets hit with a double whammy: thimerosal, plus a dysregulated immune response to the MMR. The resulting gut infections and autoimmune problems can then contribute further to food reactions.

The theory that childhood vaccinations can contribute to allergy was demonstrated in a recent study, in which children who had actually contracted measles were found to suffer approximately 50 percent less atopic disease, including food and inhalant allergies, than those who had been vaccinated against measles.

Another similar study, conducted in England, showed even more dramatic results. In this study, children who had been vaccinated were fourteen times more likely than others to be diagnosed with asthma, and 9.4 times more likely to have eczema.

Therefore, vaccinations are now considered by many researchers to be one of the factors that contribute to allergy, by influencing immunity.

Inflammatory Factors

Inflammation contributes to allergies, and allergies contribute to inflammation. This cycle can be self-perpetuating, and go on indefinitely, unless parents, patients, and doctors actively intervene.

Here's how the cycle works: 1. A food or inhalant allergy creates inflammation. 2. This inflammation causes the immune system to become overreactive and hypersensitive. 3. This overreactivity and hypersensitivity then causes the immune system to attack normally harmless substances, such as molecules of milk or pollen. This immune attack is the allergic response. 4. Then allergies create even more inflammation.

Distant inflammation is one root cause of allergy that is often overlooked. For example, many doctors fail to realize that airway allergies are often exacerbated by distant inflammation, in the gut. However, this happens quite often. Therefore, patients can frequently overcome airborne allergies when they resolve their intestinal inflammation.

It's easy for inflammation to affect distant areas of the body. When one part of the body is inflamed, it sends out immune cell messengers, or cytokines, that travel throughout the body. These messengers then trigger inflammation in many different areas of the body, including the joints, the mucus membranes of the airways, the lining of the gastrointestinal tract, and even the brain. Each of these areas then sends out its own inflammatory messengers, creating even more inflammation, in a feed-forward phenomenon. All of this inflammation contributes to allergies. And the allergies, of course, then cause even more inflammation.

One disturbing example of the far reach of inflammation was revealed recently by researchers at Johns Hopkins University Medical Center, who had performed autopsies on the brains of a number of autistic children who had died in accidents. The brains of almost all of these children showed signs of neuroinflammation. Researchers concluded that this inflammation had probably contributed to some of the autistic symptoms of these children.

Widespread inflammation now appears to be a common denominator in virtually all atopic disorders, including eczema, hay fever, and food allergies, and is also a major component of bowel dysbiosis, immune dysfunction, autism, ADHD, and asthma. Inflammation is one of the ties that bind all these problems together.

Therefore, all of the various elements that contribute to inflammation must be recognized, and remedied. These contributors include:

Food. It is often a major contributor to inflammation, specifically if it is high in saturated fat and low in essential fatty acids.

Childhood vaccinations. They can trigger inflammation, by creating subclinical chronic infection, and also by contributing to heavy metal overload.

Stress. It contributes to inflammation by promoting production of pro-inflammatory immune system messengers, such as interleukin-6. These messengers create further inflammation, and this inflammation harms children with autism and ADHD. Unfortunately, when this harm occurs, it makes the children feel even more stressed out, thereby causing even more inflammation, in an endless cycle of destruction.

Infection. This is another common cause of inflammation. Many children who suffer from the 4-A epidemics have persistent infection, particularly in their gastrointestinal systems. These infections can last for years, because so many 4-A kids have impaired immunity.

To intervene in the cycle of inflammation-disorder-inflammation, parents and doctors must remove as many of the sources of inflammation as possible, and must also counteract existing inflammation.

Nutrients are among the very best treatments for inflammation. The most powerful nutritional anti-inflammatories are:

Anti-Inflammatory Nutrients

• **EFAs,** including omega-3 (such as EPA and DHA) and GLA (such as borage oil, black currant seed oil, or evening primrose oil).

• **Quercitin,** which is a natural antihistamine, and an anti-inflammatory plant chemical.

• **Pycnogenol,** which many people take in relatively high doses for allergy symptoms, due to its anti-inflammatory and anti-allergic properties.

• **Curcumin,** the active ingredient in the spice turmeric, which has powerful anti-inflammatory effects.

• **Transfer factor,** which helps modulate immunity (by promoting Th-1 activity). This helps stop inflammatory immune overreaction, particularly when it is related to Th-2 skewing.

• **Zinc,** another immune modulator, which enhances cellular immunity.

• **Vitamin E,** an antioxidant that helps prevent oxidation of the EFAs.

• **Vitamin A,** an antioxidant that is typically low in children with the 4-A disorders.

In addition, some pharmaceutical drugs can decrease inflammation, including the medication Actos, a drug that improves insulin sensitivity. Actos is most commonly used for diabetes and metabolic syndrome, but appears to soothe inflammation. Extensive research is now being done to look into its far-reaching anti-inflammatory effects in the treatment of colitis, psoriasis, and neurological disorders. Another medication that appears to be promising in the treatment of autism is Namenda, which is FDA approved for the treatment of Alzheimer's disease. Although Namenda does not decrease inflammation directly, it may be helpful by acting upon the glutamate receptors on the cells to block the activity of glutamate, an excitatory amino acid that may act synergistically with inflammatory mediators. Additionally, Spironolactone, a generic potassium-sparing diuretic, has been shown to have anti-inflammatory properties and is currently being researched in the treatment of autism spectrum disorders.

For some time, physicians believed that the popular Cox-2 inhibitors, which are used for rheumatoid inflammation, would help with neuroinflammation. However, they have not proven to be particularly effective. They appear to be more active peripherally than in the brain.

Ultimately, as always, there is no single medication, supplement, food, or lifestyle alteration that can fully halt the force of inflammation. A comprehensive anti-inflammatory strategy, applied as part of a larger restorative program, is the only viable solution.

The same principle governs the entire scope of therapy for allergies. Patients should employ a broad program, which addresses: (1) the nutritional factors; (2) the immune factors; and (3) the inflammatory factors.

Programs *must* be comprehensive, since the destructive forces arrayed against our children are so massive, complex, and deeply embedded within the structure of our modern industrial society.

Sometimes, however, the forces are just too strong. Some children work hard but just don't succeed.

Those who do, however, are usually very heroic young people. I admire them very much. They inspire me, one at a time, day after day, to keep struggling against the new childhood epidemics.

At night sometimes, after seemingly endless days of work, as I drift toward sleep, I can see the faces of these children. These are the kind of kids that you just can't forget.

My Kids

Do you remember Paul Avram? Poopy Pauly? When I first told you about Paul, he was still in diapers, still unable to utter a word, chained in loneliness. It seemed almost certain that his life would always be like this, until the day he died. But after two years of struggle, Paul Avram was able to tell his mother, "When you're lonely, it means you love someone. I love you, and you will always be right here, in my heart. And you love me, and I will always be in yours."

Do you remember when Kyle Olson punched his nanny in the face, and was so proud that he'd finally learned to communicate properly? He bashed kids over their heads with a broom handle to try to make friends. All that he ever felt was "the snarling dog feeling." He couldn't hold a crayon or even walk across the room without stumbling. He ended up reading all the Harry Potter books, reading C. S. Lewis, going swimming with his buddies, and playing golf with his father, who had given up the glory of pro golf for the greater glory of helping to heal his son. "Dad," Kyle said, "I was born to play golf."

Remember Alisa screaming on the airplane, as her parents heard whispers of "spoiled brat" and "crazy"? Remember the time she tore apart her entire room? "I'm just a bad person," she told her mother. I'll always think of her skating at Rockefeller Center.

I remember Matthew Smith, who didn't make it. I think of his parents.

I remember Teia O'Connor, whose mother refused to lose her to Ritalin. Teia's "goopy feeling" dulled her eyes and made her feel half-dead. She was sure she was doomed to a life of special-ed, lethargy, and feeling like a failure, before we finally figured out that her problems had nothing at all to do with the symptoms of classic ADHD. I can still see Teia's diamond-bright eyes shining, the time she told me what to say to children who were frightened: "Just tell them their *mommies* will take care of them."

And the million-dollar smile of the Million Dollar Kid—who could forget that? That's the kind of smile you can see in your sleep, the kind that brings light to your dreams.

Who could forget the day that the doctors told Loukas Renieres' mom, as he was wasting into a skeleton with severe allergy, that the best possible treatment for him was more ice cream? Loukas was spindly and whimpering the first time we met. But now when I think of him, I see him in his bright white tae kwon do uniform, ready to take on the world.

And I can still see, and I will always see, the beautiful face of Priya, on the first day I met her, as she looked up at her mother with that open-eyed gaze that reflects the purest, most whole love that any of us will ever find in this life.

And I will always remember something that Anju once told me. It was not long ago, at a DAN conference, after an exhausting day of lectures, science, and learning.

"The parents of my kids at the clinic," she said, "they're desperate. And they're willing to do anything to help the children they love. So they start on this long journey of healing. And when you start on that journey, miracles happen.

"But the greatest miracle of all is the love that you start out with."

Memorial Day, 2006

Aniyka, finally healthier now, still on an aggressive, proactive program of healing, spent the day playing. Having fun. Remembering.

Hugo Frank, his cancer in remission for several years, spent the day with his father, Ron.

For Aniyka and Hugo, the struggle to be well, and the struggle to rise beyond the pain of the past, goes on. Their lives go on.

And the love of their families, made eternal by each new generation, undefeated by epidemic, and even by death, heads toward the horizon of time.

PART THREE

THE HEALING PROGRAM

CHAPTER SIXTEEN

THE HEALING PROGRAM
How to Begin

WELCOME TO THE HEALING PROGRAM

THE HEALING PROGRAM IS A COMPREHENSIVE COMBINATION OF four elements:

1. **Nutritional therapy:** changing the diet to optimize physical and neurological health, and rebalance the metabolism.

2. **Supplementation therapy:** using nutritional supplements to maximize the benefits of dietary changes, to compensate for nutrient deficiencies and nutrient dependencies, and to support the immune system, gastrointestinal system, and nervous system.

3. **Detoxification:** eliminating toxic materials from the body, to stop the biochemical assault upon the nervous system, immune system, and gastrointestinal system, and thereby help to restore proper function of these systems.

4. **Medication:** using appropriate pharmacologic and natural medications to eliminate pathogens, to enhance neurological function, to support the immune system, and to help control various physical dysfunctions, such as bowel dysbiosis.

Three Important Principles

As you begin to apply the Healing Program to your child, you must follow three important principles. They are:

Healing Principle 1: The four elements of this program are synergistic. They are dependent upon one another to achieve optimal results.

Nothing is more important than engaging in all four aspects of the program simultaneously, after each is added in an appropriate sequence. Avoiding participation in even one of the four aspects can severely diminish the power of the program. Therefore, do not be lulled into complacency if just one aspects seems to be providing positive results. This is not a good reason to ignore the other aspects. It is, in fact, a good reason to embrace the other aspects, because each will amplify the effects of the others. In some cases, though, pharmacologic medications will not be needed.

Healing Principle 2: This is a lifelong plan for optimizing health. It is not intended to be a temporary, symptom-suppressing, stopgap measure. It is intended to be a permanent, ongoing set of improvements in basic habits and lifestyle.

Many of the disorders and conditions that cause the symptoms of the 4-A disorders are chronic and intractable, and will remain indefinitely. Improvements in metabolic function and general health do occur, but even then, underlying weaknesses may remain. For example, IgE allergies tend to remain throughout life, regardless of treatment. Therefore, to lock in recovery, your child will probably also need to lock in some permanent changes.

Healing Principle 3: The Healing Program is highly individualized. It is not a cookie-cutter, one-size-fits-all therapy. Treatment modalities, from each of the four basic aspects of the program, can vary a great deal from one child to the next. For example, your child's diet may include the anti-yeast diet, or it may not, simply because some kids need treatment for yeast overgrowth, and some do not. Similarly, some children may have harmful levels of heavy metals in their systems, and some may not.

BEGINNING THE HEALING PROGRAM: LABORATORY TESTING PROCEDURES

To begin, you must start by testing your child, to see what treatments are necessary, and what treatments might prove to be most effective. Throughout the next four chapters on the Healing Program, you will find information about treatments that can help your own child, and you'll also find information about treatments that are probably not necessary for your child. To determine which treatments can help your own child, you will need to do some initial testing, and also some ongoing testing, to monitor positive effects, as well as adverse effects.

Some of this testing will involve trying various therapies, to see if they help. For example, I recommend that almost all of my patients try the gluten-free, casein-free diet, because I have found it to be helpful for the majority of the children I treat. However, it doesn't help everyone, and the only way to know if it will help is to try it.

The other type of testing you will probably need to do is laboratory testing. Lab testing does have its limitations. For example, there is no absolutely reliable laboratory test to determine the possible need for the gluten-free, casein-free diet. Testing for gluten and casein sensitivity can be helpful, but that test does not reveal every element of gluten and casein sensitivity, such as the presence of the abnormal partial proteins that gluten and casein can create. Therefore, that diet is just something you'll have to experiment with, to determine its value for your own child. Nonetheless, there are many lab tests that provide extremely important clues about function and dysfunction, and about the body's strengths and weaknesses. As a medical detective, I rely very much on these tests. They not only indicate the need for various therapies, but they also monitor the effectiveness of the therapies that are used. As a parental detective, you'll need to learn about the tests that will help your child begin to recover.

Laboratory Testing for the Healing Program

You will probably need to do a number of lab tests to begin the Healing Program. In all cases, it is far better to do these tests than to proceed without them. Nonetheless, some families just can't afford to do a significant number of them, or even any of them. This is definitely a problem, but it is not always insurmountable. Children can be helped without always knowing the specifics of their conditions and metabolisms. This is always more difficult, though. It requires more trial and error, and a closer observation by parents of the child's reactions to various healing modalities.

It is always best to do as many of the appropriate tests for your child as you can reasonably afford. Money, however, is a very practical consideration, and parents should never feel guilty or be discouraged about not being able to do everything they wish they could. As a parent, you should do what you can do, without fixating upon what you cannot do.

If you do this, you may be surprised at how much progress you can achieve by relying mostly on just common sense, mother's intuition, careful observation, and perseverance.

Finding a Doctor

To perform the tests, you will need the assistance of a physician.

The best possible choice would be a physician associated with Defeat Autism Now, because these are the doctors who have expertise in the biomedical treatment of the 4-A disorders. Many of them are brilliant clinicians who will someday probably be remembered as the pioneers of an important medical movement. To reach these doctors, contact DAN (see Appendix 2). One of these physicians may live near you, and be able to accept new patients, or to at least place you on a waiting list. Like most CAIM organizations developing professional support for these emerging therapies, credentialing standards are currently under development. As a result, pursuing a DAN physician is a good beginning, but I cannot guarantee the approaches used by the physicians they list, and you should use your own good judgment when considering a new physician.

Another good alternative would be to contact the other physician group noted in Appendix 2, the American College for the Advancement of Medicine. This group, one of the largest organizations of physicians who practice integrative medicine, offers a doctor referral service on the Internet. Most of its doctors will be very familiar with the various tests that I recommend, and some of them will be familiar with the biomedical treatment of the 4-A disorders. I have long been a member of this organization, and was president of it in 2006.

You should not try to arrange for and evaluate these tests on your own, without a doctor's guidance. The tests can be difficult to interpret, and may occasionally suggest contradictory courses of action, which your doctor must evaluate.

When you do find a doctor, you should be aware that various doctors have differing levels of expertise, and perhaps differences of opinion, in the often baffling areas of the 4-A disorders. It is difficult to stay abreast of all of the emerging research, and some doctors are simply better informed than others. It may be wise to consult with more than one doctor, before you decide upon one with whom you wish to work.

It may be necessary for you to travel, in order to consult with the doctor you choose. Most of my own patients, in fact, must travel to meet with me. This can be difficult, but don't let it discourage you. It is quite possible that you will need to meet with your doctor only periodically once your child has become an established patient.

As a rule, it is inadvisable to rely upon the administration of the Healing Program by a doctor who is not well versed in integrative medicine. This, unfortunately, probably includes a great many of the doctors in your area, whom you may now trust and like. It might well include your own family doctor or pediatrician. If so, these are probably not the best people to administer the Healing Program. I mean absolutely no disrespect to these physicians, and to their training, because it's quite possible to be an excellent doctor without being well versed in all of the many aspects of medicine, particularly the emerging areas discussed in this book. In fact, the entire system of medical specialization rests upon the premise that focusing on specific areas of expertise can have great value. Therefore, I believe it's wise to work with a doctor who has expertise and experience in integrative medicine. The Healing Program is a highly integrated therapeutic system, and requires the stewardship of a doctor who is familiar with, and accepts the value of, its various intricacies.

Furthermore, some physicians who don't really understand integrative medicine can be dismissive of important factors, such as dietary change or detoxification, and they may even be hostile about their implementation. Consulting with this type of doctor could be extremely discouraging for you. After all, this will probably be a person who has a great deal of expertise in his or her own medical approach, and he or she will undoubtedly be very articulate and persuasive—even when he or she is misinformed.

However, even if your child's current pediatrician or family practitioner is not familiar with integrative medicine, it can still be very helpful to include them in your child's therapy, in consultation with a physician who is familiar with integrative medicine. If you and your child already trust and like your current doctor, it is important to retain them as part of your team.

Although I work mostly with M.D.'s, I also generally respect the integrative medical expertise of naturopathic physicians. Most N.D.'s are very familiar with nutritional therapy, detoxification, and the application of supplementation therapy. One drawback is that they are not generally licensed to prescribe pharmaceutical medications.

Taking This Book to Your Doctor

It may be of some value to bring this book with you to your first appointment with your doctor.

He or she may be familiar with the book, if he or she is a DAN doctor, or an integrative physician who stays abreast of the latest trends in the treatment of autism, ADHD, allergies, and asthma. If so, your doctor might wish to use some of the material in this book as a resource guide for your child's program of healing. Various elements of the book, such as the chapters on nutrition and supplementation, are quite thorough, and your doctor may choose to use some of this material to augment his or her own written materials, patient guidelines, and handouts.

Of course, this book is not intended to replace your own doctor's advice or treatment, but to add to your knowledge about the biomedical approach.

Furthermore, the book might be of value as an entry point into various discussions about treatment options. Most doctors appreciate it when their patients are well prepared for their visits, and the book can be used not only for your own preparation, but also as a communications aid in your presentation of your thoughts and concerns. For example, if you have prepared for the doctor's visit by learning about various supplements, you might use some of the lists of supplements in the book, as you converse with your doctor, to refresh your memory about what you have learned.

If you do choose to do this, please be sensitive about your doctor's own position as the manager of your child's treatment program. Your own doctor has the best vantage point from which to direct your child's healing, and encroachment upon your doctor's guidance could create tension in your relationship. In other words, don't say, "The book says to do this," or "The book says to do that." Patients, parents, and doctors must all be partners in healing, and grant one another the deserved and proper respect.

This conveyance of respect may be even more important if your physician is not a DAN doctor, or another type of integrative physician. If your doctor is a notably conventional physician, he or she may be unfamiliar with some of the protocols in this book, and may even be skeptical about the efficacy of some of them. Many doctors, for example, are not convinced of the value of nutritional therapy. If this is the case, it is important to be particularly polite and receptive, because discord and confrontation generally tend to create only more discord and confrontation. This is not the atmosphere that your child needs in order to heal.

If your doctor is unfamiliar with some of the protocols in this book, you may wish to share some of what you have learned. This book was written for people who are not medical professionals, but the technical information in it will stand up to scientific scrutiny. Your doctor may be particularly interested in the book's bibliography, because all of the scientific material in this book has been derived from research that was reported in respected and well-known medical journals.

Another thing that's very important is to not imply to your doctor that you fully expect him or her to heal your child, insofar as this book contains reports about many children who have been healed. In fact, not all children can be healed. Some, sadly, don't even improve very much, no matter how hard everyone works. This is simply reality. Don't burden your doctor, and compromise your relationship with him or her, by imposing unrealistic expectations. Hope is a great thing—it is a vital element in the long, difficult healing process—but expectation is the enemy of satisfaction, and therefore an obstacle to the many incremental gains that must be made, and celebrated, in order to finally achieve recovery. If you keep your hopes high and your expectations low, you will be better able to travel this journey of a thousand steps, which may one day take you to a destination that now lies even beyond your hopes.

This is most likely to occur, though, in a spirit of partnership.

Of this I am certain: Your doctor wants to help you—and your doctor wants your help.

Now is the time to build a team. When you do this, your feeling of aloneness—which is often overwhelming in the parent of a sick child—will begin to lift.

IT BEGINS WITH TESTING

To start this process, you and your doctor will begin with testing. These tests will determine the direction that your journey of healing will take.

In my own practice, I recommend four essential tiers of testing, moving from the most basic tests to the more uncommon tests. Of course, without obtaining a detailed history and performing a comprehensive physical examination, I cannot recommend which tests you should pursue for your child. That is a decision for you and your doctor to make. I can tell you, however, which ones I generally tend to recommend, after meeting with patients. These tests are as follows:

Tier One Testing

These tests consist essentially of basic body chemistry profiles. They are the common tests that almost all doctors routinely perform. These tests offer clues to frank pathologies. They also help to establish a baseline level of body chemistries, so that you can monitor your child as treatment progresses.

They include:

- Complete blood count.
- Basic urinalysis.
- Basic blood chemistry.
  - Liver function.
  - Kidney function.
  - Electrolytes (including CO_2 levels).
  - Calcium levels.
  - Magnesium levels.
  - Blood sugar.
- Lipids.
  - Cholesterol.
  - Triglycerides.
- Thyroid function (including T_3, T_4, and TSH).

As you can see, even these very basic tests can be confusing to people outside the medical profession. Therefore, it is absolutely essential that you consult with a doctor.

The Healing Program is, for the most part, administered at home, under the direct supervision of parents, working in partnership with their doctors. The Healing Program is not a do-it-yourself treatment plan. The conditions it addresses are complex, stubborn, and dangerous, and they demand the attention of a skilled, experienced physician.

Tier Two Testing

These include nutritional and metabolic tests that I generally recommend to almost all patients. These tests reveal the presence of the nutritional deficiencies and excesses that are often the root causes of serious problems. They also reveal metabolic dysfunctions that can cause troubling symptoms.

Unlike the Tier One Tests, these tests are not always routinely performed or ordered by most conventional physicians. These tests often require the evaluation of a doctor who is experienced in nutrition, and in the other aspects of integrative medicine.

These Tier Two Tests are frequently performed during the first office visit, but they also may be ordered at subsequent visits.

The tests include checking the following:

- Minerals.
  - Red blood cell minerals, or whole blood minerals.
  - Plasma zinc.
  - Serum copper.
- Urine organic acids.
- Plasma amino acids.
- Essential fatty acids.
- Fat-soluble vitamins.
- Reduced glutathione.
- Lipid peroxides.
- Plasma cysteine.
- Plasma sulfate.
- Comprehensive digestive stool analysis (or CDSA).

In addition, as part of the Tier Two Testing, I almost always order:

- Food allergy and sensitivity testing (for IgE and IgG reactions). This is usually done by blood testing, but IgE reactions can also be determined by skin testing.

Tier Three Testing

These are tests for more individualized problems. Therefore, many of them may not be necessary for your child. Your physician can help you to determine which ones are necessary. You will also be guided by your child's own unique signs and symptoms, such as chronic bowel problems, chronic infections, recurrent tics, or obsessive-compulsive behaviors.

These tests include the following:

- Immune testing panels, which evaluate the following:
  - IgA levels.
  - IgM levels.
  - IgG levels.

- IgG subclass levels.
- Lymphocyte subsets.
- Natural killer cell activity.
- Vaccine titers.
- Viral titers.
- Thyroid antibodies.
- Anti-myelin basic protein (MBP) antibodies.
- PANDAS profile.
  - ASO titer.
  - Anti-DNAse B titer.

Tier Four Testing

These tests, like those in Tier Three, may be done as treatment progresses. Not all patients will require these tests. However, most patients will receive challenge testing for heavy metals. The tests consist of:

- Provoked urine testing for heavy metals.
- Urinary porphyrins.
- Genetic polymorphisms.

As I've indicated, I never begin a program by dictating to parents the tests that I insist they do. Instead, I sit down with them in a spirit of partnership, and usually ask them two specific questions, at the very beginning of our quest for healing. I ask them, "What would you like to see me do?" and, "What is your understanding of what I may do?" Their answers to these questions help guide me toward the creation of their child's individualized program. During this initial meeting, I begin what I sometimes refer to as the dance of medicine, in which the patient, the family, and the doctor all begin to move together, in harmony. We all determine, together, the goals that are the most desirable, the most necessary, the most achievable, the most practical, the most helpful to the family as a whole, and the most affordable to the family. Sometimes our mutual goals are grand, and sometimes they're modest. Sometimes the goals are very incremental—we start small, then move on to greater goals as the healing takes traction.

All goals are good.

Ultimately, though, the Healing Program is less about achieving far-reaching, future goals than it is about doing the best that you can for your child each day, every day, and celebrating every victory, no matter its size.

The Healing Program can take years to fully unfold. It is a journey, even more than a destination, and as my friend Anju Usman has said, it's a journey of love. Your participation in this program is a reflection of your love, and the possible healing of your child will be a reward for this love. In the final analysis, however, love is its own reward.

BEGINNING THE PROGRAM

We begin by performing the various first-tier laboratory tests.

Then, guided by these tests, we move immediately to the first element of the program, nutritional therapy. Changes in diet usually come before anything else. They can create astonishing improvements. (However, since it is difficult for some parents to make changes in their child's diet, we sometimes start with supplements, as the parents ready themselves for the necessary dietary changes.)

Then we generally move to supplementation therapy. This often supercharges the improvements created by nutritional therapy. It can also trigger tremendous improvements by itself.

Shortly after the introduction of supplements, we proceed to detoxification. For many children, this adds an even greater boost to recovery. Sometimes recovery is slow until detoxification begins. However, the process of detoxification needs to be implemented carefully and safely, to minimize any possible adverse effects, such as uncomfortable healing reactions.

The medication element of the program can be used throughout the program, according to the child's specific needs. Early in the program, medication can help control troubling symptoms, such as extreme behaviors, while the other elements provide deeper, more fundamental healing. It can also be added later in the program, after the other elements are in place, to provide a powerful stimulus that can carry your child to the final level of healing.

All four elements, working together, have remarkable clinical power, and can change your child's life. This has happened in my practice, with my patients, many, many times.

Now it's your turn.

CHAPTER SEVENTEEN

THE HEALING PROGRAM

Element #1:
Nutritional Therapy

STARTING YOUR CHILD'S NEW DIET

VIRTUALLY ALL CHILDREN ON THE HEALING PROGRAM MUST MAKE significant changes in their diets. Dietary factors invariably play a major role in the onset of symptoms of the 4-A disorders, and alteration of diet can play a primary role in healing.

There is no single, one-size-fits-all diet in the Healing Program. The diet must be carefully individualized. There are six basic dietary plans that comprise nutritional therapy in the Healing Program, and you should evaluate each of them to determine if they are appropriate for your child.

It may be possible that just one of these six basic diets will be sufficient to help heal your child. However, it is far more likely that you will need to combine two or more of the diets.

The six diets are:

The Six Essential Healing Program Diets
1. The Gluten-Free, Casein-Free Diet, or GF/CF Diet.
2. The Specific Food Reaction Diet.
3. The Anti-Yeast Diet.
4. The Anti-Hypoglycemia Diet.
5. The Specific Carbohydrate Diet.
6. The Low-Oxalate Diet.

You probably became familiar with most of these dietary plans earlier in this book, and now recognize the remarkable healing effects that they can trigger. If you are familiar with most of these approaches, you probably also realize that they all fit together quite effectively, and are not mutually exclusive of one another. For example, you may have noted that many of my young patients have gone on a diet that was a combination of the gluten-free, casein-free diet, plus the anti-yeast diet, plus the anti-hypoglycemia diet. Often, healing depends upon combining these diets. After all, this is a comprehensive program, based on the belief that isolated therapies are not as effective as combined therapies.

Furthermore, most 4-A kids have combinations of diet-related problems. They may have food reactions to gluten and casein, plus various allergies to specific foods, plus yeast overgrowth, plus hypoglycemia. You simply can't overcome these combined problems with just one diet. It requires a combination of associated diets.

The first four of these diets address four extremely common problems, but the last two address less common problems. It is very possible, therefore, that your child will need to go on a combination of the first four diets, but not the last two. The last two—the specific carbohydrate diet, and the low oxalate diet—are generally applied only when kids don't respond adequately to the first four diets.

As a rule, the various diets are implemented one at a time, beginning with the gluten-free, casein-free diet; followed by the specific food reaction diet; followed by the anti-yeast diet; and then the anti-hypoglycemia diet. Implementing the diets in this sequence has three basic advantages: (1) It helps indicate which diets are helping, and which are not; (2) it's easier for kids, and for parents; and (3) it can moderate the speed of healing, and thus minimize the uncomfortable healing reactions that are often a part of recovery.

Sometimes, though, two of the diets can begin at the same time. For example, if yeast is a big problem, I often address it at the outset; at the same time, I implement the GF/CF diet.

There is no one, single approach for all children.

I know that dietary change can be intimidating, to both kids and to parents. Many 4-A kids are notoriously picky eaters. Their resistance to eating more than just a few favorite foods decreases significantly, however, as they overcome allergic addictions, yeast overgrowth, and hypoglycemia.

When this occurs, cravings subside considerably. For example, kids tend to love macaroni and cheese, and autistic kids are sometimes really hooked on it, as if it were the best tasting food in the world. But this desire for mac-and-cheese is driven at least as much by the food's biochemical effects as by its intrinsic tastiness. Mac-and-cheese provides a double-hit of gluten and casein, and not only satisfies allergic cravings, but also dampens the discomfort that many kids begin to feel when it's been several hours since their last serving of gluten and casein. These cravings, and the need for relief from discomfort, subside dramatically once gluten and casein are eliminated from the system. When the cravings subside, most kids start to perceive mac-and-cheese in much the same way that adults do—as just another side dish.

The same goes for sweets. Almost all kids like sweets, but only hypoglycemic kids go crazy for them. Once your kids overcome their hypoglycemic tendencies, their cravings will recede, and they won't be driven nearly so much by their sweet tooth.

Therefore, it's important for parents to be patient, consistent, and firm. Learn to trust the wisdom of your kids' bodies. As their metabolisms become stable, that wisdom will shine through much more brightly.

Another important element in nutritional therapy is the use of organic foods, whenever possible. Many children with 4-A disorders are already burdened by heavy metals and other toxicants, and the pesticides and herbicides in inorganic foods can add to the total toxic burden of these children. Many of these children have difficulty with detoxification, and can be affected more strongly by food toxins than most other children.

Furthermore, many inorganic foods, such as inorganic meat or milk, also have other components that can be harmful to children with delicate systems. These components include hormones, antibiotics, and various toxins, such as the arsenic that is sometimes present in inorganic chicken.

Another reason to buy organic food is that it often contains higher levels of nutrients than food that is derived from the mass-production agribusiness system.

Organic foods often cost more, but for most kids the expense is a worthwhile investment in recovery, if it's financially feasible for the family.

In the remainder of this chapter, let's examine the six diets, one at a time.

Don't be overwhelmed by the amount of information. It's mostly all just good common sense. For the most part, it's the same basic advice your own mom probably gave you: Eat your fruits and vegetables, go easy on the sweets, keep the junk food to a minimum, eat enough protein, and if a certain food doesn't seem to agree with you, don't eat it. In a very real sense, that advice covers all six of these diets. As I've often said, *Moms know.*

THE TWO FOOD REACTION DIETS

You should start your child's new diet by removing the foods that don't agree with him or her. By this, I mean the foods that cause food reactions: allergies, sensitivities, and intolerances. These problems are enormous contributors to the 4-A disorders.

Two diets accomplish this:

• **The gluten-free, casein-free diet,** which removes the two most commonly reactive foods, gluten and casein.

• **The specific food reaction diet,** which removes the particular foods to which your own child is uniquely reactive.

I generally first start patients on the gluten-free, casein-free, or GF/CF diet. It's a great way to begin.

However, if there are glaring food reactions that a patient's mother already knows about, I almost always continue those restrictions at the same time that I start the GF/CF diet.

Together, these two powerful diets can generally eradicate the many symptoms of food reactions. This can set your child on a course toward healing.

Signs and Symptoms of Food Reactions

Food reactions include:

• **IgE allergies,** the most severe, but least common, type of food reaction.

• **IgG sensitivities,** which are much more common than classic allergies, but usually less severe.

• **Intolerances,** which are not caused by the immune system, but by chemical reactions. They are very common, and can cause serious symptoms.

What to Look for in Your Children

The signs and symptoms of each of these three food reactions may be similar, and may include the following:

• **Congestion** of the nose, sinuses, and throat. Infection may accompany chronic congestion.

• **Gastrointestinal problems,** including bloating, gas, heartburn, burping, ulcers, diarrhea, constipation, nausea, or vomiting.

• **Watery, glassy eyes;** puffiness around the eyes; dark circles under the eyes; or a horizontal crease just under the eyes.

• **Perspiration,** for no apparent reason, or night sweats.

• **Ear infections,** triggered by congestion; or red, warm earlobes.

• **Dizziness,** vertigo, or poor balance.

• **Headaches,** migraines, or tension in the neck and shoulders resembling that of stress tension.

• **Eczema,** skin rashes, or canker sores.

• **Swelling** of the hands, feet, face, or other areas.

• **Coughing,** sneezing, wheezing, asthmatic symptoms, or tightness in the chest.

• **Muscle aches,** leg cramps, or twitchy legs.

• **Cognitive problems,** including poor focus, poor memory, or brain fog.

• **Emotional problems,** including depression, anxiety, or anger, accompanied by associated behaviors.

• **Lethargy,** or low stamina.

• **Insomnia,** restless sleep, feelings of distress while trying to sleep, or chronic bedwetting.

• **Excess salivation,** spitting during speech, or drooling.

• **Negative behavioral symptoms associated with autism and ADHD,** including hyperactivity, disassociative behavior, stimming, or tantrums.

This is obviously a wide range of signs and symptoms, almost all of which can be caused by factors other than food reactions. However, food reactions are generally the *most common single cause* of practically all of these signs and symptoms. Food reactions are a common denominator of the 4-A disorders.

Following is a detailed account of the two most effective diets for preventing food reactions: The gluten-free, casein-free diet, and the specific food reaction diet.

Let's start with the GF/CF diet.

(1) THE GLUTEN-FREE, CASEIN-FREE DIET

It's possible that one of the best things you can do for your child in the Healing Program may be one of the hardest things: Ask him or her to stop eating gluten and casein.

This can be difficult, but this one element of dietary intervention has consistently had remarkable effects.

I put virtually all children with 4-A symptoms on this diet, for at least a trial period of a month or more.

In my practice, at least 60 percent of children with autism improve when they go on the gluten-free, casein-free diet, or GF/CF diet. The diet also achieves a high rate of positive response among kids with

ADHD and asthma. It is not at all unusual to see major improvements in symptoms within a relatively short time, after children begin the GF/CF diet. The GF/CF diet has become the single most popular dietary intervention for autism, ADHD, and asthma. Because it's an anti-allergenic diet, it is also, of course, appropriate for kids with classic allergies to foods with gluten and casein, such as wheat and milk.

The symptoms that often begin to improve on the GF/CF diet are: poor language skills, bowel disorders, mood disorders, hyperactive behavior, skin problems (particularly eczema), insomnia, fatigue, cognitive disorders, and various metabolic disorders, such as thyroid dysfunction. Many common symptoms of food reactions also improve, including swelling, bloating, and food craving.

The GF/CF diet turns lives around.

The bad news: It's relatively hard. It's hard for kids to give up many of their favorite foods, and it's hard for parents to enforce these food restrictions.

As I've mentioned, giving up gluten and casein means giving up two of America's favorite staples: wheat and dairy products. These two food categories are absolutely ubiquitous in our dietary culture. In addition, these two food categories also compose many of kids' favorite fun-foods. Therefore, it can be a real struggle to put kids on the GF/CF diet. But it is eminently worth the effort.

In fact, it is sometimes almost impossible for children with pronounced symptoms of the 4-A disorders to heal unless they do go on the GF/CF diet.

Giving Up Gluten

Gluten is present not only in wheat, but also in:

* Rye.
* Barley.
* Oats (to a lesser degree).

Gluten is not present in the other food grains: rice, corn, and millet. Some nutritionists believe that it is only moderately present in oats, and food scientists are currently trying to develop a gluten-free type of oats.

Gluten, like most of the other food components that cause food reactions, is a protein, and it has a sticky, gluey texture that helps give wheat products the ability to bake properly.

Unfortunately, though, a large percentage of the American population has a deficiency of the particular enzyme that breaks down gluten. This enzyme is called DPP4. It is also involved in the digestion of milk products.

When the DPP4 enzyme fails to do its job, gluten is only partially broken down. This creates partial proteins, or peptides, that can sometimes mimic the chemical composition of opiates. These peptides are also very similar to the innate human opiates called endorphins. These opioid peptides frequently cause feelings of spaciness, and even intoxication, in kids who don't have enough of the DPP4 enzyme, and who are therefore intolerant to gluten and casein. These feelings of intoxication can become very appealing to kids, and the pleasure they create can make it hard for kids to give up gluten and casein.

Another terrible effect of partially digested gluten and casein—one discovered by my colleague Jon Pangborn, Ph.D.–is damage to the process of methylation. As you know, methylation is absolutely critical for removing toxins from the body. Methylation also helps to maintain proper levels of neurotransmitters–particularly dopamine, the neurotransmitter most often involved in ADHD, and also in obesity.

There are lab tests that can indicate whether your child will respond to a gluten-free diet. One is a test for celiac disease, which is the most extreme form of gluten sensitivity. Also, tests for IgE or IgG food reactions can indicate gluten intolerance, or reactivity to wheat, rye, oats, or barley. Even so, a child can still have this intolerance without having celiac disease, or any frank allergies or sensitivities, due to the damaging effects of opioid peptides.

Unfortunately, there is no way to adequately bolster insufficient amounts of the DPP4 enzyme. Taking digestive enzyme supplements can help, but it does not fully solve the problem.

The most virulent form of gluten intolerance, celiac disease, is known to be present in at least one in every 250 people. Celiac disease, however, may be even more common than this, and may exist in a milder form among a much larger segment of the population. Celiac disease is also closely associated with Type 1 diabetes. Approximately one in every twenty Type 1 diabetics has celiac disease. The symptoms of celiac disease are similar, in many ways, to the ancillary symptoms associated with autism and ADHD. This similarity of symptoms is one more reason to believe that gluten intolerance plays a role in autism and ADHD. It also indicates that many children with celiac disease may be misdiagnosed as having classic autism or ADHD. The symptoms of celiac disease are as follows:

Celiac Disease: Symptoms and Associated Disorders

- Weight loss, and inability to gain weight.
- Fatigue.
- Irritability.
- Failure to grow.
- Depression.
- Anemia.
- Skin rash.
- Hypoglycemia.
- Poor appetite.
- Migraine headaches.
- Encephalopathy.

- Bowel disorders, including constipation and diarrhea.
- Chorea.
- Brain stem dysfunction.
- Myelopathy.
- Peripheral neuropathy.
- Epilepsy.
- Dementia.
- Developmental delay.
- Hypotonia.
- ADHD.
- Chronic headaches.

A popular theory about why gluten intolerance is so common is that wheat was not introduced into the human food supply until relatively late in the process of human evolution. People didn't eat wheat until after the advent of agriculture, about ten thousand years ago. This, however, was preceded by at least one million years in which people subsisted mostly on wild fruits, vegetables, and game meat. This long period of living on vegetables, fruit, and meat may account for the fact that reactions to vegetables, fruit, and meat are far less common than reactions to grains.

Giving Up Casein

Casein is one of the primary proteins in milk and all milk products—including cheese, cream, and butter—and it's the hardest of these proteins to break down. An insufficiency of the DPP4 enzyme results in only a partial breakdown of casein, creating a partial protein, or peptide. My friend Sid Baker, M.D., refers to this partial protein as "a mischievous peptide" in the excellent book *Autism: Effective Biomedical Treatments,* which he wrote with Dr. Pangborn.

This mischievous protein can create caseomorphins that cause the same type of intoxication, contentment, and pleasure as the morphine-like substances that can come from gluten peptides. This intoxication can result in cravings, and in the strong attachment that so many kids have to milk.

This attachment, not incidentally, is also strongly reinforced by the aggressive marketing campaigns of the dairy industry, which generally portray milk as our society's most wholesome and harmless health food. These ads make it much harder for kids to realize that milk can be bad for them, and the ads also make it harder for parents, themselves, to actually recognize the potential for harm that dairy products hold.

Milk also often causes problems because of IgE allergies. Furthermore, intolerance to milk is often caused by a deficiency of the enzyme lactase, which breaks down milk sugar, or lactose.

Lactose intolerance, due to genetic reasons, is more common among certain racial groups. It appears to be more common among the racial groups that had the least exposure to milk during the long evolutionary process. Consider the following chart.

Lactose Intolerance Among American Racial Groups

Asian Americans	95%	
African Americans	65%	
Native Americans	65%	
Hispanics	50%	
Caucasians	15%	

Lactose intolerance can often be adequately remedied by taking supplements that contain lactase enzymes. However, these enzymes don't help kids whose problems are a result of a shortage of the DPP4 enzyme, or a result of an IgE allergy.

Therefore, the only adequate course of action for a great many children is simply to restrict dairy products from their diets. Sometimes these restrictions can be lifted after several months or years, or they can be modified to allow occasional intake of dairy products. More often than not, however, the avoidance of milk products must last throughout life, and be quite strict.

The positive response to avoiding dairy products can be relatively quick. It often occurs in just a few days. However, it can take up to three weeks. In contrast, the positive response to avoiding gluten requires at least several weeks, and usually several months, because gluten tends to remain in the system for a longer period of time.

Therefore, I recommend the following minimum time trials for restricting gluten and casein:

- **3 weeks for casein.**
- **3 months for gluten.**

By the end of this time period, positive results will appear, if the child does have a problem with gluten or casein.

Because the restriction of dairy products generally creates quicker results, many parents prefer to restrict dairy first, and then move on to gluten, after their kids begin to feel better.

Sometimes, though, restriction of gluten foods also creates fast results. If a child has a classic IgE allergy to wheat, or to the other gluten grains, he or she may feel enormously better in a very short period of time.

Before things get better, though, they often get worse.

Things can get worse immediately after the restrictions begin, due to classic symptoms of withdrawal, which can be very much like those experienced by a person withdrawing from an addiction to drugs or alcohol. Kids sometimes experience the following symptoms:

Immediate Symptoms of Withdrawal from Gluten and Casein
- Insomnia.
- Anger and anxiety.
- Fatigue.
- Night sweats and day sweats.
- Hyperactive behavior.
- Constipation, or diarrhea.
- Clinging and whining.
- Upset stomach.
- Cognitive dysfunction.
- Return, or amplification, of prior ADHD or autistic behaviors.

These symptoms generally tend to resolve in about forty-eight hours, but they can diminish more gradually. Because some of these withdrawal symptoms are similar to those of the reactive condition it-self, they sometimes do not cause a noticeable increase in a child's distress. For most kids, though, the withdrawal period is a difficult time. During this difficult transition, it's often tempting for parents to allow their children to have a slight reprieve from the restrictions, and let kids eat a food with gluten or casein, especially as a reward. But this is not a good idea. It prolongs the process, and reawakens cravings. It can also send a message to children that it is acceptable for them to sneak some of their restricted foods.

The restrictions can be especially hard to enforce among older children and adolescents, who have more freedom to stray from the restrictions, and who have ideas of their own about what's best for them. Almost every time that I place teenagers on a restricted diet as part of their Healing Program, I sit down with them, preferably alone, and try to gain their own endorsement of these often difficult restrictions. I tell them in a compassionate but clear way that I don't want to waste their time, my time, and their parents' money on a program that will be sabotaged by their unwillingness to fully participate. It's critically important that they invest their own personal sense of ownership in the program. If they feel it's being forced upon them, they will be far less likely to make the necessary commitments and sacrifices. As a rule, I get a very good response to this frank approach. Kids don't want to feel bad, and they don't want to behave badly. If you provide them with strong evidence that they can succeed, they'll usually agree to make the necessary sacrifices.

However, temptations are everywhere, and all children are fallible, so I also try to help kids realize that if they make one slip-up, it's not the end of the world, or the end of their program. If parents and doctors are too absolute in their demands, kids will adopt this all-or-nothing attitude themselves, and will sometimes abandon their efforts when they fall prey to a single, temporary failure.

Another important strategy is to embrace the tasty substitutes for gluten and casein foods. These substitute foods are readily available in health food stores, in many supermarkets, and on the Internet. For example, kids can have delicious snacks of nondairy ice cream and wheat-free brownies, and feel quite satisfied. Frequently, they even begin to prefer the GF/CF substitutes over the conventional products. Many people who go on the GF/CF diet remark that after they became accustomed to substitutes made from rice and soy, conventional wheat products began to taste gluey and gummy, and regular dairy products tasted thick and fatty. Tastes and preferences can change, and this often happens quickly when cravings go away. In fact, many of our desires for baked goods and rich dairy products stem much less from the intrinsically pleasing tastes of these foods than from the fact that these foods temporarily dampen uncomfortable cravings, and cause mild intoxication. As kids begin to recover, they often actually begin to have negative associations with reactive foods. They start to associate eating wheat or milk with insomnia, diarrhea, and agitation. This makes it much easier for them to stick to the diet.

In short, each new day gets a little easier, just as it generally does for recovering alcoholics or drug addicts.

One problem with the GF/CF diet, though, is that it can trigger hypoglycemia if a child begins to eat too many carbohydrates, particularly sugar, as a substitute for gluten and casein foods. Parents often allow this to happen, because they feel bad that their children's diets have been limited. Parents often like to reward their kids with treats, but sweets are the wrong reward. Thus, kids on the GF/CF diet may need to also be on the anti-hypoglycemia diet, at the same time. I'll give you details on that shortly.

Another very common difficulty is that parents often find it harder to prepare meals when they can't rely on wheat and dairy products. Meal planning and preparation on the GF/CF diet can be very intimidating to parents. However, most parents quickly realize that they can still cook in the traditional meat-and-potatoes fashion, and prepare wholesome and hearty meals that satisfy the whole family. In fact, parents sometimes even find that cooking becomes much easier when they create simple meals. There's nothing difficult about preparing a meal of grilled meat or fish, a salad, a potato, and a vegetable. These meals can be much less time consuming and fussy than more elaborate combinations of processed foods, sauces, and casseroles. Again, kids probably will miss their favorite sauces and complicated concoctions at first, but the human appreciation for good food is notably flexible. Furthermore, in much the same way that people on the GF/CF diet often develop a distaste for the gluey texture of wheat products, they also often learn to dislike the contrived combinations of cream sauces, breading, and fillers that are so common in America's culinary culture. This acquisition of a more sophisticated palate is similar to an adult learning to dislike traditional kid-foods, such as canned spaghetti, chocolate cereal, or Gummi Bears.

What primarily makes the GF/CF diet practical, though, are the substitutes for foods with gluten and casein. The substitutes taste really good, and are easy to find. For example, most cream sauces can be made with rice milk or soy milk, and it's easy to find great-tasting rice bread, soy ice cream, rice-flour cookies, and cakes, puddings, and biscuits made from soy flour or rice flour. If you are currently unfamiliar with these products, they may sound exotic to you, or even distasteful. But they taste great, and usually aren't much harder to prepare than their standard counterparts. Many of them are available in mixes and packages. There is a very large and growing industry that provides these foods, and that industry has made tremendous progress in giving consumers the kinds of foods they like to eat.

Parents are also often concerned that having their kids on the GF/CF diet will make it harder for them to eat at restaurants. To some extent, this is true, particularly regarding fast-food restaurants, which primarily serve sandwiches and breaded meats, such as chicken nuggets, which many autistic kids seem to crave. However, most fast-food places do serve salads now. Even so, though, taking kids with serious health problems to fast-food places is generally a poor way to help restore their health. It's wiser to spend a little more money and take them to a full-service, family restaurant. These places are usually healthier, and you can almost always find something on the menu that doesn't have gluten or casein in it.

Another frequent concern of moms and dads is that their kids won't get enough calcium if they don't drink milk. That's a legitimate concern, so take a look at the section in this chapter entitled "Sources of Calcium Other than Milk." As you'll see, the most practical way to ensure a rich supply of calcium is simply to give your kids a calcium supplement. Supplements are a very important element of the Healing Program, because they provide kids who have health problems with very specific nutrients, in the abundant amounts that these kids need, in order to heal.

When you do start the GF/CF diet, it would be a good idea to buy one or two of the many GF/CF cookbooks that are available. They will give you the details you'll need to implement this diet with ease and grace.

The other thing you need to do to start the diet is to find the best health food stores in your area, and to check out their many GF/CF food substitutes. If you aren't currently a regular shopper at health food stores, you'll probably be delighted to find out how much tasty GF/CF food is available in them.

When kids do slip up and eat some gluten or casein, it can help if they take a special kind of digestive enzyme that breaks down the partial proteins, or peptides, that gluten and casein can create. This enzyme, available at most health food stores, is known as peptidase.

It's also important to be compassionate with your kids when they do go off the diet. The GF/CF diet can be hard for kids. It's also hard for parents to keep kids on the diet, so be compassionate with yourself, too, if your kids have problems. Don't feel guilty. Guilt won't solve the problems you face, and will only make you feel worse.

After kids have been off casein for three weeks, if there have been no apparent positive responses or changes, allow them to have some, to see if symptoms return or worsen. After kids have been off gluten for three months, if there have been no apparent positive responses or changes, allow them to have gluten, to see if symptoms return.

If symptoms do return, restrict the foods indefinitely. If symptoms do not return, the diet can be modified, by allowing either occasional gluten or casein, or by completely lifting the restriction. Be cautious, though. Symptoms can be subtle, and they can be delayed, occurring several days or more after the food is eaten. Err on the side of caution.

One last word about the GF/CF diet, before I give you more of the specific details that you'll need: Be patient, be strong, and don't expect miracles. The GF/CF diet, like every other element of the Healing Program, requires time and effort. It also requires the contributing elements of the rest of the program. This is not magic bullet medicine. It is a comprehensive program with many elements, most of which must be in place before significant progress can occur.

Even so, this is a terrific place to start. You might see improvements in your child before this month is over.

Foods with Gluten and Casein

People on the GF/CF diet should avoid all of the following foods. Some may contain greater quantities of gluten or casein than others, but even small amounts can cause reactions, particularly after the body has already eliminated gluten and casein. As a rule, the foods that contain both gluten and casein, together, tend to do the most damage.

Foods with Both *Gluten and Casein*

Artificial cream
Artificial sweeteners
Baby foods
Bagels
Biscuits
Bread
Bread crumbs
Bread rolls
Cakes
Coffee creamer
Cookies

Croissants
Custards
Doughnuts
Dry roasted peanuts
Gravy
Hot chocolate
Hot dogs
Luncheon meat
Malted milk
Milkshakes
Muffins

Pancakes
Pastry
Patés
Pies
Pizza
Puddings
Sandwich spreads
Soups: canned/packet
Spam
Vegetarian cheese

Foods with *Gluten*

Baked beans
Baking powder
Barley
Barley malt
Barley sugar
Bleached all-purpose flour
Bouillon cubes/powder
Bran (except rice bran)
Bulgur wheat
Cereal
Chicken nuggets
Couscous
Crackers
Croutons
Curry powder
Durum wheat
Enriched flour
Flour tortillas
Graham flour

Ice-cream cones
Ice-cream syrup
Kamut
Malt
Malt extract
Malt flavoring
Malt syrup
Malt vinegar
Marzipan
Mincemeat
Muesli
Mustard powder
Noodles
Nougat
Oat flour
Oatmeal
Oats
Pasta
Pearl barley

Pita bread
Pretzels
Rice malt
Rye
Rye flour
Rye semolina
Sausages
Semolina
Soy sauce
Spelt
Stuffing mixes
Teriyaki sauce
Vinegar
Waffles
Wheat
Wheat bran
Wheat flour
Wheat germ
Wheat malt

Foods with Casein

Bavarian cream	Curds	Mousses
Butter	Dried milk	Nonfat milk
Butterfat	Evaporated milk	Powdered milk
Buttermilk	Fudge	Rennet casein
Butterscotch	Goat's milk	Shortening
Caseinate	Ice cream	Skimmed milk
Cheese	Lactalbumin	Sodium caseinate
Cheese powder	Lactalbumin phosphate	Sour cream
Cheese slices	Lactate acid	Sour cream solids
Cheese spread	Lactoglobulin	Toffee
Chocolate	Lemon curd	Whey
Condensed milk	Margarine	Whey protein
Cooking chocolate	Mayonnaise	Whey sodium caseinate
Cottage cheese	Milk	Whey sugar
Cream	Milk chocolate	Whey syrup
Cream cheese	Milk powder	Whipped cream
Curd cheese	Milk solids	Yogurt

Gluten-Free Substitutes

A number of excellent substitutes are available for the foods that contain gluten and casein. Following are brief descriptions of these substitutes.

Gluten-Free Wheat Substitutes

Many varieties of flour may be used in place of wheat flour. Following are some of the most popular wheat flour substitutes. Some of these gluten-free wheat substitutes may also be eaten as side dishes, rather than used as flour, by cooking them with two parts water to one part grain.

Rice can be eaten as a staple, and also produces a richly textured flour that can be excellent for baking. Some people find the texture too gritty, but it can work well in certain foods, such as brownies.

Amaranth flour is gluten-free, and is fine for baking. It is available in some packaged products, such as crackers. Amaranth tastes best if you buy it from a store that refrigerates it, and if you continue to refrigerate it at home. It mixes well with other foods, and browns quickly as a breading. When baking with it, try using one part amaranth combined with three parts rice flour.

Arrowroot is a finely ground powder that resembles cornstarch. It's great as a thickening agent in soups or cooked dishes, in place of wheat flour or cornstarch. It has very little flavor, so it won't disturb the taste of the dishes in which you use it. For baking, use one part arrowroot, combined with three parts of other nonwheat flours.

Buckwheat sounds as if it's a form of wheat, but it's not. It's actually a seed that is related to rhubarb. Popular for pancakes, it has a distinctive flavor. It can be used in noodles, and is generally well tolerated by people who react to wheat.

Teff is an African grain, widely available, that is used for flour. It can be used in most baked goods, and is also often added to soups, stews, and puddings. It has a rather sweet taste and a slightly rough texture.

Tapioca is well known as a pudding ingredient, and can also be used as a thickener.

Potato starch is also a good thickener.

Millet is a high-protein grain that has a rather bland flavor. It is not ideal for baking, because it's too crumbly. It can be good in casseroles, or mixed with vegetables. It tastes a little like couscous.

Casein-Free Dairy Product Substitutes

Goat's milk can be tolerated by some people who react to casein, because it has only trace amounts of one specific type of casein. Others who are very sensitive to casein, however, react to both goat's milk and cow's milk. Goat's milk tends to have a stronger, more distinctive flavor than the blander cow's milk. It can be used for virtually anything that cow's milk is used for. The fat globules in goat's milk are smaller than those in cow's milk, and this makes it easier to digest. Many grocery stores and most health food stores carry goat's milk. It is sometimes better for infants than other milk substitutes.

Soy milk is a popular milk substitute that does not have the heavier, more distinctive flavor found in goat's milk. A variety of soy milk products are available, including low-fat milk, regular milk, cream, or butter. Soy milk can be used in almost all the ways that cow's milk is used. It can be purchased at many supermarkets and all health food stores. The various commercial brands have a wide variety of tastes.

Rice milk is similar to soy milk, and is appropriate for people who react to both soy and dairy. It is available at most supermarkets and all health food stores. It tends to taste less creamy than cow's milk.

Nut milk is somewhat less commercially available than goat's milk, soy milk, and rice milk, but various brands can be found at many health food stores. Nut milk is creamy and satisfying, but it does not taste as much like cow's milk as does goat's, soy, or rice milk.

Oat milk is generally thick and rich. It does contain gluten, and is not appropriate for the GF/CF diet, but is acceptable for people who are reactive to milk, but not to gluten.

Soy ice cream is usually delicious. It has a slightly different taste than dairy-based ice cream, but many people like this taste as much as that of dairy ice cream. Soy ice cream is sweet, rich, and smooth in texture. Like dairy ice cream, however, it's high in calories, especially calories from sugar and fat, so it must be eaten in moderation. People who are reactive to dairy often find it easier to eat soy ice cream in moderation, because it doesn't trigger the food cravings that dairy can. Soy ice cream is available in almost all health food stores, and many supermarkets. It is also packaged as various treats, such as ice-cream bars and ice-cream sandwiches.

Rice ice cream is similar to soy ice cream, and just as good. It's sweet, creamy, and filling, and it tastes much like dairy ice cream. It is carried by health food stores, and in many supermarkets. Like soy ice cream, rice ice cream can be high in sugar and fat.

Sorbet, sherbet, and fruit ices are all good ice-cream substitutes. Sometimes these products contain a small amount of milk, though many are dairy-free. Some contain corn syrup.

Nondairy margarines are usually available at health food stores and supermarkets. Many of the low-calorie brands use soy instead of milk. These products tend to be less rich than real butter, but they are lower in calories. Many soy margarines, though, contain saturated fat and yellow dye, and many are hydrogenated, which makes them particularly unhealthy. For cooking, it is best to not use butter substitutes, but to use oils, such as olive oil or sunflower oil.

Although real butter does contain casein, as well as lactose, they are present in relatively small amounts. Some people who are mildly sensitive to casein or lactose can tolerate real butter, in moderation.

Nondairy yogurts, cheeses, and sour cream are available, and some of them are tasty and satisfying. Because individual tastes vary so much, you should experiment with various nondairy products to see which ones your children enjoy. Examples of these types of products include tofu sour cream, soy cheese, and soy yogurt. Health food stores and many supermarkets carry a variety of these products.

SOURCES OF CALCIUM OTHER THAN MILK

People who react to dairy products can ensure adequate calcium intake by taking supplements, or by eating lots of the following calcium-rich foods. Some of these foods have even more calcium than milk, and others have almost as much. As a rule, it's most practical to simply take a supplement, because they are safe, inexpensive, and provide an abundant supply. It's very important to get enough calcium, because it works in close partnership with vitamin D, which is critically important for the immune modulation that is generally needed to heal the 4-A disorders. Vitamin D deficiency can be triggered by low calcium. That's why the vitamin D deficiency disease of rickets is common in certain areas of the world where people get plenty of vitamin D from the sun, but don't get enough calcium.

I recommend a minimum of 500 mg. of calcium per day, taken in conjunction with the important cofactor of magnesium. Calcium and magnesium, working together, tend to have a calming effect, and can sometimes help provide relief from the anxiety and insomnia that are common among 4-A kids.

In comparison to the following foods, a cup of whole cow's milk contains 288 mg. of calcium.

Food	Milligrams of Calcium
Sesame butter (3 oz.)	843 mg.
Soybeans (1 cup)	460 mg.
Tofu (1 cup)	258 mg.
Lamb (½ cup)	232 mg.
Sesame seeds (⅒ cup)	220 mg.
Blackstrap molasses (1 tablespoon)	137 mg.
Navy beans (1 cup)	128 mg.
Pinto beans (1 cup)	82 mg.
Garbanzo beans (1 cup)	80 mg.
Almonds (⅒ cup)	60 mg.
Mustard greens (½ cup)	52 mg.
Swiss chard (½ cup)	51 mg.
Kidney beans (1 cup)	50 mg.
Kale (½ cup)	47 mg.
Artichoke (½ cup)	47 mg.

Hazelnuts (⅒ cup)	42 mg.
Wild rice (1 cup)	30 mg.
Green beans (½ cup)	29 mg.

The Action Plan: What to Do About Gluten and Casein

1. **Restrict** all casein foods, for three weeks.
2. **Restrict** all gluten foods, for three months.
3. **Monitor children** for symptoms during the restrictions. Kids may feel worse at first, and then feel better.
4. **Use substitutes** for foods that contain gluten and casein, such as soy milk, or rice bread.
5. **Reintroduce** gluten and casein, after they have cleared from the system–but *only* if no positive changes have occurred. Look carefully for symptoms. If no symptoms occur, the foods may be eaten, either occasionally, or often, as long as they don't cause problems. If positive changes have occurred, though, don't attempt this reintroduction.

(2) THE SPECIFIC FOOD REACTION DIET

In addition to the more general GF/CF diet, I also place virtually all children on an individually designed diet that restricts all of the specific foods to which that particular child may be reactive.

This specific food reaction diet, which is also commonly referred to as an anti-allergy diet, is of consummate importance. It is extremely difficult for most children who suffer from 4-A disorders to recover if they do not go on this diet.

Food reactions–including (1) IgE allergies, (2) IgG sensitivities, and (3) intolerances–run rampant among the 4-A population. It is rare for me to meet a child with a 4-A disorder who does not experience at least some food reactions.

These food reactions include reactions to gluten and casein. As I mentioned, reactions to gluten and casein are present in at least 60 percent of all the children with autism that I treat, and they are also common among other 4-A kids. However, even more 4-A kids have at least some mild, isolated reactions to other, specific foods. Many have severe reactions to a number of specific foods.

Food reactions, particularly sensitivities, most frequently occur when kids eat one or more of six very reactive foods. These six foods include the two most common carriers of gluten and casein: wheat, and dairy products. Most reactions to wheat and dairy occur because of the gluten and casein that's in them, but not all. For example, many people react to dairy products because of the lactose that's in them, rather than the casein.

The Sensitive Six Most Reactive Foods

1. Wheat.
2. Dairy products.
3. Eggs.
4. Peanuts.
5. Corn.
6. Soy.

A second tier of very reactive foods includes:

The Second Tier of Most Reactive Foods

7. Chocolate.
8. Yeast.
9. Various tree nuts.

A third tier of foods that also frequently cause reactions includes:

The Third Tier of Most Reactive Foods

10. Citrus.
11. Tomatoes.
12. Aspartame and MSG.
13. Vinegar.
14. Shellfish (more common in adults than kids).

However, reactions are highly individualized, and also often involve the following foods, which tend to be moderately reactive:

The Fourth Tier of Occasionally Reactive Foods

15. Bacon and other pork.
16. Cinnamon.
17. Mustard.

18. Bananas.
19. Grapes and raisins.
20. Coconut.
21. Onions.
22. Berries, particularly strawberries.
23. Peas.
24. Celery.
25. Spices, including turmeric, cloves, and curry.
26. Kidney beans.
27. Melon.
28. Pineapple.
29. Mushrooms.
30. Peppers
31. Plums.
32. Barley.
33. Beef.
34. Chicken.

In contrast, some foods are seldom reactive. These foods are a good source of nutrition for people who are trying to restrict commonly reactive foods. These foods also often constitute the diets of people who are doing elimination challenges, in which they restrict all potentially reactive foods, and then add them back in, one at a time, to see if they cause reactions:

Generally Nonreactive Foods

Rice.	Carrots.
Pears.	Beets.
Lamb.	Cauliflower.
Kale.	Squash.
Salmon, halibut, sole.	Cranberries.
Trout.	Apricots.
Turkey.	Broccoli.
Olives, olive oil.	Rabbit.
Cabbage.	Sweet potatoes.
Tapioca.	

TESTING FOR SPECIFIC FOOD REACTIONS

Testing is the first step of the specific food reaction diet. It determines the foods your child reacts to.

There are three basic ways to test for food reactions: They are: (1) skin testing, (2) blood testing, and (3) elimination challenge testing (in which a patient eats a food to see if it causes a reaction). I generally recommend that patients first do a blood test, or occasionally a skin test, and then confirm the results with elimination challenge testing. However, elimination challenge testing is the most reliable way to diagnose food intolerances.

1.   Skin Testing These tests can indicate classic IgE allergies, but IgE allergies are usually relatively uncommon. IgE allergies do seem to be relatively more common, though, among kids with the 4-A disorders.

Many allergists use the skin test called the prick test, or scratch test, in which they place a small amount of a suspected allergen in a scratch, or prick, in the skin, to see if it will cause a red, inflammatory wheal, due to the immune system's IgE antibodies.

As I've mentioned, I don't think this method is as accurate as the other type of skin test, the intradermal test. To perform the intradermal test, doctors place the suspected allergen slightly more deeply into the skin. I believe this deeper placement significantly increases the accuracy of this test. However, the intradermal test is more uncomfortable, and kids often object to it.

When I do perform the intradermal test, I sometimes restrict it to a relatively small number of suspected allergens, such as eight to ten, to limit its discomfort. This often reveals the majority of IgE food allergies, because most classic food allergies involve one or more of the sensitive six foods: wheat, dairy, corn, soy, eggs, and peanuts.

The biggest problem with skin testing, besides the discomfort of multiple needle-pricks, is that it only reveals IgE allergies, and IgE allergies represent only a relatively small portion of all food reactions.

2. **Blood Testing** I rely primarily upon blood testing, because it reveals both IgE and IgG allergies. Another advantage is that it limits discomfort to just one needle poke, during the extraction of the blood sample.

As I stated in the chapter on allergy, I think blood testing is generally very accurate, even though it's not perfect.

Many allergists don't rely upon blood testing, because it doesn't reveal the obvious, unmistakable physical signs of the allergic response, as do skin tests. Instead, it reveals the presence of antibodies, which are secondary indicators of the allergic response. I understand why some doctors would prefer to diagnose allergies from the unequivocal signs produced by the skin tests, but I think blood testing adds significantly to the diagnostic process. I think blood testing provides a very practical combination of accuracy, comfort for the patient, and broad-spectrum analysis. I also think blood testing is probably as accurate as the conventional prick test, even though it's less accurate than the intradermal test.

A very significant advantage of blood testing, as opposed to skin testing, is that it reveals the presence of IgG reactions. IgG reactions typically don't show up during skin testing, because they often don't begin to occur until a few hours, or even a few days, after contact with the food. In contrast, IgE reactions generally occur almost immediately, enabling doctors to spot them during the short duration of the skin testing procedure.

IgG reactions are very common, and very troublesome. They are extremely common among kids with 4-A disorders. They tend to create less severe symptoms than IgE reactions, but their symptoms still can be very destructive, particularly when IgG reactions to several foods occur at once, causing combined, cumulative damage, or when they combine with IgE reactions.

There are two major types of blood tests: RAST (radioallergosorbent tests), and ELISA (enzyme-linked immunosorbent assays). They are very similar, and many people are more familiar with the RAST test, so I sometimes refer to the ELISA testing that we do as a RAST test. There is strong evidence that both can be effective.

The RAST test, similar to other food reaction tests, can

screen for just a few foods, or for a great many. It's generally more clinically prudent to test for a relatively large number of foods, but the cost of the tests goes up as the number of tested foods goes up. Therefore, to hold down expense, it can be reasonable to test your child for a relatively small number of foods. I generally do an IgE screen of ten of the most commonly reactive foods. In that screen, I usually include any foods that a child craves, since craving is a strong indicator of reactivity.

After analyzing a blood sample, your doctor will receive lab results that will indicate which of the tested foods appear to be causing reactions. The results will indicate if they are IgE reactions or IgG reactions, and they will estimate the severity of the reaction. A mild IgG reaction may not cause notable damage or distress, by itself. If your child has only a minor IgG reaction to a food, he or she may be able to eat this food on an occasional basis, such as once every four to seven days. This is commonly referred to as a rotation diet. These mild IgG reactions can even go away entirely, after a food is avoided for several months, or possibly a year or two.

One problem with blood tests, though, is that they don't usually reveal food intolerances. One exception is testing for lactose intolerance, which can be done with a blood test or a breath test. Other blood tests, however, generally only reveal reactions caused by the immune system's IgE and IgG antibodies. Therefore, your child might have a significant, damaging food reaction–caused by an intolerance–that will not show up on a blood test.

The only way to spot intolerances is with the third method of testing for food reactions: elimination challenge testing.

3. Elimination Challenge Testing This method can be a very effective way to uncover any type of food reaction, if performed properly. To do one, you need to eliminate a certain food from your child's diet for seven to ten days, and then have your child eat that food again. After he or she eats it, you look for reactions.

Elimination challenge testing is necessary for most 4-A kids, since these tests are the only way to spot intolerances. Intolerances sometimes have less severe symptoms than IgE allergies and even IgG sensitivities, but they can still be extraordinarily disruptive and damaging. Lactose intolerance, for example, can contribute immeasurably to symptoms of bowel dysbiosis symptomatology.

Furthermore, elimination challenges are the best possible way to confirm the results of skin testing and blood testing. The challenges can eliminate false positives, as well as false negatives. There is a huge advantage in eliminating false positives—in which a test diagnoses a reaction that doesn't actually exist—because this can allow your child to eat a wider variety of foods. It's also extremely important to catch false negatives—in which allergies go undetected by the skin or blood tests—because these undetected allergies can cause terrible damage, without anyone knowing what's going wrong.

Therefore, I recommend to most patients that they try the elimination challenge. They eliminate a food—particularly one already labeled as reactive by blood or skin testing—and then reintroduce it in seven to ten days, challenging their systems to tolerate the food. If they don't tolerate it well, they know for sure that they are reactive to it. If they do tolerate it, without any symptoms, they can usually begin to eat that food again. To be cautious, however, you should try the challenge at least once more, because the blood and skin testing usually tend to be accurate.

When doing an elimination challenge, it's important to restrict the food for only about seven to ten days before trying it again. Less than that time period, or more, can compromise the accuracy of the challenge.

Elimination challenge testing can be done not only to confirm results of skin and blood testing, but also can be done as a stand-alone procedure, without any other form of testing.

There are two most common ways to do a stand-alone elimination challenge: (1) eliminating only the most frequently reactive foods, such as the sensitive six foods, plus any foods your child craves, and then reintroducing them; or (2) eliminating practically all foods that may cause reactions, and then trying them.

The sensitive six elimination challenge is easier, and can be very revealing, but the broader challenge, often called a total elimination challenge, is more likely to reveal more obscure, uncommon reactions, such as a reaction to potatoes.

The Sensitive Six Elimination Challenge

To do this, eliminate wheat, dairy, corn, eggs, soy, peanuts, plus any food your child craves, from his or her diet for seven to ten days. During this time, your child may start to gradually feel better, and have fewer symptoms, if he or she has indeed been suffering from reactions to any of these foods. Then add foods back in, one at a time, every two days, and look for reactions. Reactive symptoms can be quite varied, but they will usually be the same symptoms that may previously have been present, such as bloating, swelling, headaches, or behavior problems.

Unfortunately, this approach can be confusing, because so many other factors can influence how your child feels and acts. That's why I urge parents to do the blood tests first. The blood tests make the whole process much easier.

When doing the sensitive six elimination challenge, which is also called an elimination diet, it's pivotally important to include any food your child craves, since craving is usually such a dead giveaway of a food reaction. Your kids won't like this, of course, but their cravings will soon go away, and then the restrictions will be much easier to enforce.

Another reason to not rely entirely on elimination diets is because it's often hard to know when your child is eating a particular food, since foods are frequently present in unexpected sources. For example, wheat is found in some candy bars, milk is in doughnuts, and corn syrup is in hundreds of foods. Because of this, it's important that you become an avid reader of labels.

Also, when your child goes on an elimination diet, he or she will need to avoid taking antihistamines, because they can mask symptoms.

Some parents keep a diary of how their kids seem to react to certain foods. This can help eliminate some of the confusion.

The Total Elimination Challenge

This is the best approach for reducing confusion. However, it's more difficult than the sensitive six challenge. To do this challenge, you need to remove every food item from your child's diet other than those that are the very least reactive. To determine these foods, consult the prior list that specifies the least reactive foods. As you will note, these foods can comprise a satisfying diet, but they don't allow for much variety.

In addition, virtually no processed foods may be eaten, because they usually contain so many reactive ingredients.

This challenge works much like the sensitive six elimination challenge, but with many more foods to add back in, as challenges. One draw-back of the total elimination diet is that it takes so long to add back all the foods. This allows a lot of time to elapse, and this can skew the results. The skewing occurs due to the fact that after a food is eliminated for two weeks or longer, the body doesn't always react the first time this food is eaten, even though the food may still be reactive when it's eaten regularly. Therefore, even the total elimination challenge is occasionally confusing.

Because both forms of elimination challenges can be confusing, and also relatively difficult, especially for children, I believe it's much more sensible to use them mainly as secondary tests, to confirm the results of the blood or skin tests. The only advantage of not doing the blood or skin tests is to save money, and for most people, the savings just aren't worth the effort, or the risk of making a mistake, and exposing your child to further harm from food reactions.

After you do determine which foods cause problems, you will need to re-strict them almost entirely. A food reaction-avoidance diet is not at all the same as a weight loss diet, in which you can cheat on the diet one day, and make up for it the next. Cheating on this diet can reawaken cravings, and cause cascades of dysfunction that can be difficult to remedy.

Therefore, you will need to be aware of all of the possible sources of various reactive foods. You can determine this by reading labels carefully.

Reactive Food Additives

In addition to foods, many additives to foods also cause reactions. Sometimes these reactions provoke the IgE and IgG responses, but often the reactions are simple intolerances. For example, you may re-call that I placed both MSG and aspartame on my third tier of most reactive food substances, primarily because many kids are intolerant of them. These two substances do most of their damage from chemi-cal reactions, instead of reactions from the immune system. MSG, or monosodium glutamate, is known to be an excitotoxin, which can damage and kill brain cells in people who are sensitive to it, by over-stimulating these cells. Also, one of its primary ingredients, glutamate, can interfere with dopamine metabolism, which is one of the central problems of most kids with ADHD symptoms. Furthermore, MSG is one of the most common triggers of migraine headaches.

Aspartame is also an excitotoxin. Its only active ingredient, phenylalanine, is an amino acid that helps govern the function of the brain and nervous system. When too much phenylalanine hits the brain, it can cause hyperactivity and other behavioral symptoms.

Because many food additives cause intolerance, rather than IgE allergy or IgG sensitivity, you may need to perform elimination challenges to see if these additives are causing problems. Another practical approach is simply to look for reactions when your child does eat one of these food additives.

These additives can add to the confusion of eliminating reactive foods, because you may think your child is reactive to a food, when he or she is actually just reactive to an additive in that food. For example, kids might react to mustard not because of the actual mustard seeds in it, but because of yellow dye in it.

To deal with the inescapable confusion that food reactions cause, you need to be patient and observant. Keep looking for clues. You, and you alone, are your kids' most important medical detective, because you are the person who is with them day and night.

Food Additives to Avoid

You may need to restrict the following food additives from your child's diet. To help make these restrictions practical, you may need to begin buying brands of food that are labeled as being free of additives, such as foods labeled "nitrite-free," or "no MSG." Like every other element of the Healing Program, this can require effort and sacrifice, but the rewards can be vast.

Nitrites and nitrates. Bacon, hot dogs, sausage, bologna.

Sulfites. Lettuce, dried fruits, and fresh fruits and vegetables (especially in restaurants.

Sorbic acid. Cheese, frosting, dried fruit, dips.

Dyes (especially yellow dye #5). Hundreds of processed, colored foods.

Parabens. Jelly, soda pop, pastry, beer, cake, salad dressing.

Benzoic acid. Soda pop, fruit juice, margarine, apple cider.

Monosodium glutamate (MSG). Bouillon, Chinese restaurant dishes, chicken broth or flavoring, and may also be present in glutamate, hydrolyzed protein, sodium caseinate, calcium caseinate, or yeast extract.

EDTA. Margarine, salad dressing, frozen dinners, and other processed foods.

Aspartame. Artificially sweetened foods.

Propyl Gallate. Frozen dinners, gravy mix, turkey sausage.

Alginate. Ice cream, salad dressing, cheese spread, frozen dinners.

Bromates. Baked goods, bread crumbs, refrigerated dough.

Environmental and Chemical Reactions That Exacerbate Food Reactions

It's very common for kids with 4-A disorders–particularly those with asthma–to have reactions to various industrial chemicals, as well as to environmental allergens, such as dust, mold, pollen, animal dander, and dust mites. These reactions, which are generally inhalant reactions, are also relatively more common among kids with multiple or severe food reactions, because inhalant reactions and food reactions tend to reinforce one another. Sometimes it's very difficult to overcome food reactions if these inhalant reactions are still present.

These environmental and chemical reactions can consist of IgE allergies, IgG sensitivities, or intolerances. They can significantly impact the symptomatology of 4-A children, and can impede healing, if they are not addressed.

These reactions are often quite obvious, particularly if they are inhalant allergies that directly affect the airways. It's usually easy to spot hay fever, and to link it with its environmental source. It can be more difficult to recognize inhalant sensitivities and intolerances that cause a wider range of symptoms, some of which can be similar to the symptoms of food reactions. For example, inhalant allergens to grass or pollen can sometimes cause hives, a condition more commonly associated with food allergies.

Testing for common inhalant allergies, such as IgE pollen allergy, is generally relatively easy, and can be performed by most allergists. It can be more difficult, however, to determine a non-IgE reaction. Furthermore, some allergists are rather skeptical about the presence of chemical sensitivities, believing that they are quite rare. I don't agree with that perspective. I don't think they are common, but I believe they do exist in a significant subset of children who have sensitive systems.

In addition, chemical exposures, when combined with environmental allergies, may contribute to a child's problems, by adding to his or her total immune load.

The best way to deal with these reactive substances is just to avoid them. However, this is sometimes difficult. It's hard to avoid many seasonal, airborne allergens, and it can be very difficult to give up a family pet, or move away from a home that has resistant mold and mildew.

When people simply cannot avoid these allergens, allergists often achieve good results by desensitizing patients, using injections that contain very small amounts of the allergen. This is a common treatment for reactions to airborne allergens, such as pollen. This therapy can take six months or longer, but it's worth the effort when reactions are severe.

Another form of desensitization therapy can also be performed for food allergies, but this is much less common and is often not endorsed by conventional allergists. This form, Low-Dose Allergen Therapy, is a newer desensitization treatment that consists of administration of an allergy shot every two months. This shot is for multiple allergens, including foods, inhalants, and chemicals. It consists of very low doses of the allergenic extracts, in mixtures. The mixture is potentiated by an enzyme that helps ensure the proper immune response, even at a very low dose. This makes it safer, and simpler to use.

Among the most practical ways to avoid contact with airborne allergens are to institute environmental controls, such as: covering mattresses with a pad to avoid dust mites; installing air purifiers; washing away mold and mildew; and keeping animals out of the home.

In addition, you may need to help your child limit direct contact with some of the following chemicals, which are the ones most closely associated with reactions.

COMMON REACTIVE CHEMICALS THAT CAN EXACERBATE FOOD REACTIONS

Chemical	Source
Petrochemicals.	Car exhaust, gas or oil furnaces.
Formaldehyde.	New articles, including new clothing, carpets, paint, cars, or homes; hair gel, wood smoke.
Chlorine.	Tap water, swimming pools and hot tubs, bleach, household cleaners.
Phenol.	Perfumes and colognes, newspapers, glue, wood smoke.
Ethanol.	Car exhaust, perfume, household cleaners, wood smoke.
Fluoride.	Tap water, toothpaste, fluoride treatments.
Benzyl alcohol.	Solvents, perfume, artificial flavors.
Glycerin.	Makeup, soap, lotion, furniture polish.

SUMMARY: FOOD REACTIONS

Overcoming food reactions is of absolute, pivotal importance. It is often the single most significant element of the Healing Program. In many cases it's just as important as the element of eliminating toxicity. As the old saying goes, "One man's meat is another man's poison." Reactive foods can literally act as a poison within the systems of certain people.

Frequently, food reactions can be entirely overcome by avoiding the food for a long period of time, by restoring metabolic balance, and by improving the function of the immune system.

This can be difficult.

It's worth the difficulty.

The Action Plan: What to Do About Food Reactions

1. **GF/CF diet.** Do this first. Start with casein, then gluten. Or you may start them at the same time.

2. **Food reaction testing.** Do this second. The best tests are the blood tests. Intradermal skin testing can help, but it's limited. Elimination diets also work as tests for food reactions, but they're difficult, and often confusing.

3. **Do elimination challenges.** After the blood testing, you may wish to confirm the results with elimination challenges.

4. **Restrict** all reactive foods indefinitely.

5. **Determine environmental reactions** that exacerbate food reactions, because allergies are additive. Eliminate contact with environmental triggers as much as possible.

6. **Do the other elements of the Healing Program.** Many diverse aspects of health influence food reactions.

(3) THE ANTI-YEAST DIET

Throughout this book, I've demonstrated the critical importance of overcoming yeast overgrowth. This condition is extremely common among 4-A kids, and generally must be cleared for these kids to recover. Here's how to do it.

What to Look for in Your Kids

Yeast, or candida overgrowth, is generally diagnosed clinically by the child's history, as well as by a set of signs and symptoms. Some laboratories perform a stool test for candida, but I generally do not rely on this test. This test can confirm my clinical suspicion that a patient has yeast overgrowth, but I do not require the results of this test to make a clinical diagnosis. The clinical signs and symptoms, along with the child's history, are the best indicators that the problem exists. The test, however, can be helpful in choosing the proper medications.

The signs and symptoms of candida overgrowth often overlap with those of food reactions. However, some signs and symptoms, such as the presence of a white coat of thrush on the tongue, or a vaginal yeast infection, are related solely to yeast.

Here's what to look for:

The Signs and Symptoms of Candida Overgrowth

- Bloating in the belly, particularly after eating a yeast-promoting food.
- Thrush, a thick white coating on the tongue; or white patches in the mouth.
- Itching or redness in any of the mucosal membranes, or in any external body tissue that is in a warm, moist area, such as a boy's genitals or a girl's vagina.
- Recurrent vaginal infections; or "jock itch" irritation in males.
- Recurrent fungal infections of the toenails and fingernails; or recurrent athlete's foot.
- Swelling throughout the body, particularly in the hands, face, and feet; or a tendency to suffer from chronic water retention.
- Fatigue, for no apparent reason.
- Depression, for no apparent reason.
- Poor memory, poor cognitive function, and brain fog.
- Chronic nasal congestion from mucus; or swelling of the nasal membranes.
- Insomnia, restlessness.
- Joint pain, with or without swelling.
- Muscle aches; or headaches.
- Weight gain; or difficulty losing weight.
- Cravings for sweets and other refined carbohydrates, including bread and pasta.

- A history of steroid use.
- A history of frequent antibiotic use.

Overcoming Candida Overgrowth

Candida overgrowth can be overcome with: (1) diet; (2) supplements; and (3) medication. Often, all three must be applied. I almost always start with the simplest and least invasive procedure, dietary change, frequently accompanied with specific supplements. Medications can be extremely effective, but are not always necessary. In this chapter I will present the dietary therapy. I will present the treatment with supplements and medication in the following chapters on those subjects.

How to Do the Anti-Yeast Diet

This diet, which can be done at the same time as the GF/CF diet—as well as the anti-food reaction diet, and the other appropriate diets—is somewhat difficult for some people, but not very complicated. The difficulty of this diet is reduced drastically if your child is already on the GF/CF diet, because many yeast-promoting foods contain gluten and casein. This diet also goes hand in hand with the anti-hypoglycemia diet, because the same general restrictions apply to both.

The foods to restrict on the anti-yeast diet are those that:

1. Contain yeast (such as bread).
2. Contain foods that stimulate the growth of yeast (such as sugar), or that contain other forms of mold or fungus (such as cheese or mushrooms).

The worst foods are those that contain both yeast and sugar, such as cake, cookies, pastries, and pancakes.

Other extremely harmful foods are those with exceptionally high amounts of yeast in them, such as high-rising breads, or beer (among adults).

Foods to Avoid

(1) Foods that contain yeast:

- Breads.
- Bagels.
- Pastries.

- Pretzels.
- Crackers.
- Pizza dough.
- Cake.
- Rolls.
- Alcohol, especially beer (among adults).
- Cereal.

(2) Foods that stimulate the growth of yeast, or contain other forms of mold or fungus:

- Sugar and other sweets, including honey, syrup, or corn syrup.
- Raisins.
- Fruit juices (except those highly diluted by water).
- Cheese.
- Vinegar.
- Ketchup.
- Sauerkraut.
- Vinegar-based salad dressing.
- Some barbecue sauces.
- Sour cream.
- Olives.
- Mustard.
- Capers.
- Tempeh.
- Cider.
- Tea (which is made from fermented leaves).
- Mushrooms.
- Pickles.

This list may look daunting, but like every form of dietary change, it becomes easier as new habits are formed. Furthermore, candida can sometimes be overcome in a moderately short period of time, occasionally within a few days or weeks, although this is relatively uncommon. Also, unlike food allergies, yeast-promoting foods can sometimes be eaten in very limited quantities without triggering a self-perpetuating chain of metabolic dysfunction.

In addition, some of these foods are not nearly as harmful as others. For example, it's unlikely that a child would develop a serious candida problem just from eating a couple of olives, or a pickle, or a little ketchup. Of course, all three of these foods at once could aggravate the problem.

Just use common sense, and keep the intake of these foods under control. The significant problems will come from the obvious sources: breads, cake, crackers, and anything else that your child might eat in large volumes.

Furthermore, your child can get a huge boost from the nondietary elements of the anti-candida program: supplements and medication. The use of probiotic supplements, for example, can be profoundly beneficial.

One of the most important healing elements of the anti-yeast diet is its contribution to overcoming the condition of having microscopic holes in the gut, which allow undigested food molecules to escape from the gut and enter the system. In the system, the partial proteins from these food molecules often do terrible damage, particularly to the nervous system and immune system. This condition—known as leaky gut syndrome, or as intestinal hyperpermeability—is frequently caused by intestinal candidiasis. The yeast fungus decreases the ability of cells in the gut lining to adhere closely to each other, allowing food molecules to escape between the cells. Overcoming the candidal overgrowth, however, allows the cells to properly adhere, and prevents this from happening.

Some children can begin feeling better very, very quickly on the anti-yeast diet—in as little as a few days, in some cases. This is not common, but it does happen. When it does, it can provide a great boost, and amplify motivation.

It also may be prudent to try a candida challenge, by eating some yeast-proliferating foods, after there has been enough time for the candida signs to have cleared. If your child does not suffer any significant symptoms, it is possible that his or her body has corrected the conditions that allowed yeast to proliferate, and it can now be tolerated. If this is the case, your child may begin to eat yeast products again, preferably starting with small amounts. However, this challenge should only be attempted after your child has felt good for an extended period of time.

The human body is always changing, particularly as it undergoes the healing process, and it's important to be aware of these changes. They often signal a need, or an opportunity, for alteration of the Healing Program. Sometimes, though, even healing is not pleasant. Just as withdrawing from reactive foods can cause temporary discomfort, it can also cause discomfort to kill large volumes of candida during a short period. A massive die-off of yeast can trigger intensification of symptoms, which may last from a few days to one week, and occasionally longer. This will generally occur early in the anti-yeast program, rather than after a month or two. If it is particularly uncomfortable, it can be wise to temporarily discontinue any antifungal medication the child may have been taking. In addition, taking charcoal capsules may help speed the exit of the yeast toxins from the system. These interventions will help the body to detoxify itself from the dead candida cells. If and when medication is resumed, it should be restarted at a much lower dose, and be increased very gradually. Your child may continue taking the charcoal capsules, if necessary.

Work hard with your child at controlling yeast. It is an exceptionally common problem, even among generally healthy people, and in its more severe forms it can cause significant suffering.

Clearing candida from the system pays big dividends, and your child may not be able to reach the next level of recovery without doing it.

The Action Plan: What to Do About Candida

1. Restrict yeast-proliferating foods.
2. Take appropriate supplements and medications (see following chapters).
3. Slow down the anti-candida program if it becomes too uncomfortable.

(4) THE ANTI-HYPOGLYCEMIA DIET

Hypoglycemia, or low blood sugar, is very common among children with 4-A disorders, particularly those with autism and ADHD. Many of the symptoms of hypoglycemia are consistent with those of autism and ADHD, including poor cognitive function, irritability, propensity to tantrum, spaciness, lethargy, physical weakness, confusion, and inability to be consistently articulate. Therefore, I believe, as do other practitioners of biomedical treatment for autism and ADHD, that these hypoglycemic symptoms often mimic, amplify, and trigger symptoms of autism and ADHD. Thus, the symptoms of hypoglycemia can sometimes contribute to misdiagnoses of autism and especially ADHD, particularly when they are combined with symptoms of the other physical problems that so often afflict children with autism and ADHD.

Consider this following list of hypoglycemia symptoms, and note how several of these symptoms are also considered to be symptoms of autism and ADHD.

Symptoms of Hypoglycemia

What to Look for in Your Kids

- Nervousness and anxiety.
- Poor cognitive function, and poor memory.
- Confusion.
- Difficulty speaking.
- Tendency to have nightmares.
- Fatigue and lethargy.
- Spaciness and inattentiveness.
- Physical weakness, and shakiness when hungry.
- Depression.
- Excessive perspiration, or night sweats.
- Insomnia.
- Craving for foods, especially sweets and starchy foods.
- Need for frequent meals and snacks, and irritability if meals are missed or delayed.

Obviously, many of these symptoms are also similar to symptoms of food reactions and candida overgrowth. Once again, we see how all of these conditions overlap, aggravate one another, and combine to create powerful symptoms that can mimic and magnify symptoms of autism and ADHD. When these symptoms are combined with those of other common biological problems, such as hypothyroidism, chronic infections, toxicity, and nutritional deficiencies, the brain and nervous system can suffer terrible assault.

Low blood sugar in the cells can result from insulin resistance, the condition that is often triggered by inflammation. Therefore, anti-inflammatory foods and supplements can help.

The most frequent cause of hypoglycemia is a poor diet, too high in carbohydrates. Carbohydrates, which consist of either sugar or starch, travel through the digestive system very quickly, and can cause a spike of high blood sugar, which then can result in a slump of low blood sugar.

Therefore, the anti-hypoglycemia diet is based primarily around foods that travel slowly through the digestive process, such as high-protein foods and high-fiber foods.

The best foods to fight hypoglycemia are lean meats, fish, soy, beans, eggs, and fibrous, low-starch vegetables. If dairy products are well tolerated by your child, they are also acceptable. If your child has hypoglycemia, it's extremely important for him or her to have at least one of these high-protein, high-fiber foods at practically every meal.

The single most important healing element of the anti-hypoglycemia diet, though, is **avoiding sweet, sugary foods and high-starch foods.** Sugar and sweets are terrible for hypoglycemic kids. However, these kids often crave them, because sweets temporarily soothe the symptoms of the disorder. High-starch foods, such as potatoes or corn, can also be disruptive to blood sugar levels, because pure starch sprints through the system almost as quickly as pure sugar.

However, not all foods that derive most of their calories from starch are disruptive. Some of them, such as celery, peppers, or cabbage, just don't have enough starch in them to cause many problems. Most green vegetables, even though their calories come primarily from starch, are still so low in starch, and so high in fiber, that they don't trigger blood sugar spikes, followed by drops.

Grains often contribute to hypoglycemia, because they are high in starch, and are quickly digested. Hypoglycemic kids usually need to limit grains to only about two to three servings per day, or even less, and they should almost always be served as side dishes. When eaten as side dishes, with other slower-digested foods–high in proteins, fats, and oils–the grain foods are digested more slowly. Therefore, a hypoglycemic child should not, for example, have a breakfast consisting mostly of just cereal, or a muffin, or a bagel.

Furthermore, it's very important to limit grains to whole grains, which are higher in fiber. Processed grains, stripped of fiber, can have an effect similar to that of pure sugar.

All vegetables, fruits, and grains have been ranked on a scale called the Glycemic Index, which rates them according to how quickly they are digested, and according to how many carb calories they dump into the system. This rating system should be your guide to avoiding hypoglycemia.

The Glycemic Index of the Relatively High-Glycemic Foods

Foods are rated from best Glycemic Index to worst.

1. Beans.
2. Low-starch vegetables with peels intact.
3. Low-starch, peeled vegetables.
4. Moderate-climate fruits, such as apples or pears.
5. Nonrefined, bran cereals.
6. Whole rye, pumpernickel, and pita breads.
7. Wheat breads (including whole wheat and white), crackers, and pancake mixes.
8. Sweets, with nuts and fats added.
9. Brown rice.
10. Maple syrup.
11. Tropical fruits.
12. Wheat pasta.
13. Very sweet fruits (melons and raisins).
14. Potatoes, boiled.
15. Refined breakfast cereals.
16. Honey.
17. Rice cereals.
18. Rice pasta, rice cakes, and instant rice.
19. Table sugar, or pure-sugar candies, with no nuts or fat added.

The information was extrapolated from various sources.

To feel good on the anti-hypoglycemia diet, your child will simply need to focus on protein-rich, high-fiber foods that are slowly digested, relatively low in carbohydrate calories, and full of nutrients. These foods will provide the sense of satisfaction, or satiety, that helps kids feel good, and behave well. Also, your child should eat small, frequent meals throughout the day.

The Action Plan: What to Do About Hypoglycemia

The best way to beat hypoglycemia is:

1.   **Eat high-protein, high-fiber foods** at virtually every meal. Eat abundant amounts of lean meats, poultry, eggs, fish, soy, and beans.

2.   **Eat low-calorie, low-starch, high-fiber vegetables,** in abundance.

3.   **Avoid sweets** as much as possible.

4.   **Limit consumption** of high-starch, high-calorie, low-fiber vegetables, such as potatoes and corn.

5.   **Limit grains** to only a few servings per day, as side dishes. When you do eat grains, eat whole, high-fiber grains.

6.   **Limit fruits.** When you do eat fruits, eat low-calorie, low-starch, high-fiber fruits, such as apples, and avoid tropical and sugary fruits, such as pineapple, melons, and dates.

7.   **Limit caffeinated drinks,** because they contribute to blood sugar spikes.

8.   **Strictly limit fruit juices.** If they are consumed, make sure they are highly diluted with water. A good rule for the anti-hypoglycemia diet is: Don't drink your calories.

9.   **Eat frequent, high-protein meals and snacks,** to help stabilize blood sugar levels.

Your kids can feel better fast on this diet. They might not like it at first, especially when their sweets are restricted, but as they begin to feel better, they'll become more cooperative, and better motivated.

(5) THE SPECIFIC CARBOHYDRATE DIET

Some kids need an even more stringent diet than that of a combined GF/CF, specific food reaction, anti-yeast, anti-hypoglycemia diet. They need the specific carbohydrate diet, which limits even further the types and amounts of carbohydrates they may eat.

Most kids don't need this degree of restriction, but those who do can be helped very much by it. The relatively small subset of kids who do need it are sometimes referred to, within DAN circles, as nonresponders, because they don't seem to respond adequately to the more common dietary therapies, or to the other adjunctive biomedical treatments.

If your child does *not* seem to be responding robustly to his or her various therapies, including the nutritional therapies, you may need to try the specific carbohydrate diet for several months, to see if it can inaugurate the Healing Program's cascade of recovery.

What to Look for in Your Kids

• Colitis may be present, with gastrointestinal symptoms of persistent diarrhea, gas, bloating, abdominal pain, and intermittent constipation. This diet was developed by Elaine Gottschal, M.Sc., to help her child, who had severe ulcerative colitis.

• Symptoms of persistent bowel dysbiosis may occur, in conjunction with behavioral and cognitive symptoms that have not cleared, despite treatment with other biomedical therapies, including the GF/CF diet, the specific food reaction diet, the anti-hypoglycemia diet, and the anti-yeast diet.

Because this diet is somewhat more difficult than the others, Dr. Sid Baker went on it himself, to see what it was like. He was surprised to discover that it was relatively easy for him, after a period of adjustment. It gave him a great boost of energy, and helped him lose some weight. Therefore, even though this diet can be a challenge for many children, it may be helpful, and practical, for some. Dr. Baker has installed it as an important element in his treatment of autism, and has stated that it is one of the best treatments for many children who are on the autism spectrum.

The diet is based upon further, more stringent restriction of carbohydrates. These carbs are believed to aggravate existing bacterial infection, and to contribute to inflammation in the gut. This occurs when the carbs—consisting of either starch or sugar—are not fully digested, due to enzyme deficiencies. The specific type of carbohydrate that is hard for some people to digest is the disaccharide, which consists of two sugar molecules.

These undigested carbs cause further inflammation, trigger excessive production of mucus, increase bacterial proliferation, and contribute to leaky gut syndrome.

To overcome these problems, certain foods in the following categories must be restricted:

Food Restrictions on the Specific Carbohydrate Diet

Proteins. Eliminate processed meats, such as hot dogs, bologna, spiced ham, breaded fish, canned meat, and also processed cheese.

Vegetables. Eliminate canned vegetables, potatoes, yams, soybeans, and garbanzo beans.

Grains. Eliminate virtually all grains, including some that do not have gluten, such as rice, buckwheat, and millet. Eliminate wheat, bulgur, corn, oats, rye, quinoa, and tapioca.

Fruits. Eliminate canned fruits, dried fruits that have been sweetened, jams, jellies, and ketchup.

Nuts. Eliminate roasted nuts, peanuts in salted mixtures, and glazed nuts.

Beverages. Eliminate cow's milk, goat's milk, soy milk, rice milk, canned coconut milk, tea, and soft drinks.

This diet, like others that correct long-standing gut problems, typically creates uncomfortable healing reactions from time to time, as the body eliminates toxic material, and rebalances itself. It is common for regressions in health and behavior to occur soon after the diet begins, and at two to three months, at five months, at seven months, and at nine months. These unpleasant healing episodes can last for up to two weeks. If they do occur, they are positive signs of recovery, even though they may be temporarily unsettling. To ease discomfort, you may wish to increase your child's detoxification efforts during these periods (see Chapter 19).

For access to more information on the specific carbohydrate diet, which is also referred to as the SCD, consult Appendix #2.

This diet is not for everyone. Most children can recover or improve without it. However, it can be tremendously helpful for some. Although the diet is stringent, it is quite comparable to a popular nongrain, nondairy diet commonly known as the paleolithic diet. Many people have used the paleolithic diet to lose weight and feel better. Those who thrive on it quickly learn to appreciate it.

The SCD is one of the newer approaches to nutritional therapy for autism. It has not yet clinically demonstrated the broad degree of efficacy of the more established nutritional therapies. Even so, if your child is a nonresponder, this may be a fruitful approach.

The Action Plan: What to Do for the SCD

1. **Monitor** your child's symptoms for reactions to carbs, if he or she has not responded to the prior diets.

2. **Restrict** the appropriate carbohydrate foods (those containing disaccharides).

3. **Continue to monitor** symptoms, to see if this diet is helping.

4. **Discontinue it,** if it doesn't seem to be working.

(6) THE LOW-OXALATE DIET

This is one of the newest and least commonly used nutritional therapies for autism-spectrum disorders, but it has shown signs of promise. Some children have improved on this diet after having failed to sufficiently recover with other approaches.

However, it has not been scientifically evaluated, and is therefore still in the experimental stage. There is some science that suggests it may be helpful in a certain subset of children, but more testing needs to be done.

My own experience with this diet is limited, but it has proven helpful with some of my patients.

The low-oxalate diet consists solely of reducing or eliminating a common food component called an oxalate. Oxalates are found in many foods, and some people appear to inadequately metabolize them. Oxalates bind with calcium, and therefore excessive consumption of oxalates can contribute to the calcium formations in the kidneys known as kidney stones. Many people who have kidney stones go on the low-oxalate diet.

Some kids who do not thrive on the specific carbohydrate diet do better with this approach, possibly because the SCD encourages the consumption of flour made from nuts, which are high in oxalates.

Besides interfering with calcium metabolism, excessive amounts of oxalates can be toxic, and they can significantly interfere with proper function of the gut.

In addition, there are preliminary indications that this diet has been of benefit to women who suffer from vulvodynia/vulvar vestibulitis, which may be a further indication of its possible efficacy.

What to Look for in Your Kids

- GI pain within two hours of eating.
- Frequent urination.
- Difficulty with digesting fats.
- Adverse reactions to TMG or DMG.
- Chronic constipation and diarrhea.
- Cravings for high-oxalate foods.
- Inflammation of the gut.
- Symptoms of bowel dysbiosis, in conjunction with behavioral and cognitive symptoms that have not cleared, despite treatment with other biomedical therapies, including the GF/CF diet, the specific food reaction diet, the anti-hypoglycemia diet, the anti-yeast diet, and the specific carbohydrate diet.

Following is a list of high-oxalate foods.

High-oxalate beverages. Chocolate milk, cocoa, Ovaltine, any juice from high-oxalate fruits.

High-oxalate proteins. Almonds, baked beans canned in tomato sauce, cashews, green beans, peanut butter, peanuts, pecans, sesame, sunflower seeds, tofu, walnuts.

High-oxalate fruits. Blackberries, black raspberries, red raspberries, blueberries, red currants, dewberries, figs, dried grapes, purple gooseberries, kiwi, lemon peel, lime peel, orange peel, rhubarb, strawberries, tangerines, any juice made from these fruits.

High-oxalate breads and starches. Fig Newtons, fruit cake, graham crackers, grits, white corn, kamut, marmalade, soybean crackers, wheat germ.

High-oxalate vegetables. Beans, beets, celery, chives, collards, eggplant, kale, leeks, okra, parsley, parsnips, peppers, rutabaga, spinach, summer squash, sweet potato, Swiss chard, tomato soup, vegetable soup, watercress, yams.

High-oxalate condiments. Cinnabar, parsley, pepper, ginger, soy sauce.

The Action Plan: What to Do About Oxalates

1. **Monitor** your child's symptoms for reactions to oxalates, if they have not responded to the prior diets.
2. **Restrict** oxalate foods.
3. **Continue** to monitor symptoms, to see if this diet is helping.
4. **Discontinue it,** if it doesn't seem to be helping.

SUMMARY: THE HEALING PROGRAM'S NUTRITIONAL THERAPY

Here's the simplest possible summary of nutritional therapy: Restrict gluten and casein for a few months, along with any specific foods that cause reactions, and be careful about yeast-proliferating foods, excessive carbs, and nonorganic foods.

That's all most kids require, and many of them don't even need to do that much.

If you do all that and are still having lots of problems, consider the SCD, and the low-oxalate diet.

Practically every child can benefit to some degree from these basic, commonsense recommendations. Even healthy kids often get healthier.

Here's a nice side benefit: You'll inevitably begin to follow many of these new rules yourself, and when you do, you may feel better than you have in years. Wholesome, whole, nonreactive foods are good for *everyone*.

Now let's move on to supplementation therapy. An individualized program of supplementation, applied judiciously, can turbocharge the healing effects of nutritional therapy, and help your child to finally feel better.

CHAPTER EIGHTEEN

THE HEALING PROGRAM

Element #2:
Supplementation Therapy

NUTRITIONAL SUPPLEMENTS HAVE CONSISTENTLY DEMONSTRATED a high degree of efficacy in contributing to recovery from the 4-A disorders, and particularly in aiding recovery from autism and ADHD. Every practitioner of biomedical therapy for autism and ADHD now includes supplementation therapy as an integral element of his or her treatment program. Supplementation therapy is also very valuable in treating asthma and allergies.

Supplements–consisting of vitamins, minerals, amino acids, essential fatty acids, enzymes, and herbal preparations–contribute to recoveries in ways that other modalities simply cannot. They are uniquely beneficial in overcoming nutrient deficiencies, and they have an unmatched power to trigger various metabolic healing processes. Supplements are also ideal for fulfilling nutrient dependencies, the highly individualized requirements for various nutrients that vary greatly from person to person.

Autistic children, in particular, typically have an astonishing array of nutritional deficiencies and dependencies, as well as some excesses. These deficiencies and dependencies almost always contribute to their symptomatology. Overcoming the deficiencies and dependencies invariably requires supplements. The excesses can also be ameliorated, or balanced, by using specific supplements.

Among the deficiencies that I often find in autistic children are:

COMMON NUTRIENT DEFICIENCIES AND DEPENDENCIES IN AUTISTIC CHILDREN

- Calcium.
- Selenium.
- Zinc.
- Magnesium.
- Iron.
- Cysteine.
- Sulfate.
- Taurine.

- B-12.
- B-6.
- Lysine.
- Methionine.
- Essential fatty acids.
- Vitamin D.
- Vitamin E.
- Vitamin A.

In addition, autistic kids tend to have *excesses* of copper and glutamate, both of which can be directly or indirectly neurotoxic.

Each of the nutrient deficiencies among autistic children can have its own direct, negative effects. For example, low iron can cause the feelings of lethargy that are often, paradoxically, a symptom of ADHD. Furthermore, each deficiency can have indirect negative effects, by disrupting various metabolic processes. Low iron, for example, can also contribute to relatively higher levels of lead, which can lower IQ and contribute to cognitive dysfunction, and symptoms of ADHD.

Deficiencies, and sometimes excesses–particularly when present in numerous combinations–can create vast cascades of dysfunction in each of the three major systems involved in autism and ADHD: the gastrointestinal system, the immune system, and the nervous system.

These impaired systems–particularly the gastrointestinal system–then contribute to further nutrient deficiencies, in an ongoing cycle of degeneration. For example, impairment of the gut, due to nutrient deficiencies (or other factors, such as infections), can result in poor digestion, chronic diarrhea, malabsorption of nutrients, leaky gut syndrome, and other GI disorders. These disorders then aggravate and exacerbate existing nutrient deficiencies, and create new deficiencies.

4-A children are notably vulnerable to nutrient deficiencies and imbalances, due partly to the high number of gastrointestinal disorders that typically affect them. These include:

COMMON DIGESTIVE AND GI DISORDERS AMONG 4-A CHILDREN

- General bowel dysbiosis.
  - Yeast overgrowth in the gut.
  - Presence of other gut pathogens, including parasites.
  - Chronic viral and bacterial infections in the gut.
- Diarrhea and constipation.
- Abdominal bloating and excess gas.
- Excessively limited food choices during meals.
- Autoimmune disorders affecting GI function.
- Frequent presence of food reactions.

These GI problems create nutrient deficiencies that can be overcome only with the relatively high dosages of nutrients that are available in supplements.

Compensating for deficiencies, however, is not the only reason to take supplements. Supplements sometimes act as medications, triggering dormant healing processes. For example, methyl-B-12 can help trigger a restoration of the process of methylation. When the miracle of methylation is restored, the bodies of autistic kids can once again begin to detoxify themselves. Therefore, this one relatively simple course of supplementation therapy can exert an astonishing healing effect, which can change children's lives.

In addition to helping heal the brain and nervous system, supplementation therapy can also improve the function of other systems that are often involved in autism, ADHD, asthma, and allergies. Supplements, for example, can be extraordinarily beneficial to the immune system. A combination of zinc, vitamin A, vitamin C, transfer factor, and other specific nutrients can help restore the impaired immune function that is often a critical root cause of the 4-A disorders.

Some parents, however, are resistant to the concept of supplementation therapy, because they often hear presumed experts in the media saying that a healthy diet is sufficient to provide all necessary nutrients. This sounds reasonable—but it's not.

WHY DIET ALONE ISN'T ENOUGH

One reason diet alone is not enough is because kids with the 4-A disorders have specific, elevated needs. These heightened needs require full-scale, comprehensive nutritional and supplementation therapy–not just a wholesome diet. These kids need more than minimum daily requirements.

To achieve a therapeutic effect from nutrition, relatively high levels of specific nutrients are needed. These high levels are generally not attainable just from the daily diet. For example, to achieve a relatively high dosage of vitamin C, such as 500 mg.–the amount found in many vitamin C tablets or capsules–a person would need to eat ten oranges. Similarly, to get 50 mg. of B-6, which is a typical amount found in many supplements, a person would need to eat twenty pounds of liver.

Furthermore, our modern, American food supply has been stripped of many nutrients that were previously available in foods. The nutrient levels in foods have been degraded by the advent of large-scale, high-production agribusiness. Many foods are now notably less nutritious than they were in the days when small farms dominated agriculture. Forces such as monoculture of crops, hybridization, and intense fertilization have resulted in devitalized grains, fruits, and vegetables that often look large, glossy, and healthy, but are in reality only a few steps above junk food.

Another reason that some experts are also critical of people taking relatively large amounts of supplements is because of the fact that excessive amounts of some supplements may harm health. This is a reasonable concern, but it is very limited in scope. Vitamin A and vitamin D can be toxic if taken in extremely high amounts, but illness due to this is very rare. Illness from supplements is particularly rare when compared to the health damage that is consistently done by pharmaceutical drugs. For example, in one recent seven-year period, the U.S. Poison Control Centers reported that there were 2,556 fatalities caused by medically prescribed drugs, but no deaths from supplements. Other reputable agencies and organizations have stated that deaths from pharmaceutical drugs are drastically higher than this–up to 20,000 to 100,000 per year.

An exception to the safety of supplements would be gross overuse of stimulating herbs, such as ephedra, which was recently banned in the United States. Overdose of ephedra can be fatal, and it was implicated in several deaths before it was removed from the market. However, no stimulating herbs are used in the Healing Program. I do recommend a few herbal preparations for specific problems, but all of these herbs– such as garlic or oregano oil–are notably benign.

Supplements can, however, cause rather subtle and complex adverse reactions in some people. Unfortunately, these reactions are sometimes rather confusing. For example, a few kids may have a negative reaction to the substance phosphatidylcholine, the active ingredient in lecithin. This supplement is somewhat calming to most children, but some kids have a paradoxical reaction of hyperactivity, due to their own unique metabolic profiles. Thus, we again see the need for a carefully individualized program.

POSSIBLE ADVERSE REACTIONS FROM HEALING PROGRAM SUPPLEMENTS

• **Vitamin A** is a fat-soluble vitamin that can be toxic if taken in extremely high dosages. The *Merck Manual of Diagnosis and Therapy* sets the level of toxicity at ingestion of 300,000 international units per day, but I believe that significantly lower doses than this can cause at least subtle harm in some small children. Generally, children can safely take 2,500 to 10,000 i.u. per day, depending on their age, size, and their existing levels of vitamin A. However, some children appear to require higher doses, in order to return their vitamin A levels to the normal range. Their vitamin A levels should be monitored periodically to ensure that they remain within the normal range.

• **Vitamin D** is another fat-soluble vitamin with the potential for toxicity at excessive doses. It can be toxic in adults who take more than 100,000 i.u. daily for several months, according to the *Merck Manual*. Infants can suffer toxic reactions to 3,000 i.u. per day, if taken every day for an extended period. I usually recommend no more than approximately 800 i.u. per day for children. Similarly to vitamin A, I monitor vitamin D levels periodically to ensure that levels are within a safe, normal range.

• **Zinc** can partially suppress immunity at extremely high dosages, although this is contrary to its typical effect of enhancing immunity at lower to moderate doses. I usually recommend doses in the 20- to 60-mg. range, with a maximum of about 90 to 100 mg. per day for children. Zinc can also trigger a copper deficiency at very high dosages.

• **Enzymes** can contribute to diarrhea if too many are taken. For a child, even two to three per day might be too many, so be alert for this reaction. If it occurs, decrease the dose, and if it is still not tolerated, discontinue the enzymes.

• **DMG, TMG, and methyl-B-12** can contribute to hyperactivity, irritability, and emotional outbursts in some autistic children. If this reaction occurs, stop giving your child any or all of these supplements, then attempt to reintroduce them again individually, at a later date, and at lower dosages. If adverse reactions recur, you should stop them again. Another strategy is to add folinic acid, which may reduce the hyperactivity.

• **B-6 and other B-vitamins,** which are usually calming, can cause paradoxical hyperactivity and irritability in a small but significant subset of children. Also, B-6 can be toxic in exceptionally high dosages, such as 2,000 mg. or more per day, taken for two months or longer. I recommend 50- to 100-mg. doses, one to several times per day, based on weight. However, I usually do not exceed 500 mg. daily for most children.

• **SAMe** is another supplement that can cause side effects in a significant subset of autistic children. This supplement–like DMG, TMG, and methyl-B-12–is a methylator, and some kids appear to be sensitive to supplemental methylators, especially SAMe. For them, it may be helpful to use supplements that actually tone down methylation. As I've noted, no two kids are exactly the same.

• **Phosphatidylcholine** is another supplement that can exert paradoxical effects. It calms most kids down, but a few become hyperactive and irritable from it.

• **Iron** can create too much oxidation within the body at high levels, causing oxidative stress and inflammation. Many kids don't need iron, but those who do can benefit greatly from it. Because of this type of variation among children, it's important to have nutrient levels tested at the beginning of the Healing Program.

I have noticed that, as a general rule, at least 10 percent of all children may react negatively to certain nutrients, even though the other 90 percent either react positively or show no response at all. I call this the Ten Percent Rule. As medical detectives, we must always stay alert for the 10 percent of negative reactions that are the exceptions to the rule. Furthermore, some nutrients, such as TMG, may cause reactions in even more than 10 percent.

Now let's look at the specific supplements that might help your child's recovery.

For the most part, with certain exceptions, I do not recommend supplements based only upon a child's diagnosed pathology. For example, I don't recommend a single, specific set of supplements for all autistic children, or a single set for all ADHD children. That type of nonindividualized, pathology-based fragmentation is contradictory to the spirit of the Healing Program.

The Healing Program is a comprehensive strategy for the general rebuilding of health, and most of us need relatively similar things to achieve and restore health. Therefore, I recommend a somewhat similar program of supplements for most kids, and individualize these programs based upon *the unique needs of each child*. In short, as I've mentioned, I treat the child, not the disorder.

Almost all kids, as well as most adults, need certain very common supplements. Some also need extra supplements for specific problems. Still others need an even wider scope of supplements. Therefore, I have placed the Healing Program supplements that I recommend in three tiers, based upon how commonly they are needed by 4-A kids, as well as when I may add them to their supplement programs.

Tier One consists of the basic, fundamental nutrients that almost all children need to thrive, such as vitamin C, calcium, magnesium, and essential fatty acids.

Tier Two also consists of some basic, fundamental nutrients, as well as more specialized supplements that only certain patients will need. For example, some kids need the Tier Two supplement melatonin, generally as a sleep aid, and some don't. Similarly, some kids have a deficiency–or another type of need–for vitamin D, and some don't. Also, only a certain percentage of patients need extra chromium–generally for hypoglycemia, or carbohydrate cravings and intolerance.

Tier Three also consists of more specialized supplements that only certain patients will need, and which will generally be added at a later point in their supplement programs. For example, only some kids will need to take the Tier Three supplement quercitin, which may be helpful to patients with airway obstruction and allergic inflammation.

Here are the three tiers.

Tier One Supplements

- Vitamin C.
- Vitamin E.
- Zinc.
- Calcium/magnesium.
- Vitamin A (generally given in the form of cod liver oil, which also contains vitamin D and DHA).
- Essential fatty acids.
- Probiotics.

Tier Two Supplements

- Digestive enzymes.
- Vitamin B-6.
- Taurine.
- Melatonin.
- Methyl-B-12 (or methylcobalamin).
- Folinic acid.
- *N*-acetyl-cysteine.
- Amino acids, including branched-chain amino acids (consisting of leucine, isoleucine, and valine).
- TMG, or DMG (trimethylglycine, or dimethylglycine).
- Vitamin D.
- Coenzyme Q-10.
- Transfer factor.
- Selenium.
- Iron.
- Chromium.
- Multiple vitamin/mineral.

Tier Three Supplements

- *N*-acetyl-carnitine.
- DMAE.

- Silymarin.
- 5-HTP.
- Activated charcoal.
- Pantothenic acid (vitamin B-5).
- Phosphatidylcholine.
- Oral gamma globulin.
- Pycnogenol.
- Other herbal preparations, including:
  - Quercitin.
  - Curcumin.
  - Oregano oil.
  - Caprylic acid.
  - Olive leaf extract.
  - Garlic.
  - Lauricidin.
- Creatine.
- Carnosine.
- SAMe.

It's common for me to give a specific patient all of the Tier One supplements, plus a number of the Tier Two supplements, plus several of the Tier Three supplements. They may be taken in various combinations. It all depends upon the patient. I typically recommend supplements according to these three fundamental, clinical issues:

• **Deficiencies,** as established by laboratory testing, and by symptomatology.

• **Therapeutic goals,** such as the restoration of methylation; or relieving hyperactivity; or increasing cognitive function.

• **Response of the patient,** either positive or negative.

However, I also must consider the cost of the supplements. Almost no insurance companies reimburse for supplements, and some of the supplements can be rather expensive. A full regimen for a seriously ill child could easily cost $100 to several hundred dollars per month. This is a lot of money for most families, but it can be a smart investment in health care, particularly when compared to the costs of so many other therapies, such as the behavioral treatments that require one-on-one attention from therapists. Also, as recovery takes hold, it's often possible to discontinue certain supplements.

Supplements can be purchased more cheaply from discount stores and mail-order companies, and many of the supplements from these sources are of high quality–particularly for the most basic nutrients, such as vitamin C or A. However, it's often wise to buy the more specialized supplements from purveyors who have a reputation for very high quality.

It is possible that your doctor will offer a line of supplements in his or her own office. This is a relatively common practice among integrative medical practitioners, because it ensures that patients will receive high-quality, standardized supplements.

There are available to patients supplements carefully designed to improve the function of the key neurological, immunological, gastrointestinal, and metabolic systems I explain in this book. These supplements are not intended to treat autism, ADHD, asthma, and allergies, but the functional support they provide may be appropriate for your child. In general, you should feel free to investigate sources of nutraceuticals, and purchase them from whatever source you choose. For more information, please consult Appendix #2, "Resources for Help."

In addition to the cost of supplements, I must also consider the willingness of my young patients to take a relatively heavy schedule of supplements. Kids can be stubborn, and some of them have a hard time swallowing pills. If it's difficult for your child to take pills, try to find brands that are chewable, or in powder form, or liquid form, or that are relatively small in size. If necessary, you can grind them up yourself.

As you may recall, I previously noted that I generally recommend that kids start their new diets before they begin to take supplements. However, like so many other aspects of the Healing Program, the timing of this can be flexible. The sequence of the two elements can be switched, depending upon the needs and desires of the individual patient and family. Some kids do better if they take a few supplements before they change their diets, or occasionally at the same time they change their diets. The advantage of this is that the supplements often provide a pleasant boost in how the patient feels, and in how well he or she functions, and these boosts can be great motivators. For many kids, taking supplements is easier than changing their diets, so they may be able to adjust to their programs better by doing the easiest part first.

Therefore, we again see that the Healing Program is malleable, and can be based around individual preferences, and also around the progress that is triggered by various modalities.

The Healing Program is always a work in progress. Children change. Their bodies change. Their brains change. Their tastes change.

Doctors and parents need to keep up with these changes, and to direct the changes in the most positive possible directions.

Because of these ongoing changes, it can be quite helpful to continue to monitor levels of nutrients as the program progresses. *Start supplementation therapy by testing for nutrient levels–then retest again periodically, as appropriate, with your doctor's guidance.*

Now let's look in detail at every supplement, from all three tiers. The following information will probably be of great help to you over the next few months, as you begin to help your child reach his or her highest, and happiest, potential.

There's a lot of information here. Don't try to learn it all. Use this as a reference source. Also, if you would like an even more detailed reference source, you should order *Autism, Effective Biomedical Treatments* by Jon Pangborn, Ph.D., and Sidney Baker, M.D. The book is one of the finest ever written about the biomedical approach to autism, and is available from DAN.

TIER ONE SUPPLEMENTS

Nutrients Needed by Almost Every Child

Vitamin C. This nutrient is of special benefit to autistic kids, as well as other 4-A kids, for several reasons.

- *It reduces harmful oxidants.* Research shows that autistic children often suffer from excessive oxidation. This creates oxidant stress, and damages brain cells.

- *It helps balance levels of dopamine.* Dopamine is the neurotransmitter that is often imbalanced in kids with ADHD symptoms and autistic symptoms. Vitamin C helps change dopamine into norepinephrine.

- *It helps balance two important amino acids–phenylalanine and tyrosine.* These two nutrients are important for physical and mental energy, and have a direct impact upon the brain.

- *It helps form L-carnitine.* This amino acid helps metabolize fatty acids. Many autistic kids have trouble metabolizing fatty acids, and this can cause neurological and GI symptoms.

- *It helps balance hormone levels*–particularly those of oxytocin, vasopressin, and cholecystokinin, which are often imbalanced in autistic kids. Oxytocin, in particular, is important for emotional bonding. Women giving birth typically experience a surge of oxytocin.

- *It can help modulate immunity,* which is often impaired in children with 4-A disorders.

- *It can help decrease and prevent constipation,* a common disorder among 4-A kids. Magnesium also helps with this.

Parents of autistic kids rate vitamin C very favorably as a treatment. In the 2006 Autism Research Institute (ARI) survey of approximately two thousand parents of autistic children, vitamin C was rated as follows:

- **Symptoms improved: 41 percent.**
- **No discernible effect: 57 percent.**
- **Symptoms worse: 2 percent (generally diarrhea).**

My general recommendation: 250 to 2000 mg. per day, depending upon age, size, and other treatments and indications.

Vitamin E. This vitamin is occasionally deficient among autistics and other 4-A kids. It is primarily used therapeutically to boost several important metabolic functions:

- *It is an important antioxidant,* especially when the form known as gamma tocopherol is used.

• *It potentiates the effect of methyl-B-12.*

• *It boosts sulfation,* the biochemical partner of methylation, by helping preserve cysteine, glutathione, and several enzymes.

• *It helps prevent essential fatty acids from being oxidized.*

• *It helps restore damaged cells in the liver,* especially in people with low cysteine and glutathione.

• *It helps protect against the damage done by saturated and oxidized fats.* These fats can damage brain cells and blood vessels, and can impair GI function.

• *It reduces susceptibility of children to neuromuscular diseases.*

• *It helps boost immunity.*

My general recommendation: 100 to 400 i.u. per day, depending upon age, size, and other treatments and indications.

Zinc. Do you remember the phrase, "No zinc, no think?" Zinc is vital for proper cognitive function, but it is typically deficient among autistics. In one study of autistics, 85 percent had low zinc.

Zinc deficiency also impairs digestion, methylation, and the immune response. In addition, it can contribute to excessive levels of copper, which can be neurotoxic.

Zinc deficiency often occurs because of GI dysfunction, which is then exacerbated by low zinc, in a destructive cycle. This cycle is common among autistics.

One advantage of giving zinc is that it tends to increase the desire of autistic kids to eat a wider range of foods, in contrast to their usual limited preferences.

Parent ratings of zinc use, according to the 2006 ARI survey:

• **Symptoms improved: 48 percent.**
• **No discernible effect: 49 percent.**
• **Symptoms worsened: 3 percent.**

Here are some guidelines for maximizing the benefits of zinc.

- *Give zinc between meals, or give all of it at bedtime.*
- *If possible, don't give zinc at the same time as calcium, iron, folate, or lecithin.*
- *Be aware of possible urinary zinc loss during chelation.*

Because zinc is closely associated with proper digestion, zinc levels may not begin to rise until GI issues have been resolved.

My general recommendation: 20 to 60 mg. per day, and occasionally more, depending upon age, size, and other treatments and indications.

Calcium and Magnesium. I invariably give these two minerals together, because they work in tandem.

Calcium is often deficient in autistics, because of low dietary intake, and because of malabsorption, due to GI problems. Low dietary intake can be exacerbated by a dairy-free diet. Calcium is particularly low in people with celiac disease, the condition of extreme sensitivity to gluten.

Calcium is an important element in hormonal activities, which are often impaired among 4-A kids. It's good for bones, and is also known to have calming effects in some children.

In the ARI parent rating systems, calcium scored as follows:

- **Symptoms improved: 36 percent.**
- **No discernible effect: 62 percent.**
- **Symptoms worsened: 2 percent.**

If you give your child calcium in the form of calcium carbonate (from eggshells or coral), it's good to also give them some in a more soluble form, such as calcium citrate or calcium ascorbate. Calcium citrate is the most readily absorbable form of calcium, but some children show elevated levels of citrate, on urinary organic acid testing, and therefore may need to take other forms of calcium. Calcium carbonate, although not nearly as absorbable, can help avoid GI problems and can help with excess acidity. Of course, some of your child's calcium requirement of 800 to 1,200 mg. per day will be supplied by foods, such as soy or rice milk.

My general recommendation: 400 to 1,000 mg. per day, depending upon age, size, and other treatments and indications.

Magnesium should be given with calcium, and also with B-6, both of which synergistically augment and balance magnesium's effects.

Magnesium is often low in children with behavioral, cognitive, and mood disorders. Symptoms of magnesium deficiency include:

- *Depression, or anxiety.*
- *Constipation.*
- *Tics, muscle jerks, and spasms.*
- *Poor appetite.*

Magnesium is important in methylation and sulfation, the processes that can correct heavy metal overload, because it helps to activate certain key enzymes. This magnesium-assisted process of methylation is also important in neurotransmitter and hormone metabolism. Magnesium is also one of the best minerals for restoring sulfation, which is commonly impaired in autistics.

According to the 2006 ARI parent rating scale:

- **Symptoms improved: 29 percent.**
- **No discernible effect: 65 percent.**
- **Symptoms worsened: 6 percent.**

Strategies for administering magnesium include:

- *Administer it with B-6 and calcium.*
- *Start it early in the nutritional and supplementation therapy programs.*
- *Take it at meals, preferably breakfast.*
- *Test varying amounts, to determine the optimal intake.*

The primary adverse reaction to oral magnesium is diarrhea. If this occurs, try a magnesium sulfate cream, or try baths with Epsom salt (unless eczema or dry skin is a problem).

My general recommendation: 100 to 500 mg. per day, depending upon age, size, and other treatments and indications.

Cod Liver Oil. This oil is rich in vitamin D, vitamin A, and essential fatty acids (especially DHA). All of these nutrients are often low in autistic kids, and also in many children with ADHD and asthma. Because cod liver oil has so many important ingredients, all of which are present in balance, it is usually better to give cod liver oil than the isolated forms of the nutrients that are in it. However, combining cod liver oil with extra amounts of these specific nutrients can also be helpful for many children.

Vitamin A is frequently low in autistics, and this deficiency accounts for some of the vision problems that are common in autistic kids. The deficiency affects the eyes' cones and rods, and contributes to the tendency of autistic kids to rely upon their peripheral vision. This reliance–the classic autistic sideways gaze–often results in poor eye contact. This symptom is still considered by many doctors to be a purely psychological trait, indicating emotional avoidance, which has no physiological component. However, this perspective appears to be out of date, because the condition frequently improves with the administration of cod liver oil.

Vitamin A is also an important immune booster, and is often referred to as the anti-infective vitamin. Therefore, taking vitamin A–in cod liver oil, or in vitamin A supplements, or in both–is important for the many 4-A kids who have immune problems.

Vitamin A also increases the communication ability of cells, including brain cells, by stimulating the transmission of signals from cell to cell.

The 2006 ARI autism rating scale for cod liver oil:

- **Symptoms improved: 49 percent.**
- **No discernible effect: 47 percent.**
- **Symptoms worsened: 4 percent.**

Cod liver oil is sold in capsules, and also in liquid form. I generally recommend the liquid form, which may be absorbed better, and although some kids object to the taste, many will tolerate the newer flavored forms. It is important that the cod liver oil you use is free of mercury, PCBs, and other environmental pollutants.

My general recommendation: one to three teaspoons per day, depending upon age, size, and other treatments and indications.

Essential Fatty Acids. EFAs are commonly low among kids with the 4-A disorders. The particular EFAs that are most likely to be low in autistic children are EPA and DHA, the latter of which is very abundant in brain cells. DHA contributes to the function of brain cell receptors, which allow the entry of important neurological chemicals, including neurotransmitters and hormones.

EFAs are especially likely to be low in kids with bowel dysbiosis, because of poor assimilation of dietary EFAs.

EFAs are critically important as anti-inflammatories and as the primary building material for cell membranes, which let nutrients in and toxins out. When cell membranes don't have enough of the right EFAs, they become inflexible, and don't facilitate the exchange of nutrients-in, toxins-out. This can lead to nutrient deficiency, and toxic accumulation.

There are two basic types of EFAs: omega-3s and omega-6s. Omega-3s include ALA (alpha linolenic acid), EPA (eicosapentaenoic acid), and DHA (docosahexaenoic acid). The omega-6s include LA (linoleic acid), GLA (gamma-linolenic acid), DHGLA (dihomogamma-linolenic acid), and AA (arachidonic acid).

The omega-6 fatty acid GLA, which is low among many 4-A kids—particularly those with skin problems—is in primrose oil, borage oil, and black currant seed oil. The omega-3 EFAs are abundant in fish oil.

EFAs are generally very well tolerated. The most common adverse reaction is possible bowel upset in some children, generally occurring only if they take an excessive dosage. As with most nutritional supplements, however, it is best to start at a lower dose and gradually increase to the desired dose.

In the ARI parent rating scale, EFAs scored as follows:

- **Symptoms improved: 54 percent.**
- **No discernible effect: 43 percent.**
- **Symptoms worsened: 2 percent.**

My general recommendation: EPA/DHA: ¼ to 1 teaspoon liquid per day, or 2 to 6 caps per day; GLA: 80 to 240 mg. per day, depending upon age, size, and other treatments and indications.

Probiotics. Because bowel dysbiosis is extraordinarily common among autistics and other 4-A kids, probiotics are of consummate importance. It is often simply not possible to heal kids with 4-A disorders without first healing bowel dysbiosis, which is the root cause of so many of their problems, including candida overgrowth, leaky gut syndrome, chronic diarrhea and constipation, chronic gut infection, and malabsorption of nutrients.

Probiotics are healthy bacteria that promote good digestion, and help control dysbiotic gut flora, such as candida. Probiotics are abundant in yogurt, but much greater amounts are present in supplements.

Probiotics are of special importance for any child who has recently taken antibiotics. Antibiotics kill both good and bad gut bacteria, and can therefore destroy the healthy flora that the GI system needs.

Probiotics control candida by crowding out the yeast fungi, or by directly attacking it, with the probiotic constituent *Saccharomyces boulardii*.

Probiotics also promote Th-1 immunity, and can help to balance a Th-2 skewed immune system.

I strongly recommend that you use high-quality probiotics that contain large numbers of viable organisms. The amount of organisms in the probiotics, and the quality of their ability to adhere to the gut wall, are essential to their efficacy. Although products with higher numbers of organisms and better adherence quality cost more, the expense is worth the gain in this particular class of supplements, because they appear to produce superior clinical results.

When taking probiotics, it's important to support their action by first eliminating yeast-proliferating foods, and reactive foods. If this is done, probiotics can help to prevent further food reactions, and further yeast overgrowth, as gut health improves.

Because probiotics can oppose candida, they occasionally trigger an uncomfortable healing reaction during phases of rapid yeast die-off. This can temporarily increase hyperactivity, stimming, irritability, and other symptoms. These healing reactions tend to last a few days to one week, although they occasionally persist a bit longer. However, there is a relatively small subset of autistic kids who don't seem to tolerate probiotics, and probiotics should not be given if the child appears to react negatively.

If your child has lactose or casein problems, as do about 60 percent of all autistic kids, don't buy probiotics that are derived from milk. In fact, I generally do not recommend dairy-derived probiotics to any child.

My general recommendation: one to two high-potency, high-quality probiotic capsules, or the equivalent in a powdered form, per day, depending upon age, size, and other treatments and indications.

TIER TWO SUPPLEMENTS

These supplements are appropriate for a very large percentage of the 4-A patient population. Most 4-A kids take many, or most, of these supplements, at least temporarily.

Some of the supplements are in the second tier because they are either not as important for most kids as the first tier supplements, or just may not be introduced until a later time. For example, selenium is good for almost everyone, but I may not introduce it as early as vitamin C. Other supplements are in the second tier because they're appropriate for only certain children. For those specific kids, though, they may be critically important. For example, melatonin is not needed by everyone, but it's quite important for kids who have sleep problems.

Here are the sixteen Tier Two supplements.

Digestive Enzymes. In 2000, Andrew Wakefield, M.D., reported evidence of chronic colitis in 88 percent of sixty autistic children he monitored. More recently, Arthur Krigsman, M.D. (IMFAR 2004, personal communication) conducted a retrospective review of 143 autistic children and found histological tissue evidence of iliocolitis, or inflammation in the ileum, colon, or both, in 73 percent.

In other evaluations of autistic children, including upper GI endoscopy performed by Dr. Karoly Horvath, the following GI problems were present, in these percentages of patients:

Percentages of Upper GI Problems in Autistic Children
- 69 percent had reflux esophagitis.
- 42 percent had chronic gastritis.
- 67 percent had chronic duodenitis.
- 58 percent had carbohydrate enzyme deficiency.

The presence of these disorders has widespread negative consequences, including damage to the nervous and immune systems, in addition to the gastrointestinal system.

In addition to chronic infections and imflammation, an important root cause of some of these digestive problems is the failure of the pancreas to produce enough digestive enzymes. A related cause is the lack of the ancillary chemicals, or coenzymes, that allow digestive enzymes to function properly.

Among autistic kids, the most frequent enzyme problems are:

- *Deficiency of the DPP4 enzyme,* which breaks down gluten and casein.
- *Deficiency of lipase enzymes,* which break down fat.
- *Deficiency of sugar-digesting enzymes,* which break down complex dietary sugars.

Incomplete breakdown of gluten and casein, fatty acids, and complex sugars can result in the creation of partially digested molecules, including neurotoxic partial proteins, or peptides. These peptides can then trigger neurological decline and behavioral disorders.

Therefore, of special importance to kids on the autism spectrum are enzymes that contain:

- **Peptidases**–the enzymes that help complete the breakdown of peptides.
- **Lipase**–to digest fatty acids.
- **Amylase**–to digest starch.
- **Disaccharidases**–including lactase, maltase, sucrase, and iso-maltase–which help break down sugars. (However, some people must avoid these complex sugars entirely, with the specific carbohydrate diet.)

On the 2006 ARI parent rating scale, digestive enzymes were rated as follows:

- **Symptoms improved: 58 percent.**
- **No discernible effect: 39 percent.**
- **Symptoms worsened: 3 percent.**

Enzymes occasionally cause stomach upset or diarrhea, but this is rare, and usually goes away when the dosage is reduced. Some kids, however, just don't seem to be able to tolerate digestive enzymes.

As you can see, there are several different types of digestive enzymes: general, which digest many things; peptidases, which digest peptides; protein-digesting enzymes; fat-digesting enzymes; and carbohydrate-digesting enzymes. Enzymes are used in children according to what type of digestive aids they most need. One child may need more help with carbohydrate digestion, others may need help with fat digestion, some may need peptidase, and others may require combinations.

My general recommendation: one-half to two digestive enzyme capsules per meal, depending upon a child's particular needs. Dosing depends upon age, size, and other treatments and indications.

Vitamin B-6. This was one of the first vitamins ever to be employed against psychiatric disorders, and has proven to be extremely helpful in treating autism. Dr. Bernard Rimland has reviewed twenty-two studies of B-6 use in autism, and twenty-one of the studies showed positive outcomes.

Among the therapeutic effects of B-6 are the following:

• *Improvement in methionine metabolism.* Methionine is an important factor in methylation.

• *Relief from seizures,* particularly those triggered in part by an excess of the amino acid glutamate, or by a deficiency of the neurotransmitter GABA.

• *Remediation of a deficiency of decarboxylase,* an enzyme. This deficiency can result in a syndrome characterized by poor eating during infancy, irritability, sleep disturbances, developmental delays, poor muscle tone, and rolling of the eyes.

• *Relief from carpal tunnel syndrome.* This is yet another indicator of the importance of this vitamin in the proper function of the nervous system.

Some of these problems—especially impaired methionine metabolism—are common among autistic children, who tend to have a poor ability to metabolize B-6. This includes difficulty in forming its active metabolite, pyridoxal-5-phosphate. That is why P5P is frequently given with vitamin B-6 to children with autism.

The need for B-6 depends upon individual metabolic requirements, and can greatly exceed the daily intake that the government recommends for the general population. Again, we see that 4-A children have special needs for certain nutrients, which sometimes far exceed the requirements of the general public for basic health. The goal for 4-A children is not just to overcome deficiencies of B-6, but to employ B-6 as a therapeutic agent.

Because B-6 sometimes triggers adverse symptoms, such as hyperactivity, irritability, and increased stims in some children, I monitor its use closely.

Guidelines for giving B-6 include the following:

- *Give it with food,* to avoid stomach upset.
- *Ensure proper levels of zinc,* to help metabolize B-6.
- *Ensure proper levels of amino acids,* to increase the effectiveness of B-6. One way to do this is to take digestive enzymes, which help break protein down into amino acids.
- *Take magnesium with B-6,* to achieve a synergistic effect.

In the ARI parent rating scale, here's how B-6 fared:

- **Symptoms improved: 30 percent.**
- **No discernible effect: 63 percent.**
- **Symptoms worsened: 8 percent.**

My general recommendation: 100 to 500 mg. of B-6 (20 percent as pyridoxal-5-phosphate) per day, depending upon age, size, and other treatments and indications.

Taurine. This was one of the earliest nutrients to be applied in large dosages against autism. Dr. Sid Baker used it as early as 1984, and it has been an important element in the biomedical treatment of autism ever since.

Taurine has several important functions.

- *It increases the effects of magnesium,* and thereby helps prevent magnesium deficiency.
- *It is part of the metabolic process of essential fatty acid assimilation,* as well as assimilation of fat-soluble vitamins, such as vitamins A, D, and E.
- *It is a powerful antioxidant.*
- *It is an indirect component of the methylation process,* and may work synergistically with TMG and methyl-B-12.

- *It reduces seizures in some patients,* and can increase the activity of the calming neurotransmitter GABA.
- *It contains sulfur,* and may therefore help kids with impaired sulfation.

Taurine appears to frequently be low in children on the autism spectrum, particularly when they have low levels of cysteine.

Taurine can be driven even lower by poor digestion of meat, by bacterial dysbiosis, and by infection. I usually don't give it until yeast overgrowth in the gut has been addressed, because the sulfur in it can aggravate yeast proliferation.

My general recommendation: 500 to 2,000 mg. per day, depending upon age, size, and other treatments and indications.

Melatonin is one of the highest rated of all individual nutrients in the ARI parents' survey. Here are its scores:

- **Symptoms improved: 61 percent.**
- **No discernible effect: 31 percent.**
- **Symptoms worsened: 9 percent.**

The primary symptom that improves with melatonin is insomnia. Melatonin is arguably the best natural sleep aid, because it regulates circadian rhythms. Insomnia and other sleep disorders are often a significant problem in kids with autistic and ADHD symptoms.

Melatonin is also valuable as an antioxidant. In addition, it has some ability to block the activity of the pro-inflammatory cytokines, which are messengers that can spread the inflammatory response. There is also evidence that melatonin increases the activity of an enzyme in the brain, pyridoxal kinase. It also appears to aid the digestive process, by increasing the movement, or motility, of food in the GI tract.

Although I am aware of its broad spectrum of effects, I primarily employ it clinically as a sleep aid in children with sleep disorders, and have found it to be consistently effective for a high percentage of patients.

My general recommendation: 0.5 to 3 mg. per night, depending upon age, size, and other treatments and indications.

Methyl-B-12. This special form of vitamin B-12, also known as methylcobalamin, can have an extraordinary impact upon the methylation process, and is therefore often critically important for achieving detoxification from heavy metals. As you know, I believe that the presence of heavy metals—particularly mercury—is a significant contributing factor to autism and ADHD. Kids who have high levels of heavy metals generally cannot recover until these heavy metals are removed.

Unfortunately, the presence of mercury in the system blocks the body's own formation of methyl-B-12, and this often prohibits the body from solving the heavy metal problem by itself. When methyl-B-12 is administered, though, the processes of methylation and reduced glutathione formation can once again occur, and heavy metals can be eliminated.

Thus, once again we see that specific nutrients can exert a biomedical healing effect, which goes far beyond the mere ability to provide adequate nutrition.

The primary way that methyl-B-12 helps methylation is by enabling homocysteine to make methionine. Methionine is a key element in the methylation process. In addition to improving detoxification, other benefits of enhanced methylation include: improved cell membrane function, improved neurotransmitter and hormone metabolism, and improved neuronal healing.

Methyl-B-12 is very highly rated in the ARI parent survey:

- **Symptoms improved: 63 percent.**
- **No discernible effect: 33 percent.**
- **Symptoms worsened: 4 percent.**

In my own clinical experience, approximately 70 percent or more of children benefit from methyl-B-12, whereas approximately 10 to 15 percent show adverse effects, including hyperactivity, irritability, insomnia, and, infrequently, increased aggression. The adverse effects, whatever they may be, go away upon discontinuation of the methyl-B-12. It may take several days to a few weeks for these effects to fully disappear.

Methyl-B-12 can be given nasally or by injection. As a rule, methyl-B-12 is not very effective if it is given orally to a child who still has bowel dysbiosis. Therefore, if your child has lingering bowel problems, you may want to consider other routes of administration, such as subcutaneous injection. This highly effective modality, pioneered by Dr. James Neubrander, sidesteps the problem of poor absorption, and utilizes a concentrated form of methyl-B-12, injected subcutaneously, via a very tiny needle into the upper, outer buttocks. This injection is generally well tolerated, and is typically administered by parents after a training session with a doctor, or his or her nurse.

It is important to note that we are not treating a deficiency here, but a dependency. In other words, we need a higher dose of methyl-B-12 not to compensate for B-12 deficiency, but to bypass metabolic blocks, and to jump-start metabolic processes and neuronal healing.

Because of its importance, I usually recommend methyl-B-12 after a patient's second meeting. There are times, however, depending on specific circumstances, when I may recommend it after the first visit.

If you employ methyl-B-12, you must use the exact form, rather than just ordinary B-12 tablets. For access to the proper form of methyl-B-12, see the Resources listed in Appendix #2 and discuss this with your doctor.

My general recommendation: 65 mcg./kg. body weight of subcutaneous methyl-B-12 every three days, or 1,250 to 2,500 mcg. nasal methyl-B-12 per day, depending upon age, size, and other treatments and indications.

Chromium. This trace mineral helps insulin to move blood sugar into the cells, and is therefore sometimes beneficial for people who have problems with this biological action. This may include people who suffer from insulin resistance, the common disorder in which cells do not readily respond to insulin. Insulin resistance is often a cause of hyperglycemia, and is generally considered to be one of the precursor disorders to diabetes, and probably also to numerous inflammatory disorders.

There is debate over the ability of chromium supplementation to reduce hypoglycemia, and to help prevent diabetes, but many people do seem to process sugars and carbohydrates more efficiently when they take chromium. I generally use it in children with reactive hypoglycemia, or those with milder glycemic instability, characterized by an elevated desire for sweets.

My general recommendation: 50 to 400 mcg. per day, depending upon age, size, and other treatments and indications.

Folinic Acid. This is another vitally important nutrient for methylation. Many 4-A kids cannot achieve proper methylation without taking it.

Because it is only one element of methylation, though, it needs to be taken with the other nutrients that spur methylation, including methyl-B-12 and DMG.

Folinic acid is a form of the B-vitamin folic acid, or B-9. It is named after the Latin "folium," meaning "leaf," because it is abundant in leafy, green vegetables. Folic acid, when taken by pregnant women, has been proven to help prevent certain birth defects.

Folinic acid is metabolized differently than ordinary folic acid, and it is important for autistic children to take it in its exact form, instead of just taking folic acid. Also, some kids don't tolerate folic acid well.

The important contribution that folinic acid makes in the methylation process is to help produce methyl-B-12, or methylcobalamin. It helps attach methyls to cobalamine.

Folinic acid can become trapped and disabled, and this appears to contribute to a decline in methylation. When it is taken in sufficient amounts as a supplement, however, this problem can be overcome.

Sometimes folic acid levels in the blood appear to be normal, but are actually low in the specific constituents that aid in methylation. Therefore, just as with vitamin B-12, don't disregard this nutrient merely because your child has normal blood levels of folic acid.

In the ARI parent rating scale, folinic acid had the following evaluation:

- **Symptoms improved: 54 percent.**
- **No discernible effect: 42 percent.**
- **Symptoms worsened: 3 percent.**

My general recommendation: 800 to 1,600 mcg. per day, and sometimes more, depending upon age, size, and other treatments and indications.

N-acetyl-cysteine. This nutrient, abbreviated as NAC, is another supplement that can help increase the body's ability to detoxify itself. It does this by increasing the body's levels of glutathione, which boosts methylation. It also has other functions in the body. It helps with detoxification of heavy metals and chemicals, it supports the immune system, and it increases the integrity of the gastrointestinal mucosa. It is sometimes used during the process of chelation, because it can be liver-protective, and can also help detoxify the body of heavy metals.

NAC has a thirty-year history of therapeutic use, and is often applied as an antidote for acetaminophen poisoning. In addition to increasing the body's levels of glutathione, it is also an antioxidant.

It also protects enzymes that contain sulfur. In addition, it contains sulfur itself, and can thereby improve the sulfation process. However, sulfur also increases yeast proliferation, so patients who have yeast overgrowth often find that oral NAC aggravates the condition. I generally don't give NAC until candida has been cleared. I also sometimes give it in conjunction with various nutrients that decrease yeast, such as probiotics. If yeast is a persistent problem, I give NAC transdermally, instead of orally.

My general recommendation: 50 to 100 mg. transdermally, or 250 to 500 mg. orally per day, depending upon age, size, and other treatments and indications.

Amino Acids and Branched-Chain Amino Acids. Amino acids, the building blocks of protein, are often low in autistic children. Several amino acids tend to be particularly low, including taurine, lysine, methionine, and those known as the branched-chain amino acids: leucine, isoleucine, and valine.

There are twenty-one different essential amino acids that make up protein, and when any one of them is low or missing, it weakens the effects of the entire assemblage of amino acids.

Amino acids are absolutely critical for proper neurological, immunological, and gastrointestinal functions. They are used to construct enzymes, antibodies, immunoglobulins, neurotransmitters, and hormones.

They are also an important part of the detoxification process. They join with toxic substances and help escort them from the body.

Amino acids are often low in children with 4-A disorders, particularly because of restricted dietary choices, poor digestion, and poor assimilation.

Especially low are the branched-chain amino acids: leucine, isoleucine, and valine. These amino acids are known as branched-chain amino acids because one of their essential components, the carbon chain, is branched, which offers increased biochemical flexibility. These three amino acids are low in approximately one-third of all autistic children.

I often give the branched-chain amino acids in conjunction with NAC. This helps to prevent uncomfortable side effects from the movement and excretion of heavy metals. This is especially important if children are constipated, because that condition contributes to toxic build-up.

Additionally, two other amino acids often tend to be low when amino acids are measured in amino acid analysis: lysine and methionine. Lysine can help with resistance to chronic herpes-type viruses, and methionine is a critical factor in the methylation cycle. However, as with many supplements, some kids don't seem to tolerate methionine well, especially if they are not deficient in it.

One approach to increasing amino acids is to take protein products, such as rice protein. A more exact method, though, is to test for the levels of the individual amino acids, and to supplement the specific amino acids that are low.

The dosages that I recommend are dependent upon the degree of deficiency.

TMG and DMG. These two nutrients can have extraordinary effects in detoxifying the body of heavy metals, because they are intimately involved in the methylation process. TMG is an abbreviation for trimethylglycine, and DMG is an abbreviation for dimethylglycine. They are very similar, but TMG (tri) has one more methyl group attached to it than DMG (di).

The pivotal purpose of these nutrients is to increase methylation. Ultimately, increased methylation can result in enhanced glutathione, which can facilitate the removal of toxins, through the urine. Until this conjugation occurs, many toxins–including mercury and other heavy metals–cannot be excreted, and remain in the system, unable to be removed.

DMG and TMG can both work synergistically with folinic acid and methyl-B-12, so DMG or TMG are often given along with folinic acid and methyl-B-12.

Both TMG and DMG have helped thousands of autistic children to improve, with the most noticeable, initial improvements often occurring in eye contact and speech.

Relatively high dosages are generally required, but it is wise to start with low dosages and then increase them. An estimated 7 percent of children have a paradoxical, negative reaction to DMG, often characterized by increased irritability and/or hyperactivity. The percentage for a negative reaction to TMG is estimated to be even higher, at 14 percent, and may include occasional aggression.

Either of the two nutrients can be effective, and there are certain indicators that they may be needed. Indicators that DMG may be needed include:

- Low cysteine.
- High histidine.
- High serum folate.

Indicators that TMG may be needed include:

- High homocysteine.
- Low methionine.
- High serum folate.

In the ARI parent survey, TMG and DMG, rated together, were evaluated as follows:

- **Symptoms improved: 42 percent.**
- **No discernible effect: 51 percent.**
- **Symptoms worsened: 7 percent.**

My general recommendation: DMG: 125 to 1,000 mg. per day; TMG: 175 to 2,000 mg. per day, depending upon age, size, and other treatments and indications.

Vitamin D. Only in the past few years has vitamin D begun to be fully appreciated. It was previously perceived to be of peripheral importance, but now it is recognized as having a major impact upon the immune system. Many researchers believe that it can have a powerful effect upon preventing a variety of the most common cancers, including breast cancer, prostate cancer, and colon cancer, and a number of doctors are even prescribing relatively high dosages of it as an adjunctive therapy in cancer treatment.

Vitamin D also appears to have the ability to not only increase immune activity, but to modulate it, and keep it within a proper range of activity. This helps to avoid autoimmune assaults upon the body, and also helps to avoid inappropriate immune reactions, such as those involved in allergy.

Therefore, vitamin D can be of significant value to 4-A kids, who often have immune deficiencies, as well as problems with autoimmunity and allergy.

One interesting new theory is that the lack of vitamin D from sunlight that occurs in the winter may be a contributor to the typical wintertime increase in minor illnesses, such as colds and flu. It may also be possible that a lack of vitamin D from the sun is related to the autoimmune disorder of multiple sclerosis, because multiple sclerosis is much more common in the northern hemisphere of the earth, which receives less direct sunlight.

Vitamin D is found in cod liver oil, but there is almost ten times as much vitamin A in cod liver oil as vitamin D. Therefore, it may be wise for some children with immune disorders to take supplemental vitamin D, along with cod liver oil. It may also be wise to increase supplementation in the winter, and also to increase it among children who live in the northern regions of America.

As with vitamin A, another fat-soluble nutrient, levels of vitamin D must be monitored throughout treatment to avoid toxicity.

My general recommendation: 400 to 800 i.u. per day, depending upon age, size, and other treatments and conditions.

Coenzyme Q-10. This nutrient, often referred to as Co-Q-10, is a natural molecule that the body produces. It's also present in foods. It is in every cell in the body, and because it is so ubiquitous, its scientific name is ubiquinone. The reason it is in every cell is because it is needed by the energy-producing area of the cell, the mitochondria. The mitochondria turn fuel into energy, and strongly influence how people feel and function. Poor function of the mitochondria, which can occur when Co-Q-10 is low, can create symptoms of lethargy. These symptoms are often present in kids with symptoms of the inattentive subtype of ADHD. The symptoms are also often present in autistic kids.

Therefore, I often give Co-Q-10 to children who are chronically tired, lethargic, and inattentive. It can produce a notable clinical effect.

It's hard for the body to produce its own Co-Q-10, and it's also hard to get abundant amounts from food. For example, to get just 30 mg. you would need to eat a pound of sardines, which is one of the best sources of it. Therefore, many children are low in Co-Q-10.

This deficit puts particular stress on the tissues in the body that are most metabolically active, including those in the heart and muscles, and also those in the organs and glands that are associated with the immune system. Immunity is often impaired when Co-Q-10 is low, and it can be bolstered by Co-Q-10 supplementation.

Stress on the immune system typically depletes Co-Q-10. During a viral infection, the Co-Q-10 levels in white blood cells plummet.

Therefore, Co-Q-10 can help kids with immune problems, hypotonia, lethargy, and mitochondrial dysfunction.

My general recommendation: 30 to 200 mg. per day, depending upon the type of Co-Q-10 (i.e., powder, gel, or melt) as well as age, size, and type of other treatments and indications.

Transfer Factor. This is a natural substance produced during lactation. It is now available as a supplement. It helps immune system cells to communicate with one another. In effect, it enables one immune cell to teach another cell to identify pathogens.

Transfer factor is found in colostrum, the secretion from the breast that is produced immediately prior to breast milk. The function of the transfer factor in this secretion is to transfer immune information to the immune system of the offspring. By helping to transfer this information, transfer factor can enable the body to launch a more effective immune response. Transfer factor also promotes Th-1 immunity, helping to balance Th-2 skewing of the immune system, which is so common among 4-A kids.

Transfer factor supplements are usually derived from either eggs or cows. As a rule, lactose is removed from commercial preparations, so people who are lactose-intolerant can take it. There are numerous colostrum preparations available at health food stores, but these contain only a small amount of transfer factor, and often contain casein. Actual, purified transfer factor, which is free from casein and other allergens, can be obtained from a number of sources.

Transfer factor can be used to help the immune system prevent illness, or it can be used as an adjunct to medications, herbs, and nutrients. It can sometimes help remediate chronic immune dysfunction.

I frequently recommend it to children who suffer from recurrent infections, autoimmune disorders, and allergies. It may also be beneficial to children who are experiencing a lingering chronic, low-grade viral infection in the gut, or other areas.

In the ARI parent survey, transfer factor was rated as follows:

- **Symptoms improved: 39 percent.**
- **No discernible effect: 53 percent.**
- **Symptoms worsened: 8 percent.**

My general recommendation: 200 to 1,800 mg. per day, depending upon age, size, and other treatments and indications.

Selenium. This is a popular nutrient among people in the general population, because it is one of the most powerful antioxidants. It is even more valuable for 4-A kids than other people, because it plays an important role in the metabolism of glutathione, which is vital in the methylation process.

The metabolism of glutathione appears to be subnormal among autistics, partly because mercury interferes with the ability of selenium to help promote the metabolism of glutathione. This may be compensated for, to some degree, by selenium supplementation. Selenium is also an important component in the immune response. Even relatively low dosages of it appear to enhance immunity. High levels of selenium in the body are associated with reduced risk of cancer.

Selenium also protects cell membranes from oxidant damage, when taken in conjunction with vitamin E and beta-carotene, the vitamin A precursor.

Excessive selenium can cause subtle negative reactions, so it should be taken rather cautiously, and levels should be monitored.

My general recommendation: 100 to 400 mcg. per day, depending upon age, size, and other treatments and indications.

Iron. This supplement isn't for everyone, but it can be very valuable when applied according to individual needs.

Iron supplements can trigger profound benefits among kids who are deficient in iron. These kids may have symptoms of lethargy, fatigue, and listlessness. These symptoms often precede frank anemia, and may be present even when serum iron is in the low-normal range. Sometimes children are misdiagnosed as having the inattentive subtype of ADHD when they are actually just low in iron. If these kids are given Ritalin, it can mask their symptoms, but the root problem remains.

Iron is also important for proper immune function, so kids with chronic infections should be tested for low iron. Deficiency of iron causes lymphocyte depletion, decreased antibody and cytokine production, and depression of T-cell activity. If iron is low, supplementation can boost the power of other immune stimulants.

Iron is also necessary for the proper activity of many enzymes. Thus, we see once more that many nutrients are valuable not only for their direct effects, but also for indirect effects, including their effects upon other nutrients. Nutritional therapy is a puzzle of many pieces, and if any one of those pieces is missing, the puzzle might never be solved.

Iron is harmful, though, if taken in excess. Too much iron is immune-suppressive, and can also stimulate the production of free radicals. In addition, excess iron can be used by bacteria and yeast for replication, and can contribute to bacterial infection, and to candida overgrowth. Because of this, iron supplementation should be administered only when there are clear signs of deficiency, including symptomatology, confirmed by appropriate laboratory testing.

My general recommendation: 10 to 80 mg. of elemental iron per day, depending upon age, size, and other treatments and indications.

Multiple Vitamin/Mineral. It's generally wise to give a multiple vitamin/mineral supplement to many children, because a multiple is good at correcting a relatively wide array of mild deficiencies, some of which may be so subtle that they are not clinically discernible.

Multiple vitamin/mineral supplements are also helpful for kids who are extremely resistant to taking large numbers of individual supplements.

One drawback of multiples, though, is that they can make it harder to determine exactly what nutrient is helping. Individual supplements are better for revealing the responses that are related to specific deficiencies or dependencies that may exist.

Also, there are so many ingredients in multiples that if one ingredient causes an adverse reaction, it can be hard to determine the specific nutrient that is causing the problem.

I generally only give multiples if the child has already demonstrated an ability to tolerate a number of supplements without any negative reactions.

It's usually best to give multiples that do not contain copper, because copper can be toxic, and because a relatively high percentage of 4-A kids are already high in copper. You may also wish to limit vitamin A, iron, or B-6, depending upon your child's needs.

There are big differences in quality among the many brands of multiples, so look for one with relatively high, but balanced, levels of individual nutrients. You may wish to check the Resources section for information about supplements.

My general recommendation: The dose of the liquid, powder, tablet, or capsule depends upon age, size, and other treatments and indications.

TIER THREE SUPPLEMENTS

The third tier of supplements consists of those that are intended for much more specialized, discrete needs. Many of my patients use some of these supplements, at least during certain periods, but others never use them at all.

This tier includes herbal preparations, which I use in certain situations. Herbal supplements are applied as natural medications for particular pathologies, such as airway congestion, inflammation, or infection.

For some patients, though, these third tier supplements are pivotally important. They are the special supplements that bring certain patients to their final level of recovery.

DMAE. This nutrient, dimethylamine ethanol, is a relatively recent addition to the natural pharmacopeia, but it is proving to be very helpful for some patients. It is especially beneficial for any child who has cognitive impairment, characterized by poor memory, or inability to focus. This problem is often seen in children with the inattentive subtype of ADHD.

DMAE helps the body to produce acetylcholine, the neurotransmitter that is the primary carrier of thought and memory. When acetylcholine levels are low—as they are in many autistic and ADHD kids—it can be very difficult for children to maintain coherent streams of thought. When levels are increased, it can result in relatively sudden bursts of cognitive improvement.

DMAE produces acetylcholine when it is combined with phosphatidylcholine (derived from lecithin), and with vitamin B-5, or pantothenic acid. Therefore, DMAE should be given with these other two nutrients, or it may not have the desired effect.

DMAE is especially valuable for increasing short-term memory, because short-term memory, in contrast to long-term memory, is less hardwired into the brain, and is instead completely dependent upon adequate levels of acetylcholine.

In some kids, use of DMAE also results in improved mood, and in heightened feelings of well-being.

Increasing the levels of acetylcholine generally has a calming effect, but some children experience the paradoxical effect of stimulation. If this occurs, it can sometimes trigger insomnia. The nutrient is also generally not appropriate for patients with epilepsy or bipolar disorder, because it has been known to exacerbate both conditions.

My general recommendation: 100 to 500 mg. per day, depending upon age, size, and other treatments and indications.

Creatine. This amino acid is often low in autistic children, partly because its metabolism can be blocked by mercury.

Creatine is widely known as a muscle builder. That's why so many products for athletes and bodybuilders contain high amounts of creatine. Many kids on the autism spectrum, and a number of kids with ADHD symptoms, have notably poor muscle tone, sometimes because of creatine deficiency. This can even show up very early in life as the "floppy baby" condition.

Creatine is also involved in energy transfer, in both brain and muscle. Therefore, it can aid in multiple cellular processes, all of which require energy. Detoxification is one of the cellular processes that is most notably energy-dependent. Restoring low creatine levels can help kids who are weak, due to low muscle mass and poor muscle tone.

Creatine is also very important in the communication abilities of one cell to another, including cells in the brain. Because of this, low creatine is believed to be part of the cause of deficient expressive speech among some autistic kids.

Here are some clinical clues to creatine deficiency:

- *Poor muscle development,* including low muscle mass and poor muscle tone.
- *Low blood serum creatine.*
- *Deficient urine creatine.*
- *Elevated levels of the amino acids ornithine and beta-alanine.*

My general recommendation: 750 mg. to several grams per day, depending upon age, size, and other treatments and indications.

Gamma Globulin. This supplement, a powerful booster of immunity, was previously available only as an injectible, but is now available in an oral form. It is a processed form of concentrated IgG antibodies, which have been selectively derived from serum. The IgG molecules from this serum are so large that they don't get absorbed, essentially confining their action to the gastrointestinal tract.

Oral gamma globulin is appropriate for children with pronounced, resistant immune dysfunction. It is especially valuable for those with persistent GI dysfunction, particularly dysbiosis. Sometimes it produces benefits that could not be achieved by more common substances that enhance immunity and improve GI function.

Healing reactions occasionally occur during a course of oral gamma globulin, as they do with other treatments that suddenly increase immune function. These reactions can include headache, nausea, or flu-like symptoms.

Oral gamma globulin can be particularly helpful to patients with the forms of persistent gut dysbiosis that are related to infection.

I occasionally use this supplement, and in certain cases it has been quite effective.

My general recommendation: one to two scoops of oral IgG powder per day, depending upon age, size, and other treatments and indications.

N-acetyl-carnitine. This nutrient carries fatty acids into every cell's energy-producing area, the mitochondria. It has demonstrated positive effects among autistics, who often appear to suffer from mitochondrial dysfunction.

N-acetyl-carnitine is preferable to the more common L-carnitine, because it tends to be more neuroactive.

The supplement has been shown to improve cognitive function, and some researchers believe that it heightens the communication ability between the two hemispheres of the brain. It is a potent brain antioxidant, and is frequently used by people who suffer from age-associated memory impairment, or from Alzheimer's.

Indicators that it may be needed include the following:

- *Elevated blood triglycerides.*
- *Low levels of carnitine in the blood.*
- *High urine or blood levels of the fatty acids adipic, suberic, and octene-dioc.*
- *Presence of any muscle disease, including hypotonia, or low muscle tone.*
- *Chronic fatigue.*

It is generally best to administer this supplement after nutritional therapy has already begun, and after the resolution of GI problems.

My general recommendation: 500 to 2,000 mg. per day, depending upon age, size, and other treatments and indications.

Activated Charcoal. This supplement, which is usually in capsule form, is generally used for a single, specific purpose. It binds with toxins in the GI tract, and helps remove them from the system. It can be of value when pharmaceutical medications and nutraceuticals trigger a rapid die-off of pathogens, such as yeast or bacteria. These die-offs can overwhelm the systems of elimination, and create uncomfortable healing reactions. These reactions can be ameliorated by speeding the exit of necrotic material from the system.

Activated charcoal should be taken by itself at a different time than other supplements, medications, or food, to prevent it from interfering with the absorption of other medications, supplements, or nutrients. It tends to cause temporary darkening of the stools, because it is black, but this is a harmless effect. Adverse reactions to it are extremely rare.

My general recommendation: one-half to two capsules, two to three times per day, depending upon age, size, and other treatments and indications.

Silymarin. This nutrient, which is popular among the general public, is another supplement with a very focused function: protecting liver cells. It protects them from many liver-poisoning, hepatotoxic chemicals, and there is a great deal of evidence that it is valuable in the treatment of cirrhosis and hepatitis. It also protects the liver from the toxic effects of certain medications, and even from some poisonous mushrooms.

Silymarin can be helpful for protecting the body from toxins that are not captured and eliminated by activated charcoal. These toxins often target liver cells, and create discomfort, and further dysfunction.

Silymarin helps protect liver cells by stimulating DNA and RNA synthesis, and by blocking receptor sites on liver cells that allow the entrance of toxins. It is also a potent liver antioxidant, it promotes glutathione production, and it helps prevent oxidative stress on the liver.

Silymarin is derived from the herb milk thistle, and is sometimes sold commercially under this more common name, in capsule, tablet, and liquid form.

There is no established need for this supplement as a nutrient, but it can be very effective when used medicinally. It is generally applied only when medications, illnesses, or healing reactions threaten the integrity of the liver.

My general recommendation: 80 to 525 mg. per day, depending upon age, size, and other treatments and indications.

Phosphatidylcholine. This is the active ingredient in the common nutrient lecithin, and it is the main building block, or nutritional precursor, for the neurotransmitter that is the primary carrier of all thought and memory, acetylcholine. Any deficit of this important nutrient can have a strong impact upon cognitive function, and supplementation with it can dramatically improve cognitive function in patients who have a deficit.

The average daily diet generally provides about 1,000 mg. of this nutrient, so a multiple of this amount may be necessary to achieve noticeable improvement in cognitive function.

As I've mentioned, to produce acetylcholine, phosphatidylcholine must bond with DMAE and with vitamin B-5, so it may be necessary to also take extra amounts of all of these nutrients to achieve a noticeable boost in cognition.

Phosphatidylcholine not only helps manufacture the neurotransmitter acetylcholine, but also helps to repair and maintain neurons. In addition, it is used outside the brain in the metabolism of fats. It is also used in the regulation of cholesterol, and in the production of the sheaths that surround all nerves, which are constructed of myelin. It is also a vital component of cell membranes, which participate in cell receptor function and in signal transduction, carrying messages across the cell membrane into the cell. In addition, it is an important liver protectant and detoxifier.

This nutrient is notably benign, generally contributing to calmness, but a small subset of children appear to have the paradoxical reaction of stimulation.

My general recommendation: 1,500 to 9,000 mg. per day, depending upon age, size, and other treatments and indications.

5-HTP. This nutrient is a form of the amino acid tryptophan, which is the primary nutritional precursor of the calming neurotransmitter serotonin. Serotonin levels are frequently low in children with ADHD and autism, and this supplement can sometimes help increase these low levels.

5-HTP is considered by some to be a reasonable natural alternative to the pharmaceutical drugs that increase serotonin activity. These drugs, the selective serotonin reuptake inhibitors, or SSRIs, are known more commonly as antidepressants. In some people, 5-HTP has an effect that is similar to SSRIs, although SSRIs generally have stronger and more reliable actions.

Some studies have indicated that 5-HTP can be effective for depression, anxiety, panic attacks, insomnia, and weight management. As a rule, it tends to cause fewer side effects than the SSRIs, which are typically applied to mood disorders.

Although 5-HTP is generally well tolerated, some people experience the paradoxical effect of increased agitation. This may be due to the fact that these people already have an excess of serotonin. An excess of serotonin can cause mood disorders, just as a deficiency can. Serotonin, like all neurotransmitters, works best in a limited bandwidth.

I often recommend 5-HTP for insomnia, depression, and irritability. It may also help reduce carbohydrate cravings.

My general recommendation: 50 to 200 mg. per day (usually taken at night, but occasionally in divided doses), depending upon age, size, and other treatments and indications.

Carnosine. This is a partial protein that is of special value for the subset of autistic children who suffer from seizures. It appears to have a unique ability to not only decrease the incidence of seizures, but to also improve general cognitive function among children who have seizures. One of the symptoms that is most frequently improved is impaired speech. It is theorized that carnosine exerts these effects primarily by enhancing the activity of the neurotransmitter GABA, which is present in the brain and in the central nervous system, and can have seizure-alleviating actions.

Carnosine is also often helpful for improvement of muscle mass, and has been used in the treatment of muscular dystrophy diseases.

Carnosine is not indicated for a significant subset of autistic children, however, who may already have an excess of it in their systems. Carnosine levels appear to be elevated in as much as 20 percent of the autistic population. This elevation probably occurs because of a deficit of zinc. Zinc helps break down carnosine, and zinc is often low in autistic kids. When carnosine is given to children who already have an excess of it, they tend to become hyperactive, and this trait can last for several days after the carnosine is discontinued. Therefore, we again see the need for careful individualization of supplementation therapy. Proper supplementation therapy can not be achieved with a cookie-cutter approach. Doctors and parents must be good medical detectives, and stay alert for adverse reactions, even though these reactions may occur in only a relatively small percentage of children.

My general recommendation: 200 to 800 mg. per day, depending upon age, size, and other treatments and indications.

SAMe. This is another of the nutrients that is helpful only in certain, individual cases. It can be beneficial in the methylation process, but because of complex individual variations, only about one in five children benefit from it. More often than not, it has no effect.

This limited value is reflected by the ARI parent survey:

- **Symptoms improved: 19 percent.**
- **No discernible effect: 66 percent.**
- **Symptoms worsened: 15 percent.**

Even so, it helps some patients. All patients are different. In adults, for example, it has been shown to be helpful in the treatment of depression and arthritis.

However, in children with autism-spectrum disorders, I rarely use SAMe. I prefer to enhance methylation with other nutrients, such as methyl-B-12, folinic acid, DMG, and TMG, because of the higher possibility of adverse effects from SAMe.

My general recommendation: 200 to 800 mg. per day, depending upon age, size, and other treatments and indications.

Pycnogenol. This botanical antioxidant is one of only a few antioxidants that can cross the blood–brain barrier, and directly enter neurons. It is a powerful scavenger of free radicals, and therefore can help relieve the oxidative stress that is common among children with autism, ADHD, and the other 4-A disorders. Studies have indicated that it is a more powerful antioxidant than even vitamins C and E. It can also act as a powerful anti-inflammatory, when used in higher dosage.

Because free radical damage and inflammation are components of so many diseases and disorders, pycnogenol is used as an element of nutritional therapy for a wide array of problems, ranging from asthma, to arthritis, to ADHD, to heart disease.

It does not appear to have significant side effects, and is generally well tolerated.

My general recommendation: 25 to 200 mg. per day, depending upon age, size, and other treatments and indications.

Other Herbal Preparations. People have been using concentrated extracts of herbs for many centuries as natural medicines, and many pharmaceutical medicines are still derived from, or patterned after, various herbs.

I frequently recommend herbal preparations, but usually for specific conditions, because most of them have limited, targeted actions.

Most commonly, I recommend them for infectious disorders. One of the most important attributes of a number of herbs is that they can be equally effective at helping to overcome a variety of pathogens, including bacteria, viruses, parasites, and fungi. This is in contrast to most pharmaceutical drugs, which are generally effective against only single categories of pathogens. For example, antibiotics kill only bacteria, and not viruses, parasites, or fungi. Furthermore, they may be effective against only particular strains of bacteria. Similarly, antiviral medications are only effective against viruses, and generally just specific viruses. By the same token, antifungals are only effective for fungi.

Another advantage of herbal preparations is that they tend to have milder actions than most pharmaceuticals, with fewer side effects, and this makes them more appropriate for children. It especially makes them more appropriate for children who have the delicate systems that typify many kids with 4-A disorders.

Among the herbal preparations that I most frequently recommend are the following:

Curcumin. This is a powerful antioxidant, but its most effective action is as a natural anti-inflammatory. It also has nerve protectant properties, and can aid in colon health. A reasonable daily dosage is in the range of 500 to 1500 mg., depending upon the patient and circumstances.

Quercitin. This is often helpful for asthma patients, as well as people with eczema and allergies, because it blocks the release of histamine and reduces inflammation. In effect, it is a natural antihistamine, as well as a natural anti-inflammatory. A reasonable daily dosage is in the range of 600 to 1,800 mg., depending upon the patient and circumstances.

Oregano oil. The primary component in it, carvacal, can be effective against bacteria, fungi, and parasites. A reasonable daily dosage is in the range of one to two drops, mixed in olive oil, or taken as capsules, depending upon the patient and circumstances.

Capryllic acid. This fatty acid has been shown to be effective against viruses and bacteria. Some clinicians believe it is also an effective antifungal, and apply it against yeast overgrowth. A reasonable daily dosage is in the range of 800 to 1200 mg. per day, depending upon the patient and circumstances.

Olive leaf extract. This herbal extract is effective against a range of infectious conditions that are caused by viruses and bacteria. It has the unique ability to stop viral replication. It can also be helpful for allergies. A reasonable daily dosage is in the range of 500 to 1500 mg. per day, depending upon the patient and circumstances.

Garlic extract. The active ingredient in garlic, allicin, can help quell infections due to bacteria, viruses, parasites, and fungi. It is also an anti-oxidant. Due to its sulfhydryl groups, it even has some ability to act as a natural detoxifying agent, and helps flush heavy metals from the body. A reasonable daily dosage is in the range of 500 to 3,000 mg. per day, depending upon the patient and circumstances.

Lauricidin. This medicinal oil, derived from coconut, is believed to help eradicate bacteria, viruses, fungi, and parasites. A reasonable daily dosage is in the range of 10 to 40 pellets, in divided doses, depending upon the patient and circumstances.

SUPPLEMENTS FOR TARGETED SUBSETS OF PATIENTS

Although all patients must take their own unique combinations of supplements, tailored to their own needs and their own metabolisms, there are certain subsets of patients who may have somewhat similar supplement programs. These programs may include a core group of supplements that are targeted to impact specific conditions, such as inflammation, or immune dysfunction. These core groups of supplements can also be targeted to achieve specific goals, such as improved cognition, or improved methylation.

Following are core groups of supplements that apply to these specific conditions, and goals. They are not used to treat these conditions, but rather to improve function.

However, these core groups of supplements will rarely compose a patient's entire program of supplementation. In almost all cases, other supplements will also be helpful. Most frequently, for example, the Tier One supplements are given in conjunction with these various core groups of supplements. Supplements from the other two tiers may also be taken.

Supplements to Enhance Cognition

- Methyl-B-12.
- DMAE.
- Phosphatidylcholine.
- N-acetyl-carnitine.
- B-spectrum vitamins, including pantothenic acid.
- Zinc.
- Iron.

Supplements to Enhance Immunity

- Zinc.
- Cod liver oil.
- Vitamin A.
- Essential fatty acids.
- Probiotics.
- Vitamin C.
- Vitamin E.
- Vitamin D.
- Transfer factor.
- Oral gamma globulin.
- Specific herbal supplements.
- L-Arginine.
- L-Glutamine.

Supplements to Reduce Inflammation

- Essential fatty acids.
- Antioxidants, including vitamins C, E, and selenium.
- Chromium.
- Quercitin.
- Pycnogenol.
- Melatonin.
- Magnesium.
- Curcumin.

Supplements to Reduce the Autoimmune Response

- Essential fatty acids.
- Vitamin C.
- Vitamin E.
- Vitamin D.

- Anti-inflammatory nutrients and flavonoids, including quercitin, pycnogenol, and others.
- Transfer factor.

Supplements for Hypoglycemia

- Chromium.
- Zinc.
- Magnesium.
- Niacin.
- L-Glutamine.

Supplements for Viral Infection

- Garlic.
- Lauricidin.
- Transfer factor.
- Vitamin A.
- Vitamin C.
- Selenium
- Olive leaf extract.
- Zinc.
- Arabinogalactan.

Supplements for Leaky Gut Syndrome

- Probiotics.
  - Acidophilus.
  - Bifidus.
  - *Saccharomyces boulardii.*
  - Cobiotic Companion (a supplement which is a combination of all three).
- Zinc.
- L-Glutamine.
- Pantothenic acid.
- Gamma oryzanol.
- Evening primrose oil.
- Permeability Factors (a supplement containing many of the above).

Supplements for Fungi

- Paramicrocidin (grapefruit seed extract).
- Capryllic acid.
- Garlic.

- Lauricidin.
- Oregano oil.
- Probiotics.
- Cobiotic Companion (a combination of acidophilus, bifidus, and *Saccharomyces boulardii*).
- Zinc.
- Vitamin C.
- Transfer factor.
- Biotin.

Supplements for ADHD, Inattentive Subtype

- DMAE.
- Phosphatidylcholine.
- Magnesium.
- Zinc.
- Iron.
- L-Tyrosine.
- Methyl-B-12.
- Vitamin C.
- Pantothenic acid.
- Taurine.
- Omega-3 EFAs.

Supplements for ADHD, Hyperactive Subtype

- Magnesium.
- 5-HTP.
- L-Theanine.
- Taurine.
- GABA.
- Inositol.
- Methyl-B-12.
- Omega-3 EFAs.

Supplements for Asthma

- Magnesium.
- Vitamin C.
- Gamma-linolenic acid (GLA).
- Vitamin B-6.
- Pantothenic acid.
- Quercitin.

- Pycnogenol.
- Fish oil (EPA/DHA).
- L-Arginine.

Supplements to Enhance Methylation

- Methyl-B-12.
- Folinic acid.
- DMG.
- TMG.
- Zinc.
- *N*-acetyl-cysteine (NAC).
- Glutathione.

SUMMARY

Supplementation Therapy

Do not allow all of this information to overwhelm you. This is not information that you must commit to memory, or even fully understand. Instead, it is a reference guide, which you can consult over the next few months, or years, as you work with your doctor to individualize your child's supplement program.

I have described almost fifty different nutrients in the prior material, but your child will probably be taking only a relatively small portion of them, perhaps as few as ten.

If your child is not accustomed to taking supplements, even ten might seem daunting, but I am confident that you and your child can adjust to this.

As your child begins to improve, I believe that your family will embrace this program of supplementation therapy. Getting children to take supplements can present some challenges, but most parents can find a way to make this happen, because supplements typically trigger profound, lasting, positive changes. As these positive changes accumulate, motivation will build.

Now we move on to the third component of the Healing Program: detoxification. As toxins clear from your child's body, he or she will emerge as a happier, healthier child, and your hopes for the future may become closer than ever to coming true. Detoxification can take your child to the next level of healing.

CHAPTER NINETEEN

THE HEALING PROGRAM

Element #3:
Detoxification

IT'S TIME TO DETOX

TOXINS, MORE THAN ANY OTHER SINGLE, ISOLATED ELEMENT, APPEAR to be the primary root cause of the 4-A epidemics.

In specific, toxic heavy metals, along with environmental chemicals, are the two most destructive toxic forces. Heavy metals and environmental chemicals are the greatest contributors to the epidemic of autism. In addition, they often play an important role in ADHD, and can also be involved in asthma and allergies.

Even more specifically, the toxic heavy metal mercury, from environmental and other sources, lies at the heart of the autism epidemic. If it were not for toxification from mercury, autism would probably not currently exist in epidemic proportions.

Many other factors contribute to the 4-A epidemics, including poor nutrition, immune dysfunction, gastrointestinal distress, genetic vulnerabilities, and assaults by viruses, bacteria, and fungi. However, many of these factors could be overcome or successfully endured by most children if it were not for the role played by toxins, and especially heavy metals.

Toxins, particularly toxic chemicals and heavy metals, may well have inaugurated the cascading process of disease and disorder in your own child.

Now it's time to reverse that process. You can reverse it by employing a number of detoxification measures, including administration of glutathione, boosting the process of methylation, and engaging in chelation therapy.

IMPAIRED DETOXIFICATION

Toxins would not be as destructive as they now are if everyone had the capability of adequately detoxifying their bodies. Unfortunately, everyone can not. 4-A children, in particular, often have impaired detoxification.

From my clinical experience, it sometimes appears as if autism is more a result of impaired detoxification than any other single contributing factor. Impaired detoxification creates:

- **Oxidative stress,** which damages and destroys cells throughout the body, including cells in the brain and nervous system.

- **Chronic inflammatory conditions,** including neuroinflammation, and inflammation in the gut and the immune system.

- **Toxic build-up,** in cells and in the bloodstream, which creates vast cascades of cell dysfunction and death throughout the body and brain.

When impaired detoxification is reversed, though, kids commonly experience dramatic bursts of healing.

The toxins that make kids sick and miserable consist of two types:

- **Exogenous toxins,** or toxins that come from outside the body. These include heavy metals, pesticides, and pollutants.

- **Endogenous toxins,** or toxins that come from inside the body. These include metabolic waste, bacterial by-products, and necrotic matter in the gut.

These exogenous and endogenous toxins can be grouped in five general categories. It is quite possible that every single day your child is exposed to every one of these categories of toxic material.

The Five Primary Sources of Toxins

1. **Metabolic end products.** These are the toxins that are formed by the natural functions of the body. They include such diverse toxicants as ammonia that is excreted in the urine, hormones that require metabolism and expulsion, and acetaldehyde created in the yeast cycle. All children have some of these toxins in their bodies, but some kids can't adequately get them out.

2. **Microorganisms.** These are the bacteria, viruses, fungi, and parasites that invade the body, and then sometimes proliferate within the body. Their presence is unavoidable, but their impact must be kept within healthy limits through the process of detoxification.

3. **Contaminants.** These are the exogenous toxins that surround us in our environments. They include heavy metals, pesticides, insecticides, and a variety of pollutants, such as PCBs. These toxins can lodge in cells and tissues in the brain and body, if they are not properly expelled. Mercury, in particular, has an affinity for brain cells.

4. **Drugs and alcohol.** This category includes not just recreational substances, but also common pharmaceutical and over-the-counter drugs. These medications are generally nontoxic when taken in the proper dosages, but they can build up in the system during long-term use, if not adequately metabolized and detoxified.

5. **Food additives.** This includes food colorings, preservatives, and common excitotoxins, such as MSG or aspartame. These additives are often eaten in excess by kids who overindulge in processed foods and junk foods. This category also includes hormones and antibiotics that are added to foods.

Your child's exposure to all five of these categories of toxins must be minimized. When exposure does occur, though, you can help your child to detoxify, and stay healthy.

Getting Toxins Out

The body has a four-phase line of defense against toxins. When each of these four phases is functioning properly, toxins can be adequately eliminated. However, a breakdown in even just one phase can derail the entire process and enable toxins to begin their attack upon children's bodies and brains.

Each of these detoxification phases requires the expenditure of considerable energy. This energy is required twenty-four hours a day, seven days a week. We tend to think that the body is completely at rest if we are just sitting around, or sleeping, but the internal functions of the body are always at work, and one of the primary, 24/7, internal functions of the body is to get rid of toxins. Unfortunately, though, just having toxins in the body makes it harder to get rid of them, because toxins drain energy, even at the cellular level. They do this by interfering with the energy-producing mitochondria in each cell. This can render each cell less capable of detoxification. This can create a spiral of increasing toxicity and decreasing energy. Sometimes this spiral can be overcome only by active intervention with various detoxification measures. These measures can improve the function of all four phases of detoxification. Following are the four phases.

The Four Phases of Detoxification

Detox Phase 1 consists of keeping ingested toxins confined to the GI tract, where they can safely exit the body, instead of allowing them to be absorbed by the system. This first phase of detox can fail, though, if the gut wall is excessively permeable, due to conditions such as yeast overgrowth. This hyperpermeability allows toxins to escape from the gut and enter the system. Another problem that can allow toxins in the gut to enter the system is impairment of the IgA antibody system, which is designed to disable toxins, as they undergo the process of elimination. One other factor that can allow toxins from the gut to enter the system is an exceptionally slow transit time through the GI tract. When the gut is functioning sluggishly, because it doesn't have enough dietary fiber, or isn't contracting strongly because of nutritional deficiencies, food moves slowly through the GI tract, and toxins have more time to escape from the gut.

Detox Phase 2 is focused on the liver. In this phase, toxins are moved from the gut to the liver, primarily through the portal tract, which connects the gut and the liver. In the liver, toxins, which are often fat-soluble, are converted into water-soluble toxins, because water-soluble materials are much easier to excrete. During this process, the toxins can be temporarily converted into intermediate substances that are often more toxic than the original toxins. Even though they are more toxic, this conversion process makes them, as my colleague Sid Baker describes it, "more sticky," with an increased ability to stick to other substances that can be readily excreted.

During this phase, it's important to help the liver do its job, and to protect it from toxic overload. One of the best ways to support the function and health of the liver is with supplementation therapy, consisting of B-vitamins, antioxidants, vitamin/mineral cofactors, and the liver-protecting herb silymarin.

Detox Phase 3 consists of joining, or conjugating, toxins with specific detoxifying nutrients. These special nutrients have the particular action of helping to remove toxins from the body. They are the nutrients that I have mentioned many times as being among the most valuable for 4-A kids. The nutrients include glutathione, glycine, cysteine, taurine, and sulfate.

These nutrients attach to toxins, make them less toxic, and allow them to be eliminated from the system. Without these nutrients, this elimination might never occur.

Because toxins are being actively eliminated during this phase, through the bowels and also the urinary tract, it's important to keep the bowels and urinary tract functioning strongly, by drinking plenty of fluids, eating fiber, and avoiding dehydration or constipation.

It can also help to eat certain unique, detoxifying foods during this phase, because particular foods also help conjugate toxins. These include foods with sulfated phytochemicals, such as garlic and cruciferous vegetables such as broccoli. Sometimes kids don't like cruciferous vegetables, so it may be necessary to give your child capsules or powder that contain concentrated vegetable nutrients.

Detox Phase 4 consists of supporting the body's natural detoxification processes by adjusting the body's acid-alkaline balance, or pH. As a rule, a state of alkalinity is more efficient for detoxifying than is a state of acidity. I have found that most of my autistic kids, however, are acidotic.

Dr. Jeffrey Bland and others have shown that people can overcome toxicity better by engaging in some simple techniques that increase the body's alkalinity. These techniques include eating more green vegetables, eating less high-fat meat, eating less sugar, and sometimes taking potassium citrate supplements.

Because alkalinity promotes detoxification, most of the common herbal detoxification formulas, such as green juice, are alkalinizing.

It can be a challenge for parents, of course, to help administer some of these measures. Kids usually don't like to drink green juice or eat lots of fiber.

However, one of the most powerful of all detoxification measures can be relatively easy to apply. This measure is the administration of glutathione. Of all the therapies that help kids recover from autism and the other 4-A disorders, giving glutathione stands out as among the most potent. The importance of glutathione has been demonstrated in research performed by my colleague Jill James, Ph.D.

Glutathione for Detoxification

Glutathione is especially valuable because it does so many things, unlike some of the other detoxification procedures, which have much more limited effects.

Here are all the things that glutathione does.

- It conjugates and detoxifies not just heavy metals, but also chemical toxicants.

- It is a very powerful antioxidant, and stops free radical damage.

- It protects proteins from oxidation.

- It helps preserve mitochondrial integrity, and protect the mitochondria from toxic free-radical damage.

- It promotes the production of the energy units that are formed by the mitochondria, called ATP.

• It protects the epithelial lining of the gut, and thereby helps prevent toxins from entering the system, due to leaky gut syndrome.

• It promotes normal T-cell function, and prevents the destruction of T-cells through the process of programmed cell death.

• It helps prevent the oxidation of antioxidants, such as vitamins C and E, thereby preserving their antioxidant activity.

• It activates an important enzyme in the methylation process that results in the formation of SAMe.

As you can see, glutathione supports the function of all three of the systems that are most involved with the onset of autism symptoms: the immune system, the gastrointestinal system, and the nervous system.

When glutathione is low, as it often is among 4-A children, kids are much more vulnerable to the 4-A disorders. Low glutathione can create disastrous consequences.

Consequences of Low Glutathione

1. **Reduced ability to detoxify.** Low glutathione reduces detoxification of both environmental toxicants and heavy metals. This can result in increased neurotoxicity, and immunotoxicity.

2. **Altered cell membrane function.** Cell membranes allow wastes to be released from cells, and nutrients to enter. Low glutathione interferes with both processes.

3. **Poor nerve conduction.** Without enough glutathione, nerve cells, including brain cells, cannot effectively transmit messages from one cell to another.

4. **Vulnerability to toxins in the brain.** Low levels of glutathione in brain cells create heightened sensitivity to heavy metals, and to other toxicants.

5. Absorption of neurotoxic proteins. Low glutathione that results in leaky gut syndrome allows harmful peptides to enter the brain.

6. Increased autoimmunity and allergy. When low glutathione skews the immune system toward Th-2 overactivity, it prompts the immune system to launch autoimmune attacks upon the body, and to attack food and inhalant substances with the allergic response.

7. Reduced methylation. Last but certainly not least, low glutathione decreases the body's natural ability to detoxify itself, through the essential process of methylation.

When glutathione is returned to normal levels, it can trigger great improvements in kids, at times quite swiftly. These include improvements in calmness, focus, presence, eye contact, receptive language, expressive language, and social interaction.

Glutathione can cause side effects in some kids, including increased stimming, hyperactivity, irritability, and on occasions, increased obsessive-compulsive behaviors.

Because of this possibility of side effects, I administer laboratory tests before I give glutathione. The lab results that generally support the administration of glutathione are low glutathione, low cysteine, low sulfate, and high lipid peroxides. If kids are high in cysteine, it could be an indication that they might have an adverse reaction to glutathione. If the lab reports are not sufficiently clear, I sometimes start with a low dose of glutathione and watch closely for side effects.

When I administer glutathione, I generally do it as a slow push, or sometimes a slow drip. I occasionally give glutathione as a stand-alone treatment, but I also frequently administer it just before or after intravenous administration of another therapeutic agent, such as vitamin C, phosphatidylcholine, or the chelating agent calcium EDTA.

I first became aware of the intravenous administration of glutathione for neurological problems many years ago, when a Florida neurologist, Dr. David Perlmutter, began giving it to patients with Parkinson's disease. He achieved success with this approach, and also reported successes in treating other neurodegenerative disorders with

IV-glutathione. Because autism shares some characteristics with neurodegenerative disorders, I theorized that IV-glutathione might help autistic children.

I implemented this approach in my practice, and the response to it was so favorable that I performed an informal, unpublished retrospective review of the first fifty-nine children whom I had treated with IV-glutathione. I noted improvements in approximately 75 percent of this group of autistic children. The kids responded with increased calmness, language development, eye contact, and focus. Of the remaining 25 percent, about half of them showed no response, and the other half responded negatively, with increased stimming and agitation. (*Please see disclaimer, page vii.*)

Since that time, a number of other doctors have begun to use IV-glutathione for autism, with similar positive results.

Although administering glutathione intravenously appears to be the most effective method of administering it, it can also be applied transdermally, or it can be inhaled in a nebulized form. It is possible to administer it orally, but oral glutathione is usually not absorbed very well. However, a new oral, liposomal form may be absorbed more efficiently.

In addition to directly administering glutathione itself, it is also possible to increase its levels in the body by taking other nutrients.

The appropriate nutrients are:

• **Vitamin C.** A dosage of approximately 500 mg. per day was shown in one study to increase glutathione levels by 50 percent. Raising the dosage to 1,000 mg. had no additional benefit, although higher doses of vitamin C may have other benefits, including positive effects on the immune system. In combination with vitamin C, I give kids approximately 100 to 400 i.u. of vitamin E per day, which also bolsters glutathione.

• **N-acetyl-cysteine.** This is a nutritional precursor of glutathione, and blood levels of it are low in about 60 percent to 70 percent of my autistic patients. Administering it can have significant positive effects. However, it may also create potential side effects, which may be similar to those seen with glutathione. Also, this nutrient, when taken orally, can contribute to gut dysbiosis, particularly if kids already have yeast overgrowth. In these situations, we sometimes need to consider other routes of administration, such as transdermally, intravenously, or via neb-ulization.

• **Methyl-B-12.** This also helps increase glutathione levels, and powerfully boosts the methylation process. It is also effective to give methyl-B-12 in conjunction with folinic acid, TMG and/or DMG, plus zinc. The levels of glutathione can sometimes also be raised even further by adding vitamin B-6. (For more details, see Chapter 18.)

Administering glutathione can be a terrific way to help clear the toxins from your child's body, but there are also other ways. Some can be quite effective.

Other Methods of Detoxification

Another important detoxification approach is to rev up the natural detoxification process of methylation, and to engage in other detoxify-ing processes, such as saunas. These natural modalities can be done in conjunction with chelation, the medical process of removing heavy metals. These modalities boost the power of chelation, and help the body excrete heavy metals. In some cases, these natural modalities can be successfully used without engaging in chelation, if the total toxic bur-den is not particularly severe.

I have repeatedly mentioned the nutrients that boost methylation, but they're worthy of repetition. They are:

- Methyl-B-12.
- TMG.
- DMG.
- Folinic acid.
- SAMe (sometimes).
- Vitamins C and E.
- Glutathione.
- *N*-acetyl cysteine.

These nutrients can help the body get rid of toxicants, including mercury, which is often the toxin that disrupted the methylation process in the first place. Therefore, the more mercury your child eliminates, the better his or her body will become at eliminating it. Your child can build a positive cycle of healing.

In addition to helping your child to eliminate heavy metals, you should also do your best to help him or her get rid of other toxins, including pesticides, herbicides, and industrial chemicals. Various nutrients help achieve this, including the following:

- Vitamin C.
- Vitamin B-6.
- Taurine.
- Vitamin A.
- Phosphatidylcholine.
- Silymarin.
- *N*-acetyl cysteine (NAC).
- Alpha-lipoic acid.
- Glutathione.

A few other natural approaches also help to rid the body of toxins. These are all commonsense methods that are widely used. They include drinking plenty of fluids, exercising, engaging in deep breathing, avoiding constipation, and sweating.

Sweating can be of particular benefit for some kids, because toxins are invariably removed through perspiration. In fact, the skin is sometimes referred to as "the third kidney." A number of 4-A kids have reported positive responses from taking regular, far-infrared saunas. I generally recommend that kids do some exercise first, such as bouncing on a mini-trampoline, to open up their pores and to stimulate toxin-removing lymphatic flow. They should also drink extra fluids, to prevent dehydration. Sometimes they may also benefit from taking a small dose of the B-vitamin niacin before the sauna, because niacin dilates the capillaries. Some kids don't like niacin, though, because it causes the skin to flush. Others, however, seem to enjoy taking it, possibly because it increases the activity of the calming neurotransmitter GABA.

I also recommend that kids use saunas that incorporate far-infrared heat lamps, if possible. Recent evidence indicates that infrared rays may be of some benefit in stimulating immunity, and providing a mild anti-inflammatory effect.

Saunas may also help in another way. In addition to helping remove toxins through perspiration, there is a growing belief that saunas also help detoxify the body by increasing the breakdown of fat cells, where toxins tend to be stored. This enhances the removal of these toxins by the liver. Fat cells can also be broken down during exercise, or by any other factor that causes loss of adipose tissue.

If your physician decides sauna use is appropriate for your child, he or she should monitor its course for any possible adverse effects.

Another method of detoxification is administration of IV-phosphatidylcholine, which can have several different effects. Phosphatidylcholine is important in cell membrane function and liver detoxification. It is also the primary nutritional building block for the main neurotransmitter of thought, acetylcholine. In addition, it tends to be calming. (*Please see disclaimer, page vii.*)

Other nutrients that can aid detoxification when administered intravenously are vitamin C and magnesium. IV administration of these nutrients and others can be a helpful method of delivery for kids with touchy GI tracts.

A relatively recent innovation in the approach to autism-spectrum disorders is the use by some physicians of hyperbaric oxygen therapy, or HBOT. Although this therapy is still in its early stages as a treatment for autism, preliminary studies tend to indicate that it can be helpful. An increasing number of patients have undergone the therapy, with generally good results reported.

HBOT consists of placing a patient in an airtight chamber, and then increasing the air pressure, generally while the patient is breathing pure oxygen. In milder forms of the procedure, concentrated oxygen may be used. The experience of mildly increased air pressure is usually not uncomfortable and is similar to the air pressure increases that occur while flying on airplanes. However, pressure-related trauma to the middle ear is the most common side effect of HBOT, but is minimal in the milder forms of the procedure.

HBOT was first used when scuba divers needed extra oxygen to overcome decompression sickness, but now it has a wide range of applications. Because HBOT increases perfusion, increases oxygenation in all body tissues, and decreases swelling, it is used rather commonly for wound healing and as an off-label use for strokes, brain injury, cerebral palsy, and vascular disease.

In autistic children, it is believed that HBOT helps to reduce inflammation, increase perfusion to the brain, and may alleviate oxidative stress in some cases. Some physicians, including Jeff Bradstreet, M.D., who uses it extensively, have reported positive results among autistic patients, including improved language, cognitive ability, and social skills. However, more research needs to be done and is currently in progress.

Now let's look at another of the most powerful detoxification measures, chelation therapy.

CHELATION THERAPY

Chelation is generally believed to be the most powerful and reliable biomedical method of removing heavy metals, including mercury, from the system. Chelation (key-lay-shun) is a procedure in which a patient is given a medication that attaches to heavy metals, and helps the body to excrete them.

Chelation therapy has been successfully applied to thousands of children on the autism spectrum, under the supervision of DAN doctors and other integrative physicians. The results have generally been gratifying and promising. The positive response rate, as quantified in the ongoing series of Autism Research Institute parent evaluations, is as follows:

- **Symptoms improved: 76 percent.**
- **No discernible effect: 22 percent.**
- **Symptoms worsened: 2 percent.**

These parent evaluations represent a 38-to-1 ratio of improvement of symptoms compared to worsening of symptoms. Worsening of symptoms was generally mild and temporary. It most frequently consisted of increased hyperactivity, irritability, and increased stimming.

No other single element in the biomedical treatment of autism has been rated this highly.

Of course, this rating system is not based strictly upon quantifiable, objective markers, and therefore cannot be considered to be a scientific analysis. Nonetheless, parents are generally quite astute at monitoring improvements and declines in their children's behavior, cognitive processing, general health, and daily function. Parents typically recognize changes in their children—both subtle and profound—more accurately than does anyone else in the treatment milieu, and their subjective evaluations of their children tend to correlate strongly with various objec-

tive, scientific measures. For example, parental reports of improved behavior tend to coincide with measured excretion of heavy metals. As
I've said so many times, *moms know* (and dads, too).

Most of the parents of my own young patients have generally reported significant improvements to me when their kids began to be
chelated. Not all kids respond positively to chelation, of course. No single modality works for everyone. The presumption that a particular
therapy will have a 100 percent positive response rate is a reflection of
an outdated, magic-bullet approach to medicine.

Chelation is so consistently helpful, however, that biomedical practitioners typically test most autistic children for heavy metals by performing a test called a provoked heavy metal urine challenge.
Physicians use the results of this test to determine possible need of future treatment. Generally, a full course of treatment can trigger at least
moderate improvements in symptomatology, and sometimes the improvements are remarkable.

The possible success may depend, in part, upon the relative severity
of the heavy metal overload that is originally present in the child's system. When there is a great deal of heavy metal in the system prior to
chelation, improvements tend to more often be notable. Success can
also sometimes depend upon the age of the child. Younger children generally respond more positively than older children, whose damage may
be more deeply embedded by years of physical and neurological deterioration. Furthermore, success can depend upon how actively the child
is participating in the other aspects of the Healing Program, which synergistically support chelation.

Success can sometimes occur even when children do not excrete
large amounts of heavy metals in their urine. Sometimes a small amount
can make a big difference. Improvement also occasionally occurs relatively quickly because of factors that cannot be attributed to metal excretion. The improvement may be due to improved sulfation, or to
decreased oxidant stress.

Chelation is nonsurgical, painless, and safe when administered and
monitored appropriately. It has been medically proven to be an effective
way to flush lead out of the system. It is commonly used in the treatment of autism, but is much less commonly used by biomedical physicians in the treatment of ADHD, asthma, and allergies.

Even though chelation is not commonly used for kids with ADHD, asthma, and allergies, it can, in limited cases, be helpful to these children, *if they have evidence of heavy metal burden.*

Chelation has been used by many doctors throughout the world to treat people with a wide variety of diseases and disorders, including Parkinson's disease, multiple sclerosis, hardening of the arteries, chronic fatigue syndrome, fibromyalgia, arthritis, and lead poisoning. It can be of help to a broad spectrum of people who carry excessive heavy metals in their systems.

Chelation has for many years been approved by the U.S. Food and Drug Administration as a safe and effective therapy for lead poisoning. Currently, not enough research supports FDA approval of chelation for other, more diverse disorders, such as treatment of cardiovascular disease. However, this status may change in the future, as more studies are performed that support the efficacy of chelation for conditions other than lead poisoning. For example, I am currently participating in a $32-million, five-year, multicenter study on using chelation therapy in the treatment of cardiovascular disease, sponsored by the National Institutes of Health. Positive outcomes from this study and others may widen the FDA approval of chelation as a treatment for a variety of disorders.

Even though chelation has not been approved specifically as a therapy for autism, it is still often applied for this use by physicians employing a biomedical approach to autism. It is a standard medical practice for physicians to use various drugs and procedures for purposes other than those for which they have been specifically approved by the FDA. This practice is referred to as off-label usage. For example, the procedure of Botox injections is approved only for facial tics, but it is used primarily as a cosmetic procedure for wrinkles. Similarly, it's estimated that approximately half of all cardiac medications are used for off-label purposes, as well as about 42 percent of all asthma drugs, and 34 percent of all allergy medications.

Upon occasion, you may hear people remark deprecatingly that chelation has not been approved for autism, but as you can see, this statement of fact can be used as a rather contrived way of inferring that this application is inappropriate, or arcane. Chelation is, in fact, a well-accepted treatment for autistic children among physicians using a biomedical approach.

Furthermore, you may hear that chelation is an "unproven" treatment for autism. Again, this is true, but this statement can be used to mislead people. To many people, "unproven" sounds as if it means the same thing as "disproven"–but it doesn't mean the same thing at all. "Unproven" is a specific medical term that means that a medication or procedure hasn't yet been approved by the FDA for a particular, specific application, based upon extensive studies. For example, Botox is an unproven treatment for wrinkles.

At some point, it's quite possible that chelation will be approved specifically as a treatment for autism, after more studies have been completed. However, if your physician does recommend chelation, it would probably be unwise for you to postpone this treatment for your child until after the procedure has been approved specifically for autism. That approval process may take many years. Meanwhile, your child may lose ground by waiting, since younger children appear to respond more quickly and completely than older children to chelation therapy and other biomedical interventions.

Even if chelation does become approved specifically for autism, chelation will still not be appropriate as a single, stand-alone therapy. Autism is a multifactorial disorder, and responds adequately only to a multifactorial program. Chelation can be an important component of that program, but it will never be more than just one element.

To be approved specifically for autism, chelation would have to meet the two standard FDA criteria for approval: safety and efficacy. At this time, only the issue of efficacy, or effectiveness, remains open to scientific debate. The safety of chelation has already been accepted by the FDA. If it had not been accepted, chelation would not have been approved as a treatment for lead poisoning, nor would it have been approved for the NIH study on chelation therapy and cardiovascular disease.

However, even though chelation has been scientifically proven to be safe, there are still rumors about possible dangers of chelation that sometimes circulate among the general public. These rumors are medically unfounded, because chelation, when performed properly, has a compelling clinical record of safety. It must be performed properly, though, with sensitivity to safety issues. As a clinician who has administered chelation to many children, I am particularly sensitive to safety issues.

Safety First

The primary reason that there are some rumors circulating among the public that chelation might be dangerous for kids is because two children died during recent years when they were mistakenly given the wrong drug during chelation treatments. Some news reports, particularly those that appeared immediately after the deaths, gave the mistaken impression that the deaths occurred because of the procedure itself, rather than because the wrong drug was used.

Chelation, like every medical procedure, must be done properly. If it is not, it can harm patients. Many thousands of chelation treatments have been performed properly, with no adverse effects, but mistakes can, unfortunately, occur.

In the two fatal incidents, the cause of death, according to the U.S. Centers for Disease Control and Prevention, was administration of the wrong drug. The specific problem was that the two children both experienced a sudden gross deficit of calcium, which resulted in cardiac arrest. This deficit of calcium occurred because the patients were given the wrong chelation drug—disodium EDTA. Instead, they should have been given calcium EDTA. If they had been given the proper chelating agent, they would not have suffered the sudden calcium deficit, and the resulting cardiac arrest.

The drug that they were given, disodium EDTA, is an FDA-approved drug for certain conditions, including hypercalcemia and digitalis toxicity. However, as a general rule, disodium EDTA should not be administered to children. I do not administer disodium EDTA to children in my own practice.

Adults generally respond well to disodium EDTA, though, when it is administered correctly. In fact, disodium EDTA is the medication we are currently using in the large NIH study that is evaluating chelation therapy for cardiovascular disease.

Another reason the two deaths may have occurred from the administration of disodium EDTA was that the chelation medication was not administered as a slow intravenous drip. Instead, it was administered as a relatively fast intravenous push. The slow IV drip method minimizes the possibility of sudden adverse reactions. We are employing the slow IV drip in the NIH study on chelation therapy.

When chelating medication is given intravenously, the push method is more convenient for patients, because the drip method in children may take from one to one and a half hours. Also, some doctors feel that the push method may be somewhat more effective. However, as an extra precaution, when most biomedical practitioners administer chelation therapy, they use either oral medication, such as DMSA, or a slow IV drip, using calcium EDTA.

Another precaution that they take is to frequently administer extra minerals to patients prior to and during their courses of chelation, even if their mineral status appears to be normal, according to laboratory testing. Many children show evidence of multiple mineral deficiencies, and these need to be addressed prior to embarking on a course of chelation therapy. This is yet another mechanism to ensure maximum safety. Prescribing extra minerals before chelation is also wise simply because chelation can sometimes have a moderate effect of decreasing minerals.

This moderate decline in minerals is among the most common side effects of chelation, along with a few other generally mild negative reactions, including hyperactivity, irritability, and increased self-stimulating behaviors. Doctors must monitor for these side effects on an ongoing basis. Other possible side effects include: mildly lowered white blood count; elevations in liver enzymes; exacerbation of yeast overgrowth; elevated BUN (blood urea nitrogen) and creatinine, indicative of decreased kidney function; a moderate decline in bone marrow function; hypoglycemia; and, rarely, a sufficient drop in calcium levels to contribute to tetany (which virtually never occurs with an IV-calcium EDTA drip).

All of these possible side effects are meaningful concerns, but they can all be adequately addressed through proper care and vigilance. Even so, unlike the more naturalistic elements of the Healing Program—such as dietary modification and supplementation therapy—chelation is a moderately invasive medical intervention that holds some risk for harm, if it is performed improperly. Therefore, chelation is usually considered to be significantly more controversial than the most notably benign elements of the program, such as good nutrition. Nonetheless, chelation's safety record, as evidenced by its FDA approval for the treatment of heavy metal toxicity, is acceptable. However, chelation must be monitored, and administered appropriately, by physicians who are experienced in administering chelation to children.

Now let's address the specifics of chelation therapy. This material will help you understand the procedures that your child may participate in, under the guidance of a physician.

Before beginning chelation, all patients undergo laboratory tests to see if the therapy is necessary and advisable for them. All testing must be supervised by physicians.

Testing for Heavy Metal Overload

Three types of tests can be done to determine the presence of excess heavy metals in the system. The most reliable test is the provocation test. The three tests are:

- Blood tests.
- Hair and urine tests.
- Provocation tests

Blood Tests

Blood tests are the least effective way to test for heavy metals. Sometimes, though, blood tests do reveal the presence of lead, mercury, arsenic, aluminum, or other heavy metals. Blood tests aren't very effective for finding most heavy metals because heavy metals generally don't remain in the blood for very long. They quickly move into tissues. Lead exposure, however, is frequently ongoing, so sometimes lead is still in the blood during the testing procedure. Mercury, on the other hand, is rarely found in high levels in the blood. Unfortunately, most mercury travels quickly to tissues and cells, including brain cells.

Technically, the presence of these metals in the tissues and cells does not meet the generally accepted diagnostic criteria for heavy metal toxicity. The only condition that meets the conventional definition of heavy metal toxicity is an elevated level of heavy metal, such as lead, in the blood. Therefore, a more precise term for the presence of excessive metals in tissues and cells is heavy metal overload, or heavy metal burden. This definition may seem rather arbitrary to nonmedical people, though, so in this book, which is intended for the layperson, the terms "toxicity," "overload," and "burden" are used interchangeably.

Hair and Urine Tests

Urine testing for heavy metals shares the same basic problem as blood testing. Urine testing is only accurate for revealing recent excretion of heavy metals, of no more than about three days. Therefore, it is not a very reliable method of determining heavy metal overload that is locked into tissues and cells. This heavy metal is not being excreted into the urine. If it were, toxicity probably wouldn't be as much of a problem.

Hair analysis is used by some physicians to screen for heavy metals, but this method is controversial, and not widely accepted. This method is also not effective for determining the types and quantities of heavy metals that are trapped in tissues, but only the presence of heavy metals that have been expelled from the tissues, into the hair.

As you can see, tests that only detect recent excretions of heavy metal are generally not accurate for determining the presence of heavy metals in tissues. The bodies of the kids who have the most severe accumulation of heavy metals in their tissues are usually not adept at excreting heavy metals. If these kids' bodies were more adept at this metabolic function, the kids probably wouldn't have significant heavy metal accumulation.

Children have varying natural degrees of the ability to excrete heavy metals, through processes such as methylation and sulfation. Two different children can be exposed to the same amounts of heavy metals, but one child may excrete them successfully, while the other may not. The child who can *not* excrete them successfully through these natural detoxification processes of methylation and sulfation may be the child who can benefit most from chelation.

Provocation Tests

These tests are usually considered by the majority of integrative physicians to be the most accurate tests for the presence of heavy metals in the tissues and cells. This testing method is taught at medical workshops that cover heavy metal detoxification and chelation therapy. These workshops are presented by groups such as Defeat Autism Now and the American College for Advancement in Medicine.

The testing method is very straightforward. First, urine is checked for heavy metals. Then a chelating agent is administered, as a challenge test, and the urine is checked again for the presence of heavy metals. Some physicians may also check a fecal sample for heavy metals. If significant amounts of heavy metals have been excreted, it is evidence of probable heavy metal overload. If little or no metal was excreted on the first urine challenge test, it may indicate that little or none is present. However, it's also possible that none was excreted because the heavy metal was so tightly bound to tissues. Because some children do not excrete heavy metals on the first challenge, some clinicians still administer a few courses of chelation, and then rechallenge.

The results of the provocation test can not only reveal the presence of heavy metals, but can also indicate that chelation can be a successful method of removing these heavy metals.

Some heavy metals can initially be missed, because they are not as easily excreted as others. They may remain in the system, while other types of heavy metals come out. This happens because certain heavy metals bind preferentially with chelating agents. Mercury, in particular, might not be excreted in the early chelation challenge. Sometimes mercury will not be excreted until many of the other heavy metals have already been excreted. Therefore, it's wise to be patient, and to refrain from jumping to the conclusion that no mercury is present, just because it was not excreted during the first several chelation challenges, or treatments.

Furthermore, the rate of excretion of heavy metals varies for each individual, and so does the clinical response to the removal of heavy metals. Certain patients show some positive changes early on, while others may require many treatments before they show bursts of improvement. Therefore, it is important to move slowly, patiently, and—most important, safely—during this process. Usually, chelation therapy must be continued for months, or even up to a year or two, to achieve maximal clearance of heavy metals, and clinical improvements.

Waiting for improvements during this long period of time, however, can be hard for parents and kids. Sometimes, unfortunately, improvements never happen. Not all autistic kids have heavy metal overload. Heavy metal overload is very common, but it's by no means universal. This is yet another reason why individualization of therapy is so important.

COMMONLY USED CHELATING AGENTS

The most common pharmaceutical chelating agents are DMSA (dimercaptosuccinic acid), DMPS (dimercaptopropanesulfonate), and calcium EDTA (ethylenediaminetetraacetic acid).

DMSA works well for lead, mercury, arsenic, and other metals. DMPS works especially well for mercury. Calcium EDTA is used for lead, cadmium, aluminum, and other metals.

A provocation test with DMSA is the most commonly used test, and it is the one that I most often employ. DMSA is an FDA-approved drug for lead toxicity. It is an effective chelator for heavy metals, and has an extremely good safety record among children.

DMSA provocation testing has been studied by Dr. Jeff Bradstreet and others. Dr. Bradstreet tested 221 autistic children and eighteen normal children. His study showed that the autistic children excreted three times as much mercury as the normal children. This confirmed the presence of heavy metal overload in these autistic children.

DMPS and calcium EDTA are also employed by some doctors for provocation tests, but they are used less frequently than DMSA. Calcium EDTA is FDA-approved for lead toxicity, but DMPS is not FDA-approved for general distribtion, but may be obtained on an idividual prescription basis from compounding pharmacies.

Many children excrete more than one heavy metal. These heavy metals can vary, but lead, mercury, arsenic, tin, nickel, and aluminum seem to be the most common. Sometimes mercury does not come out until a child has excreted a significant amount of lead.

A relatively small subset of children, however, can react negatively to DMSA and DMPS, because they contain a form of sulfur. These chelators can cause some kids to become more hyper, irritable, and stimmy. When this happens, the appropriate response is to stop the treatment temporarily, and then reintroduce the chelating agent at a lower dosage level, safely and slowly.

However, if gut dysbiosis is present, and is persistent, adverse reactions may recur until the GI problems are effectively resolved.

Also, it is important to ensure that minerals are repleted, because mineral deficiency can contribute to unfavorable symptoms.

If your physician determines, through testing, that your child has heavy metal overload, it is extremely important to eliminate these heavy metals. If heavy metal toxicity is severe, it is very possible that your child will not be able to reach the next level of healing. Therefore, your child will in all likelihood need to engage in a program of chelation, supervised by a physician. Other methods of detoxification can help, but chelation is by far the most effective modality for removing heavy metals.

Before beginning chelation therapy, however, it is important to address four issues, which will enhance the effects of chelation therapy, and help protect your child from any possible side effects.

These four issues are:

1. **Reducing** further exposure to toxins.
2. **Improving** nutritional status and overcoming any nutritional deficiencies.

3. **Resolving** intestinal dysbiosis.

4. **Monitoring** liver and kidney function and checking complete blood count.

Here are the details of the four issues:

PRE-CHELATION ISSUE #1

Reducing Further Exposure to Toxins

This is vitally important, because the benefits of toxin removal can be decreased if more toxins are added in their place. Following are the most damaging sources of potential new toxins.

• **Mercury Amalgam Dental Fillings.** To avoid further exposure to mercury, some children may need to have mercury amalgam dental fillings removed. If the child's fillings contain mercury amalgam, the fillings can cause ongoing toxification, because these fillings can release small amounts of mercury into the system on an ongoing basis. This occurs through the normal wear and tear on amalgams that occurs through eating, and grinding of the teeth.

The possibility of harm that dental mercury may do is a controversial subject. The majority of dentists do not believe that mercury amalgams cause any appreciable problems, but many other dentists and physicians do not agree with that perspective. In my opinion, these amalgams *can* be harmful, depending primarily upon the metabolic status of each individual, and secondarily, upon the number and amount of fillings. Many people can tolerate exposure to low levels of mercury in dental fillings, partly because their bodies are adept at excreting mercury, and partly because they have not been exposed to significant amounts of mercury from other sources.

Another reason some people may be able to tolerate mercury in fillings is because they do not suffer from notable degrees of toxification from other heavy metals, or other toxins. All toxins have a cumulative effect. For example, if a person has high or even moderate levels of lead, arsenic, aluminum, or other toxins, he or she may not be able to tolerate even low exposure to mercury.

The harm that comes from the *cumulative* effect of toxins is another reason that some health experts underestimate the damage that toxins can do. Some experts believe that a person can be free from the harm of heavy metals if he or she has only a slight accumulation of mercury, and a slight accumulation of lead, and a slight accumulation of cadmium. However, the scientific literature suggests that the combined effect of these metals is synergistic. Their net effect is an elevated total toxic burden, beyond the sum of their individual effects.

My colleague John Green, M.D., has likened the cumulative effect of heavy metals to the cumulative effect of various types of cocktails. If a person drinks a martini, then a Bloody Mary, then a mint julep, he or she might not consume very much of any one liquor, but the net effect might be a hangover.

Therefore, if your child has been toxified by mercury in vaccinations, or from environmental sources, or from food, he or she may not be able to tolerate any additional mercury from dental amalgams.

Unfortunately, it's not easy to replace dental fillings, but it can be well worth the effort. Replacement should be done only by an experienced expert, though, to minimize the chance of the mercury entering the body during the replacement process. This procedure should be done before a child is treated with chelation therapy.

• **Mercury in Seafood.** Another important aspect of avoiding further exposure to mercury is to stop eating fish that are contaminated with it. Tuna is by far the most commonly eaten fish in America, particularly among children, but it contains such high levels of mercury that the federal government now recommends that it should not be eaten more than once per week and that it should not be eaten by pregnant women at all.

Other fish that contain high levels of mercury are large fish such as swordfish, shark, and sea bass. These fish are not appropriate for children.

• **Other Foods with Toxins.** It is also important to eat a clean, wholesome daily diet that is as free from all other toxins as possible. Most foods don't have heavy metals in them, but pesticides and herbicides on foods can add to the body's total toxic burden. If children are known to be toxic, they should be given organic foods whenever possible.

Furthermore, inorganic chicken often does contain the heavy metal arsenic. Therefore, it can be important to eat only organic chicken, which is generally free from arsenic. Lots of 4-A kids seem to love chicken nuggets, so it might be difficult for your child to give up this food. A simple alternative is to prepare chicken nuggets at home, with organic chicken and a gluten-free breading.

You should also be sure that the water your child drinks is pure. Much of America's tap water now contains impurities, including trace amounts of heavy metals. It may be necessary to buy a water purifier or to drink bottled water.

• **Environmental Pollutants.** Kids should also be protected as much as is reasonably possible from other common sources of toxins that are present in their daily, immediate environments. This includes toxins in air pollution, and particularly toxic air emitted from coal-burning plants, which contains high levels of mercury. It also includes toxins that are present in common lawn and garden herbicides and pesticides, as well as toxic products used in commercial agriculture. Even treated lumber on an outdoor deck can cause problems, if kids frequently play on the deck. Also, kids shouldn't be exposed to aluminum cookware, or to nonstick cookware that may be eroding.

There's no easy way to deal with these widespread sources of toxins, but seriously ill children should be spared from the further damage that these toxic chemicals can inflict.

• **Vaccinations with Mercury.** A final element of toxification that children should not be exposed to is mercury that is in vaccinations. Most flu vaccinations still contain mercury, and those that do contain mercury should not be given to children or pregnant women.

PRE-CHELATION ISSUE #2

Improving Nutritional Status and Overcoming Any Nutritional Deficiencies

Many autistic children have nutritional deficiencies that should be remedied prior to chelation. If they are not resolved, they can hinder the process of detoxification, and can also make children somewhat more vulnerable to further metabolic problems.

Chelation tends to lower the levels of necessary minerals at the same time that it is lowering the levels of unhealthy heavy metals. Because of this, it's important to boost mineral status prior to chelation. Mineral levels should be tested, and deficiencies should be addressed. It can be prudent, though, to increase the intake of your child's minerals, even if no deficiencies appear to exist. A mineral that definitely should be supplemented is zinc, which is typically low among autistic kids. It can also help to give kids extra calcium, magnesium, and selenium, even though chelation does not significantly lower these minerals. Copper should generally be avoided, unless it has been demonstrated to be low, because it usually tends to already be too high in autistic kids. Therefore, giving a multimineral supplement that contains copper is generally *not* a good idea. Give minerals individually, or in a copper-free multiple-mineral supplement.

As extra minerals are administered, it's important to periodically monitor their levels during the chelation process.

In addition, it's important to use specific nutrients to activate the body's own detoxification process of methylation. This will assist the process of chelation. Methylation, once activated and reinvigorated, will also continue the process of detoxification after the effects of chelation stop. If methylation remains impaired, the gains achieved during chelation can soon be lost.

Methylation also frequently needs to be boosted in autistic kids, and in kids with ADHD symptoms, whether they are chelated or not. For most of these kids, poor methylation may have contributed to their problems in the first place.

To boost methylation and other detoxification processes, it's usually quite helpful to enhance the activity of glutathione, the antioxidant that is formed from three amino acids: cysteine, glycine, and glutamic acid. Glutathione, as I've mentioned, is a very powerful antioxidant and detoxifier, and is a natural chelator. For the details on increasing glutathione, and boosting methylation, please review the prior sections on those subjects.

PRE-CHELATION ISSUE #3

Resolving Intestinal Dysbiosis

Many autistic children have GI problems, which should be resolved before they begin chelation. If these problems are not taken care of, they can impair the process of chelation, and chelation can also make these GI problems even worse.

Of particular importance is overcoming constipation, a very common problem among kids on the autism spectrum. Remediating constipation is important because some heavy metals are excreted fecally. These metals need to be excreted from the system as quickly and efficiently as possible, so they won't be reabsorbed.

Other GI problems that should also be resolved include diarrhea and dysbiosis–especially yeast and bacterial overgrowth. Chelation can exacerbate these problems, especially if N-acetyl-cysteine or alpha lipoic acid are taken orally during the chelation process. These conditions can generally be resolved with nutritional therapy, supplementation therapy, and medication. It is important to clear up these problems before beginning chelation. Sometimes, when these problems linger, it can be frustrating to have to postpone chelation, since chelation can be so valuable. Even so, it's important to do things in the right order. The timing of the Healing Program can be of critical significance.

PRE-CHELATION ISSUE #4

Monitoring Liver and Kidney Function and Checking White Blood Count

The doctor who performs chelation for your child should do it only after checking kidney function (with tests for BUN and creatinine) and liver function (with tests abbreviated as AST, ALT, GGT, and bilirubin). Your child's physician will be familiar with these tests. These tests will assure the physician that your child's liver and kidneys are functioning well enough to accommodate the extra stress of heavy metal excretion, and the stress of the medications used in chelation.

In addition, your physician should monitor your child's complete blood count, or CBC, including the platelet count, prior to detoxification. This will help determine proper eligibility for a chelation program.

These tests should also be periodically repeated, as chelation continues, to be certain that your child is not experiencing any adverse reactions.

PERFORMING CHELATION THERAPY

The chelating agent that is most frequently used is DMSA, so we will look in detail at performing chelation therapy with DMSA. To avoid redundancy, I will present relatively less information on other, similar approaches of performing chelation. These approaches include using DMPS and calcium EDTA. They also include the use of alpha lipoic acid, which can act as a mild chelator, and TTFD, another sulfur-containing substance that can help detoxify heavy metals, especially arsenic.

If your physician does choose to use one of these other methods, or to combine several, that choice, when applied and monitored appropriately, is within the realm of responsible integrative medicine. Sometimes different patients respond more positively to one chelating agent than another, and your child's own physician will be in the best position to recommend the most appropriate medication.

Administering DMSA

DMSA, like all chelating agents, attaches itself to heavy metals, which enables the body to eliminate the metals. Without the benefit of these chelating agents, heavy metals are frequently not removed from the body, and remain lodged in tissues and cells, where they wreak havoc upon normal function. They are particularly damaging to the sensitive neurons in the brain, and the cells in the immune system.

DMSA is generally administered orally, but can be given via rectal suppository, or transdermally, which is a newer route of administration.

DMSA is FDA approved for lead poisoning, but its off-label use to help excrete other heavy metals is extremely common among integrative physicians.

Although DMSA is generally quite safe when used appropriately, it is a powerful medication that can create side effects and metabolic disruptions, especially in 4-A kids with delicate systems and high loads of metals. Therefore, DMSA needs to be administered and monitored by a physician who is trained and knowledgeable in chelation therapy.

DMSA has been demonstrated to bind with a variety of heavy metals, including lead, mercury, arsenic, tin, nickel, and antimony. Although mercury appears to be a common contributor to autism, the other metals can also cause grave harm. Lead, in particular, has been repeatedly shown to lower IQ, even at relatively low levels, and to contribute to ADHD. As I've mentioned, many of these other heavy metals may be excreted before mercury, since mercury can be resistant to excretion, because it is very tightly bound to tissue.

As your child undergoes chelation therapy, over a period of several months or longer, he or she should be periodically retested, with some of the same tests that are given at the outset of therapy. These include:

- **Urinalysis, BUN, and creatinine tests,** to monitor kidney function.

- **Complete blood count tests,** including platelet count, to rule out any possible bone marrow suppression.

- **Liver tests,** particularly for the liver transaminases, ALT, AST, and GGT.

- **Mineral level tests,** particularly for zinc, because DMSA can double zinc excretion.

Copper should also be checked, although some decrease in copper may be helpful.

Treatment periods typically last for three days, followed by eleven days of no chelation treatments. This creates a convenient two-week cycle of treatment, and helps ensure that a cumulative, excessive amount of medication is not taken. Excessive amounts can cause excessive heavy metal excretion, which can result in stress upon the organs of elimination.

These two-week cycles can, in most cases, be safely continued for at least several months, and often longer, depending upon the individual patient and his or her response.

The complete course of treatment is intended to last until only a small or negligible amount of heavy metal is being excreted.

The side effects of DMSA, as compiled by *The Physician's Desk Reference,* are based upon patients taking it for nineteen consecutive days, which is the length of a course of treatment for classic lead poisoning. This nineteen-day period, however, is approximately six times longer than the more conservative three-day periods that my colleagues and I recommend. These side effects include the following:

- GI upset, in 12 percent of patients.
- Body aches, in 5 percent.
- Increase in serum transaminases, in 4 percent.
- Sore throat or cough, in 4 percent.
- Rashes, in 3 percent.
- Drowsiness, in 1 percent.
- Eye or ear irritation, in 1 percent.
- Elevations in liver enzymes, in 1 percent.
- Bone marrow suppression, in 1 percent.

Combinations of these side effects often occur in the same patient.

The occurrence of these side effects is notably less in patients who use the schedule of three days on, followed by eleven days off.

Two other significant side effects may occur, but they are extremely rare, and have only been reported a few times. One is an inflammatory condition of the mucus membranes, referred to as erythema multiforme, or Stevens-Johnson syndrome. The other is a serious skin disorder, which is referred to as toxic epidermal necrolysis, or TEN. Both can be expected to abate when the medication is withdrawn. These side effects are extremely uncommon, but physicians and parents must still be alert for them.

However, when administered and monitored appropriately, chelation therapy with DMSA generally has a good safety profile, and its side effects are usually mild and transient. In addition to the side effects just listed, I have also noted behavioral changes in some children, such as hyperactivity, irritability, and increased stimming. Exacerbation of gut dysbiosis, as well as mineral deficiencies, may contribute to these symptoms.

Other Chelating Agents

Besides DMSA, another chelator that is increasingly being used is calcium EDTA. Calcium EDTA is very effective in the excretion of lead, cadmium, antimony, aluminum, nickel, and tin, but seems to be less valuable for excreting mercury. Calcium EDTA is particularly effective for removing lead when it is used intravenously. Some kids have significant amounts of lead, in their tissues, even when it is not elevated in their blood. This lead can interfere terribly with their cognitive function. It can lower IQ, shorten attention span, and increase behavioral problems. These problems are frequently diagnosed as being symptoms of ADHD, and also autism. Lead can also cause serious damage to the kidneys, nerves, and red blood cells.

Some people think that eating lead-based paint chips is the only way that kids become toxic from lead, but that is an outdated notion. Lead can also be found in dust, water, certain industrial sites, and contaminated soil. It can be carried into the home by people who work in construction, demolition, painting, in radiator repair shops, or in battery stores. Lead is no longer present in auto exhaust or in recently manufactured paint, but it's often found in the paint that is in older homes, and in dust and dirt along roadways, where it may have settled many years earlier.

Lead and other toxins not only add to the body's total toxic burden, but they also have a synergistic effect, making one another even more harmful.

When integrative physicians use EDTA for lead and other heavy metals in children, they virtually always use the calcium form of it, instead of disodium EDTA. Kids are somewhat more vulnerable to dangerous fluctuations in their calcium levels, and these fluctuations can occur with disodium EDTA, if the procedure is performed with a fast intravenous push, instead of a slower intravenous drip. Although these reactions are quite rare, they have occurred, and, as mentioned earlier, this inappropriate administration apparently caused the deaths of two children in recent years.

Therefore, responsible biomedical practitioners give kids only calcium EDTA after proper testing procedures, and not disodium EDTA. The calcium version of the medication will not create calcium fluctuations. For extra safety, they may also administer it in a slow drip.

This does not mean that disodium EDTA does not have appropriate uses. It is, as I mentioned, the medication that we are using in the NIH study on cardiovascular disease in adults.

DMPS is another relatively popular chelating agent. DMPS is a chelator that is used much less frequently than DMSA in America, but a number of doctors have reported good results with it. DMPS is not FDA approved, and must be made specifically for each patient, with a doctor's prescription, at a special type of medication-creating pharmacy that is referred to as a compounding pharmacy. DMPS is widely available in Europe, however, and is sold in Germany over the counter, as a nonprescription drug.

DMPS is an effective chelator for mercury, and can help rid the body of arsenic, tin, antimony, and lead. It is administered in various treatment protocols, including orally, rectally, intravenously, or transdermally. It has the same basic potential for side effects as DMSA, but its use in children has not been studied as extensively as has that of DMSA.

Another less commonly used detoxifying agent is TTFD (thiamine tetrahydrofurfuryl disulfide, a fat-soluble form of vitamin B-1). It is, strictly speaking, not a classic chelator, but it does help enhance the excretion of a variety of toxins, through the liver's bile, and to a lesser extent, through the urine. It enhances the process of sulfation, as do other sulfur-containing substances, such as taurine and methionine. TTFD can be given to patients with low sulfate levels, or to those who have evidence of heavy metal overload, especially with arsenic.

The use of TTFD has been pioneered by Derrick Lonsdale, M.D., who reported favorable results with it in a small pilot study, published in *Neuroendocrine Letters*. Initial indications are that TTFD can be of benefit in ADHD, and in autistic children with ADHD features.

Another substance with mild chelating properties is alpha lipoic acid, or ALA. This natural chelator is much less efficient than others, however, so it is not generally applied as a first-line tactic against heavy metals.

One advantage of ALA is that it regenerates glutathione, which helps drive the natural detoxification processes of methylation and glutathione conjugation. Another advantage is that it's a powerful antioxidant, and can therefore help fight inflammation, at the same time that it is helping to excrete heavy metals.

ALA appears to be of some benefit when it is given in conjunction with DMSA, after a prior course of DMSA alone.

A drawback of ALA is that it can contribute to fungal dysbiosis, which can trigger behavioral symptoms. It can push yeasty kids into a state of profound agitation. It can make them extremely stimmy, and interfere with their eye contact and connectedness. When this happens, you must discontinue it and get the yeast back under control. One way around this problem is to administer it transdermally. Similarly, DMSA can be administered as a suppository, or possibly transdermally, if oral DMSA starts to kick up yeast problems.

Ideally, though, yeast should be under control before your child starts chelation. Of special importance is to resolve problems with constipation, since that can slow down the elimination of heavy metals, and allow reabsorption.

Chelation is a terrific modality. It does things that no other treatment can.

However, it is clearly more medically invasive than completely natural healing elements, such as the use of vitamin C. It carries some of the same risks as other procedures that employ pharmaceutical medications. Nonetheless, it is quite safe when administered and monitored properly.

Chelation has been the linchpin in the recoveries of a large number of children. If your child is burdened with heavy metal overload, I strongly urge you to consult with your physician about chelation.

SUMMARY: DETOXIFICATION

Toxins probably are, to a greater degree than any other single factor, responsible for initiating the negative cascade of biological processes that resulted in your child's disorder. Although this disorder may now encompass dysfunction of widely dispersed systems, organs, glands, nerves, and cells, toxification may still lie at the heart of your child's problems.

It may be extraordinarily difficult for you and your physician to correct the dysfunction in the systems most closely associated with the 4-A disorders—the immune system, the gastrointestinal system, and the nervous system—without first ridding your child's body of stored toxins. Of particular importance is the excretion of heavy metals, including mercury and lead.

Chelation is an exceptionally effective method of ridding the body of heavy metals. So are the natural processes of methylation, sulfation, and glutathione detoxification.

I have seen detoxification bring kids' lives back to normal. Perhaps it will have the same positive effect upon your child.

Now it is time to address the final element of the Healing Program: medication.

An individualized program of medication may be able to help your child vault over the final obstacles that now impede his or her quest for healing.

CHAPTER TWENTY

THE HEALING PROGRAM

Element #4:
Medication

NOT LONG AGO, A MOTHER BROUGHT HER AUTISTIC SON TO my office. She was accompanied by her father, the boy's grandpa. The poor kid had severe autistic symptoms, and was stimming and flapping around so vigorously that his mom and I could barely converse. As we attempted to talk, the grandfather tried to keep his grandson under control, but that just meant keeping him from climbing the walls. It was an uphill battle. The boy had a fiery temper and wasn't afraid to turn it against anybody who tried to thwart him, even his own grandfather. He created a constant chaos that fried everyone's nerves.

Toward the end of the appointment, I began to outline the treatment program that the child would need to adhere to. As usual, there was nothing easy about it. He would have to give up his favorite foods and go on the GF/CF diet, he'd need to start taking numerous supplements, and he would also have to participate in a long course of a behavioral therapy, such as Applied Behavioral Analysis. To get through all of this, the kid would simply have to settle down a little, and get some control over his impulses. Therefore, I also recommended that he begin a trial course of antipsychotic medication.

Mom hit the roof. No way was she going to lock her son into a chemical straitjacket! He'd be a zombie! She knew about all the potential side effects!

The possibilities for at least temporary harm were, no doubt about it, pretty dismaying, especially to a very protective mother.

Her face hardened, and she spoke in clipped tones. She was very disappointed in me. She had heard that I was different from other doctors. But here I was, offering the same tired, symptom-suppressive, dangerous advice as everyone else. She was ready to leave.

Grandpa drew his attention away from the boy, and sat next to his daughter. Quietly but firmly he said, "Honey, you came all this way. Let the doctor decide what's best."

An uncomfortable silence. Finally: "We'll give it a try, I guess." She sighed, more defeated than hopeful.

Just a few days later she called, in tears, her voice catching. "I can't believe it," she said. "He's *so* much better. He's taking his supplements. He's eating better. He's *listening* to me."

That was not the end of the boy's journey of recovery. But it was the beginning.

Sometimes using the right medication is like turning on a switch. Everything just clicks.

In this child's case, he needed a powerful, medicinal readjustment of his neurotransmitters, particularly those of his dopamine system. Without it, I don't think this little kid would have made it. The forces of chaos in his brain were just too potent. They had twisted his mind inside out, to the degree that he not only couldn't cooperate in a Healing Program, but couldn't even comprehend the concept of healing. All he understood was suffering, and acting out. He was barely hanging on, trying to distract himself day to day from the jumble of thoughts that rumbled through his brain, and then collided in shattering wrecks of confusion and pain.

Years later, after the boy had made countless sacrifices and done endless hours of hard work, he improved significantly. The final factors that made him feel and function better came from nutritional therapy, supplementation therapy, chelation, and behavioral therapy. But it was the initial boost he got from medication that made the deeper healing possible. It helped the boy see that sacrifice held the promise of better days.

And it helped his family to endure their own sacrifices. You can never forget about the family. When one member suffers, everyone suffers, and sometimes a family's love can wither. That can *not* be allowed to happen—because it's the love of the whole family that lights the way for the one who hurts most.

Medications—including pharmaceutical medications and natural, nutraceutical medications—can often ameliorate the forces that tear families apart and keep kids stuck in suffering.

Medications can provide three vital, unique elements:

1. *They can work quickly.*
2. *They can help in certain long-term situations.*
3. *They can help correct the wide variety of physical disorders that harm the brain.*

Medications definitely have their limitations. I almost never use them as stand-alone therapies, because they generally don't reverse root causes. Frankly, I believe there is far too much reliance upon pharmacology in modern medicine. Doctors and patients too often seem to be searching for the mythical magic bullet. I do not view medication as a panacea.

Even so, meds can sometimes do things that other therapies simply cannot.

The Three Unique Elements of Medication

Medications can work wonders. Pharmaceutical medications, in particular, can produce fast, robust, and lasting changes. However, some integrative physicians have a visceral distaste for pharmaceutical medications. They are irritated by the overreliance of modern health care upon pharmaceutical medications, they're tired of the side effects of medications, and they're disappointed by patients so often settling for pharmaceutical symptom suppression, instead of trying to achieve true healing. Therefore, these doctors sometimes become antagonistic to the use of almost any medication for any condition. These doctors tend to rely strictly upon nutraceuticals, such as herbal formulas, which can be extremely helpful, but usually aren't as powerful as pharmaceuticals.

I can understand these doctors' antipathy toward pharmaceutical medications, but I don't share it. I believe that pharmaceutical medications can have extraordinary effects when they are properly used. In fact, at this stage of medical evolution, I believe that integrative medicine is not truly integrative unless it integrates all necessary modalities, including pharmaceutical medications and natural modalities.

To overcome the 4-A disorders in the most effective, enduring, and practical manner, pharmaceutical medications may need to be employed. Consider the three unique elements that medications provide.

1. Medications can quickly control extreme behavioral symptoms and certain physical problems.

Medications can sometimes help kids feel better almost immediately, and can inaugurate the healing process with a flourish.

Most autistic and ADHD symptoms, such as destructive behaviors, are ultimately overcome only by long-term, naturalistic adjustments, such as changes in diet and supplementation, along with detoxification. These changes, though, often require long periods of time to achieve their full effect.

Chelation therapy often goes on for as long as a year or two, and even something as simple as restricting gluten can take three months to produce results. Resolving bowel dysbiosis can take several months, and sometimes takes much longer. As these long-term therapies take hold, medications can help keep kids from suffering, and can help give kids the self-control, executive function, and motivation they need to tackle tough things like dietary restrictions. Without this short-term relief from symptoms, lots of kids would be lost.

Meds quickly intervene in the symptoms that limit kids' function and activities, such as obsessive-compulsive behaviors, excessive stimming, and spaciness. Medications can also quickly get a handle on the extreme behaviors that harm the whole family, such as aggressive outbursts, tantrums, and self-injurious acts. Meds also save lives during acute asthma attacks.

Similarly, medications can quickly solve many of the diverse physical problems that stand in the way of long-term recovery. For example, a short course of antibiotics can help break a child's cycle of recurrent infections. Sometimes a recurrence of these chronic infections can derail the whole process of healing, and send kids back to square one. When this happens, it's not only disheartening for kids, but can also disrupt the entire upward spiral of recovery.

Nonetheless, medications are virtually *never* sufficient as stand-alone therapies in the treatment of the 4-A disorders. Medications just can't fully remediate all the root causes that cumulatively account for the complex 4-A disorders. They can be superb, though, for getting the process started.

2. Medications can help solve certain long-term issues.

Medications can serve as powerful adjunctive therapies for as long as several years at a time. Even though meds can't replace the healing power of ongoing, lifelong modalities such as nutritional therapy, they can offer a great deal of help in a supporting role for extended periods of time.

Not all of the problems that require medication as an adjunctive therapy go away quickly. Sometimes they are very intractable, and require extremely long courses of medication. On occasion, these courses of medication may last for several years, and sometimes they may even last throughout life.

Medications that may be required for prolonged periods of time include, for example, meds that are employed to fight resistant infections. Chronic infection is extraordinarily common among 4-A kids, particularly those with autism. These chronic infections, such as measles infection in the gut or strep-related PANDAS, frequently create cascades of dysfunction that result in severe neurobehavioral symptoms. These infections often occur among kids with immune dysfunction, such as those with Th-2 skewed immunity, and it can take a lot of time to solve a deep-rooted problem like that.

Ideally, the body should be able to control infection on its own, but sometimes this just doesn't happen. The body often needs the help of a pharmaceutical medication to quell a chronic infection. When the medication finally gets the infection under control, though, the natural immune response can often reassert itself, and prevent further infection.

Therefore, kids might need a very long course of a pharmaceutical antiviral medication, such as Valtrex, or an antibiotic, such as Zithromax.

Similarly, gut dysbiosis caused by yeast overgrowth can be very resistant to the body's own healing processes, and even to powerful exogenous natural modalities, such as the anti-yeast diet, and the use of probiotic and herbal supplements. When this occurs, the best thing for the child is generally to prescribe a long course of an antifungal medication, such as nystatin or fluconazole. This course of medication may last for a number of months, or more rarely, even years.

When pharmaceuticals or nutraceuticals are used over these extremely long periods of time, though, it's often necessary to balance their actions, and to protect against side effects. For example, when pharmaceutical or nutraceutical antifungal meds are taken for several months or longer, it helps to take silymarin and/or phosphatidylcholine, or transdermal *N*-acetylcysteine, in order to protect the liver. Liver enzymes can occasionally increase with some of these antifungal medications. Therefore, it's also wise to monitor liver function approximately once per month when using these medications.

Another particularly resistant chronic infective disorder is the autoimmune streptococcal condition known as PANDAS. Kids often have great difficulty recovering from this condition, which can cause symptoms that mimic those of autism, ADHD, or OCD. When this difficulty occurs, kids may need to take low-dose antibiotics for years at a time, as a preventive, or prophylactic, measure. During these extended periods, they must also take supplements, such as probiotics, that guard against the side effects of antibiotics.

Furthermore, other conditions require medication that must be taken indefinitely, and even throughout life. The most common of these conditions is imbalance of neurotransmitters. Millions of people, many of whom are generally quite healthy, have mild to moderate neurotransmitter imbalances, and take antidepressants and other psychoactive medications to help bring their neurotransmitters back into balance. This can be done safely and effectively for many years at a time, with excellent results. Many children with 4-A disorders also benefit from this. So do other kids who have problems that are related to neurotransmitter imbalance. These problems include depression, insomnia, eating disorders, and chronic headaches.

Unfortunately, some kids are overmedicated, and inappropriately medicated with antidepressants, but the blame for this lies with physicians, not the drugs themselves.

When antidepressants and other drugs that affect mood and behavior were first introduced, there was a great deal of skepticism about them, much of which was deserved. Many of the first generation of mood disorder drugs had notable side effects, such as weight gain or lethargy. Over time, though, these classes of medication have been improved, and can now generally be prescribed for long periods, without patients suffering significant side effects. This can only happen, however, when doctors and patients work together, to find the best medication for each individual.

This doesn't mean, though, that medications for mood disorders are still not sometimes overprescribed, particularly to children. Too often, antidepressant medications are given to kids who don't really have classic neurotransmitter imbalances. These kids often have relatively simple root causes of their mood problems, such as hypoglycemia or food reactions.

Therefore, we again see that medications should not be employed as biochemical Band-Aids, to mask symptoms that come from diverse sources.

Medications always work best when they are only one element of a treatment program, and are used only to treat problems that cannot be solved by more natural measures.

3. Medications can help correct the many diverse physical factors that feed into the 4-A disorders.

As you have learned, autism and ADHD are often grab-bag diagnoses that merely describe certain behavior patterns, rather than identify their root causes. The root causes of these disorders are generally found in a vast, interwoven fabric of physical dysfunctions, which may include such diverse problems as bowel dysbiosis, skewed immunity, allergies, chronic infections, inflammation, nutritional deficiencies, and metabolic imbalances.

Many of these conditions respond quite satisfactorily to appropriate medications. Therefore, kids with autism may need to be on at least temporary courses of antibiotics, anti-inflammatories, antivirals, and antifungals. These meds do not directly target the neuropsychiatric aspects of autism or ADHD, but help correct the physical problems that indirectly trigger neuropsychiatric dysfunction.

In the earlier days of autism and ADHD treatment, these underlying physical problems were considered to be unrelated co-morbid disorders—problems that often occurred at the same time as autism and ADHD, but weren't contributing to them.

These days, we know better. We know that autism and ADHD are often results of combinations of physical disorders.

Treating autism and ADHD with drugs that affect only the brain is an outdated concept. Psychotropic drugs can be helpful, but they're only one part of the overall picture of proper medication. When I medicate autism and ADHD, I do not medicate them as strictly neuropsychiatric disorders. That approach is too narrow. I must also treat the various physical disorders that underlie the psychiatric symptoms.

Physical problems also create mental symptoms in disorders other than autism and ADHD. For example, the bacterial infectious disorder of Lyme disease can have psychiatric symptoms, but doctors don't just prescribe psychotropic meds for Lyme disease. They prescribe antibiotics, to get at the root cause of the problem.

Even so, I do sometimes prescribe psychotropic medications for certain kids with autism and ADHD, in conjunction with implementation of the other elements of the Healing Program. I prefer not to use psychotropic drugs, and I generally don't need to use them. Occasionally, though, I think they are quite helpful. In this regard, I am somewhat different than the integrative physicians who have a strong disaffection for almost all psychotropic meds, including atypical antipsychotics and the newer antidepressants.

Frankly, I believe that this anti-medication approach is not always driven by pure clinical practicality, but sometimes by overly strict adherence to a philosophy of naturalism. In contrast, the only philosophy to which I am inextricably attached is the pragmatic principle of doing everything I possibly can to help the children I treat.

My philosophy of pragmatism also prompts me to avoid any stratified, rigid medication protocol for any specific disorder. Instead, I give very different medication programs to different children. Just as there is no one-size-fits-all diet in the Healing Program, there is also no standard set of meds. It's critically important to medicate children according to their individual metabolisms and widely varying needs.

One reason this is necessary is because there are so many different subtypes of 4-A kids, and especially autistic kids. There are those that I refer to as viral kids, and there are also gut-brain kids, yeasty kids, inflammatory kids, hypoglycemic kids, high-dopamine kids, and low-dopamine kids. There are a number of categories, and each one requires a somewhat different pharmacologic approach.

Meds always need to be carefully individualized, or they just won't work. Sometimes good medications work for only one particular subtype of kids. A great example is secretin. A few years ago secretin was the proverbial flavor of the month among many practitioners, because of reports that it had helped some kids achieve astonishing recoveries in remarkably short periods of time. After these reports surfaced, secretin was tested in a number of broad, lengthy studies, and the results were very discouraging. In eight out of ten controlled studies, secretin performed no better than placebo. Therefore, it fell out of favor. However, one study really caught my eye, because it confirmed a phenomenon of secretin treatment that I had noticed in my own practice. In this study, it was found that secretin produced very positive results among a subset of children who also had chronic diarrhea. That's what I'd found among my own kids. The gut-brain kids sometimes had a terrific response. For them, the drug worked great.

The same thing often happens with the commonly used psychotropic drug Namenda. Namenda started out as an Alzheimer's drug, and is now being clinically investigated in the treatment of autism. In my practice, I've found that some kids respond well to it, but it makes others have sudden meltdowns, in which they become extremely emotional for no apparent reason. Why? It's probably because Namenda decreases the activity of the neurotransmitter glutamate, and some kids are already low in the activity of this neurotransmitter. In contrast, most autistic kids generally have high glutamate activity. No two kids are exactly alike, and no two kids need exactly the same medications. As doctors and parents, we need to be good detectives, and keep looking for adverse reactions, and positive responses. If we don't look, we'll never see.

I recall being at a meeting several years ago with a neurologist from a New York City medical school, and we were discussing Namenda in the treatment of Alzheimer's disease. I mentioned that I was also achieving a positive response with Namenda in about one out of every six autistic kids. I thought he would feel this was an inadequate response, but he got really excited. To him, that meant that many thousands of children throughout the country could be helped by this drug. These were children who had a disorder for which there were *no* approved drugs. That meeting made an impression on me. It helped me realize that medications can be versatile and that no single drug or therapy has to hit a home run every time to be of value.

Now let's look at the individual medications that I most often prescribe. Many of these medications are also used by other DAN doctors, other integrative physicians, and a number of conventional physicians.

I will discuss the medications for autism, ADHD, asthma, and allergies separately, because medications are generally tied to specific disorders. However, there will be some degree of crossover among meds that are appropriate for more than one disorder.

MEDICATIONS FOR AUTISM

Medications for autism are in two categories:

- **Psychoactive medications,** which directly target the brain.
- **Co-morbid disorder medications,** which directly target various physical problems, such as infection, that indirectly affect the brain.

Psychoactive medications are the most commonly used meds for autism, but medications for the co-morbid disorders are increasingly being applied. Several years ago, only DAN doctors treated co-morbid disorders to improve brain function. However, many other doctors have recently begun to treat these physical problems. Most doctors now recognize how frequently these other problems exist among autistic kids, and many of them are aware that these problems have an impact upon the nervous system.

The psychoactive medications that are most often used to treat autism are in the following major categories:

The Psychoactive Medications for Autism

- Antidepressants.
- Atypical antipsychotics (or neuroleptics).
- Anticonvulsants.
- Stimulants (or ADHD medications).
- Anti-opioids.
- Miscellaneous medications.

The psychoactive medications for autism are not intended to be curative, but are instead employed to decrease the most troubling symptoms of the disorder.

Thus far, there has been only moderate interest among the major pharmaceutical firms in producing psychoactive drugs to treat the autism-spectrum disorders. One reason is because these drugs are intended for children, and children represent a market category that has historically been of marginal interest to drug companies. Drug companies are generally reluctant to invest in medications for kids, because there are so many difficult legal issues involved with administering drugs to children. Also, even though autism is now more common than ever before, it is still a small market segment when compared to the markets that exist for conditions such as diabetes, cardiovascular disease, cancer, obesity, and depression. This is changing, however, as the autism epidemic unfolds. The global market for autism medication was $2.2 billion in 2005, and is forecast to reach $3.5 billion by 2009.

Even so, almost all of the drugs that are used to treat autism were not developed specifically for autism, but are drugs that have been approved by the FDA for other disorders. Physicians, however, use these drugs as off-label treatments for the autism-spectrum disorders. For example, one of the major categories of medication for autistics, antipsychotic medication, was originally approved for schizophrenia and other psychotic conditions. Now these drugs are often used for children who are not schizophrenic. The off-label use of these antipsychotics to treat mental and mood disorders in children increased by 600 percent from 1993 to 2002. In 2002, doctors wrote 1.2 million prescriptions of antipsychotic medications for children, many of whom were kids with autism and ADHD.

Following are the specific psychoactive medications most often used for autism.

Antidepressants for Autism

Antidepressants are the type of medication that is most frequently used to treat autism. In one recent study, they accounted for 59 percent of all drug treatment for autism. However, although antidepressants are popular for treating autism, their effects tend to be rather limited.

Because many kids with autism, as well as ADHD, have improper action of the contentment neurotransmitter serotonin, drugs that help the serotonin system can be of value to these children. Most antidepressants are designed to improve serotonin function, and are widely used by autistics, ADHD children, and also kids with depression, eating disorders, migraines, and other problems that are related to serotonin.

The potential for positive response to antidepressants among autistics is highly variable, and in most cases low doses are best for achieving efficacy and reducing side effects.

The most encouraging responses that have been achieved by antidepressants include lessening of repetitive thoughts and behaviors. This occurred among 17 percent of kids in one study of the drug Luvox. Antidepressants have also been helpful for anxiety, panic attacks, inattentive behavior, hyperactivity, irritability, depression, and insomnia.

Antidepressants, though, like virtually all other medications, must be well tailored to the individual. For example, in some children the antidepressant Paxil, which is generally well tolerated by healthy adults, has caused agitation and even thoughts of suicide.

A note of caution before I go into the specific antidepressants that are widely used: *In this book I have not listed all of the specific side effects when describing medications, but this does not mean particular side effects don't exist. All drugs have potential side effects, and you must explore them with your child's physician. The only appropriate application of these drugs is under a physician's supervision, and I cannot intercede in that supervision in any way. Only your child's own physician can recommend specific drug treatment. I can tell you only about my own experiences, and about studies.*

Luvox, approved for children eight and over, is generally calming, and can help with obsessive-compulsive behavior. I have achieved positive responses with it in a number of kids.

Lexapro is a newer drug with fewer side effects than its predecessors, such as Prozac, Zoloft, and even Celexa. I have had good responses with this among some children. It can be effective for generalized anxiety disorder, in addition to depression, panic disorder, and OCD. Dosage, however, must be carefully tailored to the individual. In a recent study of Lexapro, 25 percent of the autistic patients who took it did not tolerate doses of the medication in excess of 10 mg. per day. My general rule is to start with low doses, and gradually increase them.

Celexa is similar to Lexapro, but is an earlier rendition that is relatively less well tolerated by some. I rarely use it.

Anafranil is another of the older tricyclic antidepressants that I virtually never use, because it has too many side effects. Other doctors, however, have successfully applied it. It is used to treat OCD, and helps some kids to avoid the unpleasant thoughts that often trigger OCD behaviors.

Zoloft. Some kids do well on it, so I use it occasionally. I consider it to be better than Prozac, but not as good as Lexapro. It's been tested in children as young as six. It can help with OCD and panic, but can be relatively sedating.

Prozac. I use it only infrequently, because the newer generations of this class of antidepressants have fewer side effects. The use of Prozac has been studied in children, though, and some have responded well to it. Various antidepressants have subtly different features, so it's often wise to do trials of several, to find the right fit.

Paxil is a shorter-acting Prozac, but I don't use it in children, because even though it's generally calming, it occasionally creates the paradoxical reaction of triggering agitation, and even prompting suicidal thoughts.

Atypical Antipsychotic Medications for Autism

After antidepressants, this type of medication is the second most frequently applied in the treatment of autism. In a recent study, 29 percent of all drugs used for autism were antipsychotics. This is notably less than the 59 percent of market share controlled by antidepressants, but is far more than the 8 percent share of the third most commonly used type of drugs, anticonvulsants.

This category of medicine sounds scarier than it really is. One reason it sounds scary is because psychosis itself is scary. Therefore, anything that treats psychosis shares some of its fear factor. Furthermore, the original antipsychotic meds, such as Thorazine and Haldol, were blunt instruments that often caused extreme sedation and other very unpleasant side effects.

In response to the problems with the older antipsychotics, the newer class of atypical antipsychotics was created. These antipsychotics, or neuroleptics, can be quite helpful for many kids, particularly those who are notably unmanageable. The drugs can help these kids come back to reality enough to participate in their Healing Programs. Also, these drugs, in low doses, can often be safely taken on a long-term basis, to help keep neurotransmitters in balance. The goal is always to eventually get kids off these drugs and others, but the greater goal is to help these kids function well, feel well, and live as normally as possible. Some of them just can't achieve this without the help of a relatively powerful medication, at some point in time.

Furthermore, although there are risks associated with this type of medication, there are even greater risks associated with self-injurious, aggressive, violent, belligerent behavior. As physicians and parents, we must be realistic and pragmatic, and not be unduly swayed by allegiance to a philosophical ideal, such as an attachment to natural therapies only.

Although the potential side effects of these drugs can be daunting, I have not yet encountered any appreciable degree of severe side effects from these drugs in my own practice. As a rule, I keep the doses as low as possible, and use the medications only to control severe symptomatology. The most common debilitating side effect of this class of drugs has been weight gain, generally related to carbohydrate metabolism. I generally attempt to mitigate this weight gain through a lower carbohydrate diet, and nutritional supplements that enhance insulin sensitivity.

Many of these atypical antipsychotic drugs have been tested for use in autism, and some of them show moderately positive effects against autism-spectrum disorders. They help control aggression, hyperactivity, irritability, self-injury, and tantrums. In one study of Risperdal—which is the only drug that has been approved specifically for autism—87 percent of the children experienced at least some degree of improvement.

Risperdal. The only FDA-approved autism drug, Risperdal can be very helpful for the kids who really need it. When these kids are self-injurious or prone to aggression, Risperdal can help restore more normalized executive function, and help children to control their impulses, and make better decisions. This drug is particularly appropriate for the high-dopamine kids, who are often put on the wrong medication. This includes autistic kids with ADHD features, and other kids with severe ADHD, who are often incorrectly prescribed stimulants. Stimulants, such as Ritalin, may help some kids with ADHD, but they're terrible for the autistic kids who already have too much dopamine activity. These kids do much better on Risperdal. Again, we see the importance of careful individualization.

The goal is always to get kids off Risperdal, but many of them seem to tolerate it well for extended periods. The biggest problem they usually develop is weight gain, but diet and supplements sometimes help with that.

Many of the parents of my kids swear by Risperdal. They say that it's enabled them to finally get through to their children, and to keep them in compliance with the more difficult elements of their programs.

Risperdal helps keep kids from developing false perceptions, and having delusional ideas about themselves, their families, and their environments. That's one reason it helps them control themselves. They don't get carried away with unfounded fears, and the anger that often follows.

Abilify is similar to Risperdal and is generally my next choice among the neuroleptics. It's good for the kids who just can't keep their feet on the ground, and stay in the real world. When kids feel like that, it can be almost impossible to motivate them to engage in a sophisticated, multifaceted program of recovery. They just feel miserable, confused, and isolated. Medications that can help these feelings go away can be good for these children.

Seroquel is another neuroleptic that can work well in some children. However, it tends to be relatively more sedating, so if I use it, I generally prescribe it to kids with sleeping problems, and recommend that they take it at bedtime.

Clozaril is used by some physicians for autism, but I don't prescribe it, because it has the potential to trigger more severe side effects than others in its class. It is often successfully used to treat severely affected schizophrenics, who have delusions and hallucinations.

Other antipsychotics. Some doctors may prescribe the older, first-generation antipsychotics to notably unmanageable autistic children, but this is something I never do. The old, major tranquilizer neuroleptics just have too many side effects, and no special benefits. These drugs include **Thorazine, Haldol,** and **Stelazine.**

Anticonvulsive Medications for Autism

A subset of autistic children suffer from co-morbid seizure disorders, including epilepsy, and these meds can be uniquely helpful for them.

However, antiseizure medications also help a number of kids who don't have seizures. This occurs because antiseizure medications typically exert their actions by modulating the neurotransmitter GABA, which is closely associated with mood. Some of these meds, therefore, have been approved for both seizure control and mood disorder.

I have achieved generally good results with antiseizure meds, which are also called anticonvulsants. These medications are particularly effective for the subset of autistic and ADHD kids who have bipolar features.

In some kids, though, these meds result in paradoxical anxiety and aggression. Because of these paradoxical reactions, some researchers are now investigating drugs that depress the activity of GABA, rather than increase it, as the anticonvulsants do. This preliminary research indicates that these GABA-antagonistic meds do appear to work in the subset of children who respond negatively to anticonvulsants.

Depakote is an anticonvulsant that I have used a number of times for autistic and ADHD kids with mood disorders, particularly bipolar disorder. Mood disorders often go undiagnosed in autistic kids, because when children are diagnosed as autistic, this diagnosis becomes their primary, overriding diagnosis, and therefore it becomes their primary area of treatment. Secondary diagnoses tend to be overlooked and undertreated. I have found, though, that successfully treating the secondary diagnoses can pave the way for more successful treatment of the primary diagnosis. Furthermore, sometimes the primary and secondary problems are interwoven, and must be treated simultaneously. The separation of them in the diagnostic process sometimes creates an artificial construct, which can lead to the use of inadequate or inappropriate medications.

Depakote is especially valuable for kids with rapid cycling mood disorders. These are the kids whose moods turn on a dime, creating confusion and anger among the people who are trying to live with them, and help them. It can also sometimes work well in conjunction with Risperdal or Abilify, the neuroleptics that frequently help kids who suffer from rapid mood changes.

Klonopin is an anticonvulsant that is also used for anxiety and panic attacks. It pushes GABA up, so it's not good for the kids who already have too much GABA. In them, it can create a paradoxical reaction of hyperactivity. Klonopin is in the class of drugs known as the benzodiazepines. This class includes the minor tranquilizers Valium and Xanax, which also increase GABA. Therefore, Valium and Xanax can sometimes trigger the same type of paradoxical reactions in some kids that Klonopin does. Because of this, I tend to avoid use of Valium and Xanax in kids who are on the spectrum. Besides, even if these tranquilizing, anti-anxiety drugs do work well, they can still be habit forming.

I sometimes give Klonopin to exceptionally hyperactive kids who have severe insomnia. On occasion this drug can also be used on a situational basis, for temporary sedation, if kids need to be sedated for a medical procedure, such as an intravenous drip.

Trileptal is another good anticonvulsant that helps improve the moods of a relatively broad spectrum of children. It has been tested in kids as young as three, and is considered effective for seizures in very young children. It is also helpful for some autistic kids with bipolar features.

Lamictal is a med I prescribe occasionally. It is generally well tolerated, with few side effects, but it can trigger potentially severe skin rashes. Lamictal has been FDA approved as a mood stabilizer, and can be used for relatively extended periods of time. It seems to help some patients who don't respond well to other mood stabilizing drugs, and is particularly appropriate for kids with bipolar features, including kids with primary diagnoses of autism or ADHD.

Tegretol is an anticonvulsant that's often applied for mood disorders. It tends to be notably fast acting, and is sometimes used for migraines, acute mania, and pain. I don't use it very often because it has more potential side effects than other similarly acting drugs. However, on occasion it has been effective.

Dilantin is an effective medication for seizures and mood disorders, but I don't use it much for mood disorders because of its potential side effects. One of the common side effects is swelling of the gums.

Stimulant Medications for Autism

This class of drugs is composed of the medications most commonly used for ADHD, such as Ritalin. This off-label use of these drugs is a reflection of the growing awareness that there is a connection between ADHD and the autism-spectrum disorders.

Several studies have indicated that the stimulant drugs for ADHD achieve moderately positive effects in some autistic children, but I don't often use these drugs for kids on the spectrum. The studies that have been done show that these medications are not as effective for spectrum disorders as they are for ADHD.

As a rule, I prefer to first treat the autistic aspects of these children, and to then move gradually into addressing their ADHD features, as their autistic symptoms subside. Sometimes, though, symptoms such as hyperactivity and impulsivity impede compliance with the Healing Program so much that certain children must be treated concurrently for both their autistic symptoms and their ADHD symptoms.

These stimulating drugs are not, of course, appropriate for the autistic subset of high-dopamine kids, because these meds push dopamine even higher.

Ritalin is in the class of dopamine-stimulating drugs known as methylphenidates. It is the most popular of the methylphenidate drugs. However, I believe it is the most popular primarily just because it's the oldest and best known. I generally do not prescribe Ritalin, particularly to autistic kids, but instead prefer the newer forms of methylphenidate, including Concerta, Metadate CD, and Focalin.

Concerta is often a more reliable medicinal tool than the short-acting forms of Ritalin for controlling hyperactive and inattentive symptoms, because its effects last longer. When short-acting Ritalin wears off, some kids react badly. Concerta does help some kids, but like even the longer-acting form of Ritalin, it's generally a poor choice for autistic children.

Metadate CD is also a long-acting methylphenidate, but it's generally more appropriate for ADHD kids than spectrum kids.

Focalin is another of the methylphenidates that I use most. It has short-acting and long-acting forms. Focalin is especially good for kids who have short attention spans. Even though I do, in very limited instances, prescribe this to a child on the spectrum, I find that this drug and others like it work best after the kids move away from the spectrum, and are left with only lingering ADHD symptoms. It generally has fewer side effects, because its developers attempted to remove the elements of the drug that caused the side effects, while leaving intact the ability of the drug to exert its therapeutic actions.

Adderall is usually not appropriate for autistic kids. It pushes dopamine too high in many of them. It works far more effectively in the subset of low-dopamine ADHD kids.

Anti-Opioid Medications for Autism

As you probably recall, there is abundant evidence that many autistic children appear to have excessive function of their sedating, contentment-related opioid systems. The leading theory is that these children literally become intoxicated by the partial proteins that occur when casein and gluten are not fully digested. These partial proteins, or peptides, are called caseomorphins and gluteomorphins (also called gliadomorphins). These peptides seem to affect some kids in much the same way that other forms of opiates affect people. This probably accounts for some of the distracted spaciness of these kids, as well as for their frequent virtual addiction to gluten and casein. In addition, this excess of opioid function also probably contributes to the indifference that some autistic children have to pain. This indifference often leads to injury, and even self-injury.

Naltrexone is the only widely used medication that is employed to negate the effects of opioid excess. Naltrexone was originally developed as a medication that could help people overcome alcoholism and drug addiction. It combats these disorders by blocking the subjective experience of intoxication. People who take naltrexone can be intoxicated by alcohol or drugs, but not feel any pleasure from it. Naltrexone is an opioid antagonist, and blocks the receptors that allow opioids to enter brain cells.

I have used naltrexone with a number of autistic children and the medication, in very low doses, does seem to have some effectiveness. Studies on it have shown mixed results. Some studies have indicated that it does reduce self-injury, but other studies have failed to corroborate this. Ongoing clinical research by Dr. Jaquelyn McCandless of low-dose naltrexone is in progress. Preliminary results indicate improvements in mood, cognition, and social relatedness in some children. A small percentage showed side effects of irritability, agitation, and restlessness.

I also sometimes employ low-dose naltrexone as an immune modulator. It appears to help keep the immune system functioning at the proper level, without becoming underactive or overactive.

Miscellaneous Medications for Autism

This is a diverse category, since so many causative factors contribute to the onset of autism symptoms, and because so many medicinal elements can be used to correct these factors.

The variety of this category demonstrates once again that autism is not a single, monolithic disorder, but is the result of an interwoven fabric of disorders.

The variety of this category also indicates the need for individualization of treatment.

Secretin. The medical community's reaction to this drug is a great example of one of the more harmful phenomena of modern medicine: the bandwagon effect. The bandwagon effect takes hold when an early study reports very positive outcomes from a medication. Many doctors, wishing to find the proverbial magic bullet, jump onboard, and prescribe the medication to a broad spectrum of patients. Then later studies are done that have more equivocal results, and doctors start jumping off the bandwagon. When this occurs, the medication can develop a bad reputation. This happened with secretin.

Initial reports heralded secretin as the wonder drug for autism, but most later studies showed mediocre results in a broad spectrum of the autism population.

Lost in the shuffle, though, was the fact that secretin performs quite well in the subset of kids who have GI problems, particularly when characterized by diarrhea. This is a relatively large subset, and many of these kids can probably be helped by secretin. The studies thus far just haven't been sufficiently substratified.

In my own practice, a significant number of the gut-brain kids have had a terrific response to secretin, and their parents swear by the drug. I've also gotten good results in some kids by administering it only approximately once every 6 to 8 weeks.

However, I generally administer it mainly to children who have already shown improvement with it, as a method of maintaining their improvements. I usually do not introduce it early in the course of treatment, due to the generally negative results of the studies.

Secretin is a gut hormone that causes the secretion of bicarbonate from the pancreas, to aid the digestive process. It also functions as a neurohormone, acting on receptors in the brain, including those in the amygdala, the brain's fear center. Its neurological function may account for the very rapid onset of the positive effects it creates in some children.

If your child has GI problems, secretin may be able to help resolve them, and to help stop the neurological assault these bowel problems can trigger. It may also help your child through its direct effects upon the brain.

Lithium has been widely applied to bipolar disorder for many years, and bipolar features are moderately common among autistic kids, and sometimes ADHD kids. In many kids, I don't see both the manic and the depressive sides of the disorder, just the manic elements. For these kids, lithium can be a good choice. Interestingly, I have also sometimes achieved good results by giving extremely low doses of lithium, which is a natural element. The doses were not quite as low as those in a homeopathic medication, but did represent only a minute fraction of a normal dose. These very low doses are extremely safe, and do not require monitoring with regular testing.

Lithium can help with aggression, racing thoughts, hyperactivity, insomnia, grandiosity, and poor judgment.

Namenda can be an effective drug among the subset of children who have an excess of the excitatory neurotransmitter glutamate. This can include children on the autism spectrum, and also those with ADHD. Excess glutamate tends to make children hyperactive. Namenda, however, blocks glutamate receptors, thereby decreasing the activity of glutamate. In one study of thirty-nine children on the autism spectrum, Namenda showed moderate success in decreasing hyperactivity and inappropriate speech. Namenda is not appropriate for all kids with neuropsychiatric disorders, but it can be of significant value to the high-glutamate kids.

Inderal is a commonly used heart medication that can help a small segment of autism-spectrum children who have rapid heartbeat, or tachycardia. It is in the class of drugs known as beta blockers, and is mostly used among adults for problems such as high blood pressure, angina pectoris, tachycardia, and migraines. I don't prescribe it very often, and when I do, I always keep looking for the root causes of the rapid heartbeat.

Actos is a diabetes medication that I have applied in off-label usage among some children with neurobehavioral disorders. It has shown signs of effectiveness in some children, probably because it is a powerful anti-inflammatory. Studies have shown that it effectively decreases levels of C-reactive protein, which is a marker of inflammation. It is currently being researched for numerous inflammatory disorders, including colitis, psoriasis, heart disease, and various neurological disorders.

Piracetam is a drug that enhances cognitive function. It is used widely in Europe but is not commonly available in America, and must therefore be purchased at a special-order compounding pharmacy, with a doctor's prescription. Piracetam has the interesting quality of improving communication between the brain's two hemispheres, via the band of connective nerves between the hemispheres called the corpus callosum. This intraneural communicative ability is often moderately impaired among children with the learning disability of dyslexia. Therefore, piracetam has been shown in studies to be an effective medication for dyslexia. It has also been shown to be an effective treatment for poor oxygen metabolism in the brain, or hypoxia, a condition that sometimes occurs in people who smoke.

Oxytocin is a natural hormone that can be administered as a medication. It is known to stimulate feelings of attachment and bonding, and is naturally secreted at high levels by women's bodies during and shortly after birth. In recent years it has occasionally been applied to autistic children. This application is still in its early stages, but the results have generally been promising. Administered as a nasal spray, it is well tolerated and appears to be of special value to children who suffer from anxiety, presumably because it dampens the activity of the brain's fear center, the amygdala. It also appears to help autistic children to establish proper eye contact, and it can also help with socialization.

MEDICATIONS FOR THE CO-MORBID DISORDERS ASSOCIATED WITH THE 4-A EPIDEMICS

The co-morbid disorders that so often accompany the 4-A disorders must generally be successfully treated in order to fully remediate autism, ADHD, asthma, and allergies. Unfortunately, the importance of resolving these conditions has generally been underestimated or overlooked by much of the medical community. Many doctors focus rather myopically, in my opinion, upon only the neuropsychiatric symptoms of autism and ADHD, in particular, and this has left the contributory roles of the co-morbid disorders shrouded in mystery.

Fortunately, though, there is nothing very mysterious about clearing up the most common co-morbid disorders that feed into autism, ADHD, asthma, and allergies. For the most part, they are merely infectious disorders, as well as inflammation, which sometimes accompanies infection, and sometimes does not.

These infections are typically caused by bacteria, viruses, and fungi.

Therefore, the proper medications for controlling them are antibiotics, antivirals, and antifungals.

Antibiotics

Treating bacterial infections is even more straightforward than treating viruses. Bacterial infections generally respond quite well to antibiotics. Sometimes, however, the infections are resistant and chronic, and must be treated considerably more aggressively.

In certain situations, it is sometimes necessary to prescribe a low dosage of antibiotics for an indeterminate period of time, to prevent infections from arising, or from becoming virulent when they do arise. On occasion, this long, preventive course of antibiotics is necessary for treatment of the autoimmune disorder PANDAS, which is triggered by streptococcal bacteria.

Many different forms of antibiotics can be appropriate for children. Treatment should generally be based upon the particular site of the infection, as well as its virulence, and the type of bacteria that is involved. Virtually all doctors are well versed in the administration of antibiotics, and your child's own physician is in the best position to recommend the specific antibiotic that your child may need.

There are a great many antibiotics that are appropriate for children, and among the mostly commonly used are **Amoxil, Zithromax, penicillin, Cefzil, Bactrim, Ceftin, and Biaxin.**

Antivirals

One common site of infection, as you know, is the gut. The small intestine, in particular, is prone to chronic infection from various sources, including live measles virus from the measles-mumps-rubella vaccination. For these gut problems, as well as other chronic viral infections that may contribute to immune dysfunction, various standard antiviral medications are appropriate.

There are currently only eleven antivirals, other than those used almost exclusively in the treatment of AIDS. By brand name, they are: Zovirax, Famvir, and Valtrex (for herpes viruses); Symmetrel, Tamiflu, Flumadine, and Relenza (for influenza viruses); Vistide, Foscavir, and Cytovene (for cytomegalovirus); and Virazole (for respiratory syncytial virus). Of these, the three most commonly used by autistic patients are Valtrex, Zovirax, and less frequently, Symmetrel.

Valtrex is most often used for common herpes virus conditions, including chicken pox and shingles. Valtrex is closely related to Zovirax, or acyclovir. It is also used relatively often among autistic children, and appears to be of benefit to many. I have used it in numerous kids, and have been satisfied with the results in some children.

No antiviral medication, however, can fully cure a chronic virus. It can only help control it until the body is capable of handling the virus by itself.

Symmetrel, which is a brand-name product of amantadine, is occasionally used in the treatment of autism, but not just because of its antiviral properties. It also modulates the activity of glutamate, the neurotransmitter that is often imbalanced in autistics. In a recent study, amantadine showed moderate success in alleviating autistic symptoms.

Antifungals

Treating fungal disorders is of extreme importance in all of the 4-A disorders, because fungi, particularly *Candida albicans,* is a primary cause of bowel dysbiosis. This bowel dysbiosis can result, directly and indirectly, in neurotoxic assaults upon the brain.

Nystatin is a good antifungal. It is not absorbed systemically, and is effective only in the gut. Due to its lack of systemic activity, it is safer than other antifungals, such as Diflucan, with a lower risk of potential adverse effects. In fact, it can even be taken by a woman while she is pregnant. At times, in certain difficult cases, combination therapy with nystatin and Diflucan can give even more positive results.

Diflucan is the most commonly used antifungal, and it has been applied with excellent results to yeast overgrowth in many 4-A kids. Known generically as fluconazole, it effectively kills fungi, and can often resolve the problem relatively quickly. However, it is not uncommon for yeast overgrowth in the gut to be quite persistent, and in these situations long-term administration is necessary, sometimes for as long as several months.

Some doctors are accustomed to prescribing Diflucan almost exclusively for vaginal yeast infections, which tend to resolve much more quickly and easily than does yeast overgrowth in the gut. These doctors often tend to undermedicate nonvaginal yeast overgrowth. A vaginal yeast infection might be cleared by as little as a single 150-mg. tablet of Diflucan, but resistant, heavy yeast overgrowth in the gut may require the medication every day for several months.

Diflucan is metabolized by the liver, so long-term usage should be monitored with liver function tests. I check these tests two weeks after starting the medication, and then once per month thereafter. However, I have prescribed long-term courses of Diflucan to hundreds of children, and thus far I have seen virtually no noticeable harm to the liver. On rare occasions, I've noted mild elevation in liver function tests, but this normalized rapidly after the discontinuation of the Diflucan. Monitoring for potential adverse effects is an important part of using prescription medication.

When an earlier version of a fluconazole-type drug known as Nizoral was introduced, there were a few reports of liver problems, but this is even more rare with Diflucan.

Anti-Inflammatories

The other condition that most often contributes to the 4-A disorders is inflammation. This inflammation can be localized in a specific area, such as the brain or bowels, or it can be spread more systemically. The treatment of systemic inflammation with pharmaceutical medications has thus far been relatively disappointing. There had previously been hope that the Cox-2 inhibitors might reduce systemic inflammation, but they seem to exert more of a localized action in areas such as the joints, where they are used to combat the inflammation of arthritis. However, there have been many severe side effects from the Cox-2 inhibitors, so it is probable that even if they had demonstrated effectiveness, they still would not be appropriate for long-term use by children.

The best medications for long-term treatment of widespread inflammation are the nutraceuticals, accompanied by nutritional therapy. For information on this, review the appropriate sections in the chapters on supplementation therapy and nutritional therapy.

Similarly, you should also review those chapters for information on nutrients and herbs that are effective against bacteria, viruses, and fungi. These natural substances, when used medicinally, in relatively high dosages, can be quite effective. Dosage is a key factor, however. For example, you would be wrong to assume that you can take one capsule per day of the anti-allergy herb quercitin and get the same effect that you could with a drug like Zyrtec. You would need to take at least three per day, or maybe even six per day.

By the same token, a nutraceutical herb such as pycnogenol is also very dose-dependent. To achieve an effective anti-inflammatory, anti-allergy effect from pycnogenol, you would need to take 25 to 50 mg. twice daily, or even 100 mg. twice daily.

However, certain pharmaceutical medications, such as Actos and Namenda, are being evaluated for their roles in quieting neuroinflammation. Another drug, Singulair, has systemic anti-inflammatory activity, and this has expanded its usage beyond its approved application for asthma.

THE ARI RATINGS FOR AUTISM MEDICATIONS

The Autism Research Institute polls parents on the effects of medication, just as it does on the effects of other therapies. Following is the ARI parent rating scale. This is a subjective analysis, not an objective, scientific analysis, and it is a relatively small sampling, of no more than a few hundred parents, in most cases.

PARENT RATINGS OF MEDICATIONS

Drugs	Got Better	No Effect	Got Worse	Better: Worse	No. of Cases
Adderall	34%	25%	41%	0.8:1	589
Anafranil	31%	37%	32%	1.0:1	386
Antibiotics	13%	55%	32%	0.4:1	1,915
Antifungals					
Diflucan	55%	40%	5%	9.7:1	409
Nystatin	49%	46%	5%	9.2:1	1,095
Atarax	22%	53%	25%	0.8:1	489
Clonidine	48%	31%	21%	2.2:1	1,363
Clozapine	19%	43%	38%	0.5:1	129
Depakote					
Behavior	31%	43%	26%	1.2:1	992
Seizures	56%	32%	12%	4.7:1	651
Dilantin					
Behavior	23%	49%	28%	0.8:1	1,087
Seizures	50%	36%	14%	3.4:1	408
Haldol	34%	28%	38%	0.9:1	1,169
Inderal	32%	51%	17%	1.8:1	265
Klonopin					
Behavior	34%	38%	28%	1.2:1	207
Seizures	16%	54%	30%	0.5:1	50

Lithium	31%	44%	25%	1.2:1	424
Luvox	34%	36%	30%	1.1:1	181
Naltrexone	34%	46%	20%	1.7:1	234
Paxil	38%	32%	30%	1.3:1	336
Phenobarbital					
Behavior	16%	37%	47%	0.3:1	1,090
Seizures	39%	43%	18%	2.2:1	495
Prozac	37%	32%	31%	1.2:1	1,181
Risperdal	55%	27%	18%	3.0:1	780
Ritalin	29%	27%	44%	0.7:1	3,921
Secretin					
Intravenous	47%	46%	7%	6.5:1	376
Transdermal	39%	50%	11%	3.6:1	157
Stelazine	27%	44%	29%	0.9:1	424
Tegretol					
Behavior	31%	44%	25%	1.2:1	1,456
Seizures	55%	32%	13%	4.3:1	794
Thorazine	24%	40%	36%	0.7:1	922
Valium	24%	41%	35%	0.7:1	834
Zoloft	34%	34%	32%	1.1:1	368

MEDICATION FOR ADHD

Medication for ADHD generally involves only a few drugs, primarily the stimulating methylphenidates, such as Ritalin. However, in a number of cases, I also apply various medications that are also used for the autism-spectrum disorders. I apply the autism drugs because some ADHD kids are former autism kids who are moving off the spectrum as they heal. Furthermore, some ADHD kids have a few autistic features, such as disassociation, even though their primary diagnosis is that of ADHD. Mostly, however, I prescribe autism drugs to ADHD kids simply because different children need different medications, and I treat the child, not the disorder.

For example, in certain ADHD children, I might prescribe the atypical antipsychotic medications Risperdal or Abilify. I don't do this because these kids are psychotic: They're not. I do it because the drugs are appropriate for the specific needs and metabolic profiles of these children. Similarly, I might prescribe an antidepressant to an ADHD child, even though the child does not suffer from clinical depression. The guide to treatment is to treat each child in a unique and effective way, without being slavish to diagnostic labels or names of drug categories.

I occasionally do prescribe the methylphenidate drugs, and most of the kids who come to me with a preexisting ADHD diagnosis are already on a methylphenidate, such as Ritalin. However, I put a lot more effort into getting kids off these drugs than putting kids on them. These meds can be appropriate in some cases, but in general they are overprescribed. It's relatively easy to understand why they're overprescribed. One reason is because of the bandwagon effect. Ritalin and the other methylphenidates are currently very popular among doctors, and also among frustrated parents and overworked educators. The drugs do generally achieve the desired effect of changing a child's behavior.

Another reason they're overprescribed is because the average American doctor's visit now lasts for seven minutes, and typically ends with the writing of a prescription. Part of the reason the visits are so short is because of the mandates of managed health care, which most doctors are generally powerless to modify. Therefore, these doctors are often forced into making quick decisions, as they attempt to achieve fast and dramatic results.

Too often, though, children get drawn into this system of overmedication and never come out. They spend their entire childhoods taking Ritalin, without ever addressing the root causes of their hyperactivity, impulsivity, or inattentiveness. Then they become adults who are still dependent upon methylphenidates.

I try to practice a different style of medicine. My appointments last far longer than seven minutes, and when I do prescribe a methylphenidate, my goal is to keep the course of this medication as short as possible, and the dosage as low as possible. I prescribe methylphenidates only to the kids with the most severe symptoms, including those kids who just can't participate in their own healing without a temporary boost from pharmaceutical medication. If their symptoms are relatively controllable, I much prefer to recommend natural therapies, including use of magnesium, omega-3 essential fatty acids, DMAE, iron, zinc, phosphatidylcholine, and other nutraceuticals that get to the root causes of the problems.

I am generally able to eventually get most kids off methylphenidates. Not always, though. All kids are different, and some seem to need long-term administration of methylphenidates to function optimally.

When kids do stay on methylphenidates for a long period, it's important to regularly monitor their metabolic functions, in order to make sure they are not suffering from any undue side effects.

Ritalin is the oldest type of methylphenidate, but I generally use the newer forms of methylphenidates.

Focalin is a methylphenidate that I more frequently prescribe. Due to its chemical structure, it has fewer side effects than Ritalin, and it comes in convenient short-acting and long-acting forms, as do other methylphenidates. The extended-release form requires only one administration per day, compared to short-acting methylphenidates that last only four hours. Therefore, the extended-release form can be more effective for kids who need to stay alert in school all day. Sometimes I discontinue it during summer vacations.

Adderall can be good for focus and attention in kids who are hyperactive. It pushes up dopamine relatively aggressively, though, so it's not appropriate for any of the autistic kids or the ADHD kids who have too much dopamine. Its use can be limited to once or twice per day, but most kids have to take it for three to four weeks to feel the full effects.

Concerta is extremely similar to Ritalin, but there do seem to be some subtle differences in the effects. Some parents report that their kids do better on Concerta than Ritalin.

Catapres, the brand name for clonidine, is one commonly used ADHD medication that is not a methylphenidate. It's a blood pressure medication. It is used rather widely to treat ADHD, though, because it helps calm kids down, without having an effect upon their blood pressures. I prescribe it to kids with the hyperactive and impulsive subtype of ADHD, and generally get positive results. On occasion, I also apply it to autistic kids who have pronounced impulsive features. In some children, however, this drug can be too sedating.

Mood stabilizers, such as Depakote, Trileptal, or Lamictal, may help some kids with severe ADHD that is unresponsive to stimulants. This may be due to the effects of these medications on the calming neurotransmitter GABA.

Co-morbid medications for ADHD are generally the same as those that I recommend for kids who have the autism-spectrum disorders, because ADHD kids tend to have the same co-morbid disorders as autistic kids. The drugs I tend to prescribe are antibiotics, antivirals, antifungals, anti-inflammatories, and antihistamines. Although many of the same co-morbid conditions that are present in autism can also contribute to ADHD, these disorders tend to be significantly milder, less frequent in occurrence, and fewer in number in ADHD kids. If this were not true, it is possible that more virulent co-morbidity might tip the balance for ADHD kids, and cause them to suffer symptoms more consistent with those of the autism spectrum.

For details on medications for the co-morbid disorders, review the information in the section on autism medications.

MEDICATION FOR ASTHMA

Asthma medications, as parents of most kids with asthma already know, consist of two categories: drugs that help control the inflammation that underlies asthma, and drugs that relieve symptoms during an acute asthma episode. Most kids must use both types of medication.

The drugs that control inflammation on an ongoing basis are either steroidal, or nonsteroidal. In addition, a relatively new class of anti-inflammatory drugs now exists that inhibits the inflammatory messengers called leukotrienes.

The drugs that help kids to get over acute asthma episodes are designed to quickly open, or dilate, the bronchioles. The bronchodilators reduce swelling, and they also help the bronchial muscles to relax.

Both of these two categories of medications can be extraordinarily effective. Of particular value are the meds that relieve severe episodes, which can be very painful, and even life threatening. Millions of children receive benefit from these medications. However, the medications don't solve the root problems.

Inflammation is the primary root problem of asthma, and there are no notably effective pharmaceutical drugs for eliminating or preventing inflammation. The existing drugs merely suppress inflammation once it has begun. Therefore, the best methods to overcome asthma are to remove the root causes of inflammation from a child's immediate environment. This can include removing anything from allergic factors such as cat hair, to dietary factors such as saturated fats. For more information on the elements that prevent asthmatic inflammation from occurring, please review the chapters on asthma.

The natural approaches to asthma are generally superior to the pharmaceutical approaches, not only because they reach root causes, but also because asthma medications tend to have significant side effects. Children who regularly use bronchodilators that increase adrenaline sometimes suffer increased long-term asthma symptoms. These bronchodilators, which contain a type of medication called beta-agonists, may do more long-term harm than good in some kids. In a study of this approach, 30 percent of patients using this medication improved over an extended period of time, but 70 percent of those using a placebo improved. This lack of improvement probably occurred because this medication increases the sensitivity of the bronchial tubes. In addition, the steroidal medications can cause even more serious side effects, including irritability, nausea, headaches, high blood pressure, cataracts, glaucoma, and bone problems.

Therefore, you should try to help your child to move beyond asthma medications. Until that occurs, though, they can be helpful, and are often essential.

Inflammation-Controlling Medications

These meds don't prevent inflammation, but they do help keep it under control. This is very important, because asthma episodes strike when inflammation causes the bronchial tubes to become clogged with mucus, and squeezed by the muscles that surround them.

Corticosteroids are the meds most often used to control inflammation. They can be taken in an inhaler, or as tablets or syrups. Inhaled corticosteroids must be taken every day. Tablets and syrups can be taken on an additional, occasional basis, if your child's air passages are very swollen, or if he or she has a viral infection, which can significantly exacerbate asthma symptoms.

The inhaled corticosteroids, which all have essentially the same actions, include **Beclovent** and **Vanceril** (containing beclomethasone); **Azmacort** (containing triamcinolone); **AeroBid** (containing flunisolide); and **Flovent** (containing fluticasone).

These medications have become the first line of drugs in the treatment of asthma, since asthma has been discovered to primarily be an inflammatory disorder. Although inhaled corticosteroids generally don't have the intense side effects of oral steroids, they can still result in relatively significant adverse effects during long-term use, including the ones listed previously. Therefore, speak to your doctor about them before making your decision.

As a rule, I try to avoid the long-term use of inhaled steroids in children, because of their potential side effects when taken on a long-term basis.

Nonsteroidals have far less side effects, but may not be quite as reliable and powerful. They also help prevent allergic reaction in the airways, and reduce the possibility of an asthma episode due to exercise. The most commonly used nonsteroidal for asthma is Tilade.

Intal, a brand of cromolyn sodium, is a medication that is in some ways similar to antihistamines. It indirectly decreases the effects of histamine, the body's own mediator of inflammation. It has a different action, however, than antihistamines, which block histamine production. Instead, it prevents the release of allergic and inflammatory substances, and blocks the effects of histamines on respiratory cells. It can be a good choice, because it achieves anti-asthma results without many side effects.

Long-acting bronchodilators take more time to have an effect, but are active over longer periods of time. They're efficient for preventing episodes that occur at night, and episodes that are triggered by exercise. The current most popular brand is Serevent. It is a long-acting medication known as a beta-agonist, which dilates the bronchioles.

Leukotriene inhibitors are a relatively new class of asthma meds that block the inflammatory chemicals called leukotrienes. They can occasionally cause some troublesome side effects, but are generally well tolerated, more so than the steroidal medications. Accolate is intended for children twelve and older, and Zyflo is for kids six and older. The one I most commonly use is Singulair.

Singulair can help decrease inflammation in the lungs, and possibly systemically. It's good for allergically triggered asthma, as well as exercise-induced asthma, and is generally very safe.

Medications for Relief During Asthma Episodes

These meds bring quick relief, and literally save some children's lives. They can be used early in an episode, to keep it from escalating, and they can also be used if the episode begins to get out of control. They're usually inhaled, but can be taken as syrups.

Beta-agonists work quickly and powerfully by increasing the action of adrenaline, which helps stop the swelling in tissues. They are used most often to stop episodes that have already begun, but can also be used prior to exercise, if there is a probability that it will trigger an episode. Among the commonly used brands are: Proventil and Ventolin (containing albuterol); Brethine (containing terbutaline); Alupent and Metaprel (containing metaproterenal); Tornalate (containing bitolterol); and Maxair (containing pirbuterol).

The side effects these products cause are generally rather manageable, such as headaches, but the side effects can become worse if these medications are used more than four times per day.

Anticholinergics are the other type of medication that can be taken when asthma flares up. They work by helping the bronchial muscles to relax, but they take longer to act than the beta-agonists. Therefore, they are often taken in conjunction with the beta-agonists. Side effects from anticholinergics taken by themselves are generally relatively mild, such as dry mouth. One of the most commonly used brands is Atrovent.

Adjunctive Medications for Asthma

Many kids also use anti-allergy and decongestant medications to help prevent asthma episodes, since most episodes are related to an allergic response. Among these are antihistamines, oral decongestants, nasal decongestants, and combination antihistamine/decongestants. For more information on these meds, see the following material on medication for allergies.

MEDICATION FOR ALLERGIES

Allergy is the least responsive of the 4-A disorders to effective remediation with medication. Allergy is the quintessentially complex internal reaction that simply cannot be contained with the highly targeted actions of pharmaceutical medicines. This is unfortunate, because allergy lies at the heart of each of the other 4-A disorders. It is the primary trigger of asthma, and is a major contributor to autism and ADHD. If allergy could be eliminated with the application of a pharmaceutical medicine, the other 4-A disorders would probably not exist in epidemic proportions.

Of particular intransigence are food allergies. They can be overcome, but the solution is generally not pharmaceutical medication. One drug, Gastrochrome, is sometimes applied, with variable results.

Similarly, inhalant allergies are also preternaturally resistant to the curative force of pharmaceutical medication.

However, both the symptoms of food allergies and those of inhalant allergies can often be managed with appropriate use of medication. In almost all instances, the symptoms can be at least partially controlled, and sometimes reduced so much that they are only minor annoyances. This, though, only applies to specific allergic symptoms, and not to the more pernicious, underlying, metabolic effects that allergies may have upon asthma, autism, and ADHD.

In addition to prescription and over-the-counter medication for allergy symptoms, nutraceutical medications can also be of considerable value. In many cases, they are more appropriate than pharmaceutical and over-the-counter meds, because they generally have fewer side effects, and can therefore be safely taken over longer periods of time. The nutraceuticals include herbal preparations, nutrients, and homeopathic medications.

Even controlling relatively mild symptoms of allergy is difficult, though. A recent consumer poll indicated the dissatisfaction that many people have with anti-allergy medication.

- 31 percent were not satisfied with their current prescription medication.
- 56 percent reported insufficient relief over an extended period.
- 60 percent were looking for a new medication.
- 42 percent were confused by medication options.
- 40 percent were dissatisfied with the range of medication choices offered by their doctors.

To explore the more effective ways of remaining allergy-free, review the material in the chapters on allergy.

Medication Options for Allergy

There are five primary options for controlling allergy symptoms: (1) antihistamines, (2) decongestants, (3) local steroidal inhalants, (4) oral or injected steroids, and (5) nutraceutical medications.

Antihistamines are the most commonly applied allergy medication. They generally reduce the side effects of inhalant allergies–such as sneezing, itching, and a runny nose–with only moderate side effects. Approximately 20 percent of people become drowsy from them, but children occasionally have a paradoxical reaction of nervousness, irritability, and nightmares. Most children, however, are mildly sedated by antihistamines.

Atarax is an antihistamine that is sometimes applied as a sedative to children, and also sometimes as an anti-anxiety agent. I have found it to be generally quite effective for itching, and also for hives, which are more common among adults than children, but do sometimes occur in kids.

Benadryl is also a sedating antihistamine, and in many kids it's so sedating that it is appropriate only for an acute allergic reaction, rather than for chronic allergy. Sometimes I give it to kids who need to calm down for a medical procedure, such as an intravenous drip. It is used for dermatitis, GI allergy, hay fever, and hives. Parents must be very cautious about giving excessive doses, which can create significant side effects.

Zyrtec is a good antihistamine that I frequently recommend, because it has a strong action without causing drowsiness. It's good for seasonal allergy as well as indoor allergy, is approved for kids as young as six months, and needs to be taken only once per day.

Claritin is another safe and reliable antihistamine that doesn't cause drowsiness. It needs to be taken only once per day, and is available as a syrup.

Gastrochrome is an oral medication used to prevent IgE food reactions in the GI tract, similar to how Intal is used in the respiratory tract, and is occasionally helpful.

Decongestants don't have any effect upon histamines, but instead narrow the blood vessels, and reduce blood flow to affected areas, which helps reduce swelling. They can be taken orally or used topically as nose drops or sprays. Oral decongestants relieve stuffy noses and promote drainage, but they do not affect itching or sneezing. Sometimes they cause mild side effects, particularly if they are taken orally, rather than used topically. Because they have a different action than antihistamines, many products combine the two medications as antihistamine/decongestants.

Sudafed, until recently, was the most popular and widely available over-the-counter decongestant, but it was abused by people who used it to manufacture the dangerous street drug methamphetamine. Therefore it is now somewhat more difficult to obtain in some states.

Singulair, which is effective against allergically triggered asthma, is also quite effective for a variety of allergic responses. Because it is a safe and effective anti-inflammatory, I have applied it to everything from allergy, to colitis, to neuroinflammation, to allergic rhinitis.

Inhaled steroidal medications can also reduce the symptoms of allergy. They are not absorbed to any significant extent, but they're still steroids, so I try to limit their use, particularly in children. One advantage of them is that they help kids avoid systemic medications.

Oral corticosteroids can be effective for kids who have severe asthma but do not seem to be responding to bronchodilators. This approach has more side effects than other asthma treatments, however, and is generally advisable only for short periods of time, due to these side effects, which can include fluid retention, mood disorders, weight gain, and impaired immunity. Another somewhat similar approach is injection of a corticosteroid known as Depo-Medrol. Depo-Medrol can control symptoms for as long as three to four weeks, and can be appropriate for children seeking short-term relief from seasonal allergies.

Flonase is an effective inhaled steroid. It shrinks swelling in the nasal membranes, and can be helpful for allergic rhinitis. One disadvantage of it is that it can dry nasal membranes during extended use.

Nutraceuticals can be valuable against allergies. These natural medications, such as quercitin and pycnogenol, can be highly effective if taken in sufficient dosages. Many people, however, tend to take doses that are too small, and then become discouraged with this approach when it does not produce robust results.

For more information on the nutraceuticals that are appropriate for allergy, review the material in Chapter 18.

SUMMARY OF MEDICATION

Medication, by itself, is not the answer to the 4-A epidemics. But it is part of the answer, when it is applied in conjunction with the other aspects of the Healing Program, as one element of a comprehensive, individualized, flexible plan.

Do not allow yourself to be overwhelmed by all of the options that medication provides. The wide scope of these options is a very positive factor. For your child to reach his or her fullest potential, several medications may be appropriate. However, it is very unlikely that he or she will need more than several, and perhaps only one or two. Even these meds will probably need to be taken for only a limited time.

Don't try to keep all of this information in your mind. It's just too much to keep track of. Use this chapter as a reference guide. Skim through it from time to time, and search for possible solutions to your child's own, unique problems. Discuss these medications with your doctor. Work in partnership with your physician, as an informed associate, and you will find yourself ever closer to helping your child to heal.

Now we have one final aspect of the Healing Program to consider: putting it all together. In the final chapter, I will share with you a number of case histories, taken directly from my own files. These case histories will show you how I combined nutritional therapy, supplementation therapy, detoxification, and medication–all into one, synergistic, comprehensive Healing Program–for a variety of children.

CHAPTER TWENTY-ONE

THE HEALING PROGRAM

Putting the Four Elements Together: Results of Fifteen Cases

SORTING IT ALL OUT

If you are like most parents, you probably feel overwhelmed now. You have seen so *much* information:

- Six variations of diets.
- Dozens of possible supplements.
- Numerous diagnostic tests.
- Several options for detoxification.
- Almost a hundred possible medications.

Don't be overwhelmed. You *can* sort it all out. This chapter will help.

Even more help will come from your child's physician. The relative complexity of this program demands the expertise of a physician who is familiar with integrative medicine.

You will learn, from your doctor, as well as from this chapter, that *you don't have to use every treatment that exists.* That would be chaotic.

Instead, you and your doctor need to carefully individualize your child's treatment program, choosing only the most appropriate treatments, and applying them at the right time.

As you'll see in the following fifteen case histories, most kids were put on Healing Programs that included only a limited number of therapeutic options. More than that would have been too much. Sometimes, in this approach to healing, less is more. Rather than to bombard your child's body and brain with a confusing and possibly contradictory avalanche of treatments, it's better to construct your child's Healing Program one element at a time and see what works and what doesn't.

It's important to apply a therapy and then stand back and monitor the reactions to it, like a good medical detective.

You will note that most of the Healing Programs that were applied in these fifteen cases unfolded over a period of months, and even years. Sometimes results came quickly, and sometimes they did not. Some children responded much more robustly than others.

As you and your doctor systematically build your child's Healing Program, it's important to realize that the program may change as your child changes. Hopefully, certain therapeutic elements, such as administration of pharmaceutical medications, can be discontinued after healing has taken traction. In the final analysis, the most profound healing that your child will experience will be self-healing, and the two most powerful forces that will direct that healing will be the wisdom of his or her body, and your love.

Following is a brief overview of the basic structure of the Healing Program. As you already know, its elements are very diverse, and are most appropriate when applied very specifically, and individualistically.

OVERVIEW OF THE HEALING PROGRAM

1. Testing Procedures

- Tier One testing (see Chapter 16).
- Tier Two testing (see Chapter 16).
- Tier Three testing (see Chapter 16).
- Tier Four testing (see Chapter 16).

2. Nutritional Therapy

- The GF/CF Diet.
- The Specific Food Reaction Diet.
- The Anti-Yeast Diet.
- The Anti-Hypoglycemia Diet
- The Specific Carbohydrate Diet (in some children).
- The Low-Oxalate Diet (in some children).

3. Supplementation Therapy

- Tier One supplements (see Chapter 18).
- Tier Two supplements (see Chapter 18).
- Tier Three supplements (see Chapter 18).
- Tier Four supplements (see Chapter 18).

4. Detoxification

- Natural detoxification procedures.
- Testing for heavy metal overload.
- Resolving pre-chelation issues.
- Chelation therapy.
- Monitoring chelation treatments.

5. Medication

- Medication for autism.
- Medication for ADHD.
- Medication for asthma.
- Medication for allergies.
- Medication for co-morbid disorders.

Now let's see how each of these elements was incorporated into a comprehensive Healing Program. As you will note, most children needed only very limited elements of the entire array of treatment options. For example, in only one of the following fifteen cases did I apply the specific carbohydrate diet, and in none of these cases did I apply the low-oxalate diet. These two diets can help some kids, but most will not require them. Furthermore, you'll note that most of the kids took only a limited number of supplements, and a far more limited number of medications.

You have seen a brief overview of the Healing Program, and now you will see how this program was applied in fifteen children. This will give you a blueprint for your own child's program. However, your child's program will be somewhat different. No two kids are exactly alike.

Your child is an unequivocally unique, special person, different from any other that has ever lived.

This singularity, among all of the many blessings your child has bestowed upon you, is among the most beautiful. Now is the time to return the blessing of individuality.

Patient #1

This six-year-old was first seen one year ago. He had developmental delay symptoms that included poor language development, poor social skills, anxiety, stimming, poor motor skills, hyperactivity, and distractibility. His weight was low, and he had chronic illnesses, including recurrent otitis and rhinitis, often seasonal. He had poor stamina, and he had persistent rashes on his lips, and redness on his ears.

He went on the GF/CF diet, and it helped solidify his bowel movements, and resolve his hyperactivity.

He had experienced an early childhood regression that appeared to have followed recurrent ear infections, which had begun within two months of his MMR/Varivax, at fifteen months old. He had received antibiotics for recurrent otitis, and his regression had appeared to follow that.

He had evidence of dysbiosis, including fungal, bacterial, and anaerobic bacterial infection, and was treated with a number of oral antimicrobials, including gentamicin, vancomycin, and Diflucan. These helped to further normalize his bowel movements. With these medications, combined with the GF/CF diet and supplementation therapy, he began putting on weight, looking much better physically, and experiencing improvement in his appetite.

He also experienced positive improvements from methyl-B-12, with bursts of energy. He became more playful with his dad after the methyl-B-12, as well as after IV-glutathione/NAC. His drawing became much better, and he became much more creative, writing letters, and drawing his first train the day after his IV-glutathione/NAC.

During his first seven months of treatment, he was healthy throughout the fall and winter, which were normally times of rhinitis and otitis.

His nutritional supplements included zinc, vitamin C, transfer factor, cod liver oil, pantothenic acid (with a glycemic stabilizing formula called Sugar Companion), essential fatty acids (including omega-3 and GLA), folinic acid, TMG, methyl-B-12, probiotics, and digestive enzymes.

After nine months of treatment, his parents reported that he was doing "great," with major improvements in his speech, and much improved peer interaction. His stamina was now "excellent." His teacher's progress report also noted good improvement with gross motor skills, although he still had some mild problems with fine motor skills. His mother noted "progress, progress, progress."

His final school reports were fantastic, noting "transformation, with incredible cognitive and academic success. He is now a class leader." Prior to the year of treatment here, his mother said he was often "cowering in the corner." His mother stated, "A kid who disappeared two and a half years ago is now back." His stimming, which used to be quite high, has pretty much stopped, the redness of his ears has greatly diminished, and the rashes around his lips and mouth have disappeared.

He will now do art, and asks to paint. Prior to the treatment, he never did any art. His thoughts and language are much more complex, and he recently asked his mother, "Mom, what's jealousy?" After her explanation, he asked, "Does jealousy have anger in it?" He now initiates conversations, and participates in long conversations. His mother stated that he is very happy, and "He is right in there now."

He is no longer hyperactive, but still has some distractibility, with decreased focus. He is being started on DMAE for his focus issues. He has some evidence of heavy metal overload, and is also being started on chelation therapy.

Patient #2

This seven-year-old boy, who is now ten years old, suffered from neurological dysfunction, with ADHD features.

He had a history of regression after his MMR, characterized by screaming and arching after his naps, stereotypic behaviors, loss of prior gains in his language, and head banging. He tended to be quite hyperactive and very loud.

He had evidence of multiple food allergies, multiple nutritional deficiencies, impaired detoxification, and increased oxidative stress.

He had a positive response to the restriction of allergenic foods, nutritional therapy, supplementation therapy, and the resultant remediation of his nutritional deficiencies and imbalances.

He was also treated with intravenous glutathione. There was much improvement in his sleep after that, as well as improvement in his verbalizations and hyperactivity.

When corn was restricted, he became even less hyper. His verbal ability increased, and he was more appropriate in conversations.

He is a child with prominent red cheeks, and sometimes we see prominent red cheeks, and red ears, with phenol sensitivity. He was taken off foods with phenols, and there was further improvement, including his ability to sleep even better. He also experienced less tactile sensitivity to his clothing.

He had very elevated ASO and anti-DNAse-B titers, which were consistent with the autoimmune disorder PANDAS, or Pediatric Auto-immune Neuropsychiatric Disorder Associated with Strep. We considered IV-gamma globulin for the PANDAS, but this was never pursued, due to the high cost. It wasn't covered by his family's insurance. Therefore, he was treated with a course of antibiotics, followed by prophylactic antibiotics. The antibiotics made a very positive difference.

School reports became very good. He continued to improve.

He also responded well to detoxification procedures. He showed significant improvement from methyl-B-12 (methylcobalamin), and transdermal TTFD, or Thiamine Tetrahydrofurfuryl Disulfide. He showed evidence of heavy metal burden during DMSA provocation testing, so he was treated with DMSA, and became much more manageable and emotionally flexible after that. He had previously been quite rigid and difficult.

He saw an experienced pediatric gastroenterologist for recurrent abdominal pain and bouts of diarrhea, and had an endoscopy. During the endoscopy, he was given secretin, and it appeared to contribute to his increased calmness, and in improvement of his stools. Therefore, we repeated courses of secretin, which the patient felt were helpful for him. He also remained on nystatin, for his fungal dysbiosis.

He was also treated with GI anti-inflammatories, which helped control his chronic diarrhea.

After the administration of Zithromax, his school reports became even better. His mother noted that since he began the antibiotic prophylaxis for PANDAS, she sees "glimmers" of a normal child, including moments in which he seems to be a different child. In addition to helping with his calmness, she also felt the IV-secretin helped with his attention, and gave him higher levels of thought for two to three weeks afterward.

He has seasonal allergies, which are helped by quercitin and Claritin.

He was having persistent bowel problems, including abdominal distention, discomfort, and diarrhea, and those problems responded to the specific carbohydrate diet, especially when he stopped eating large amounts of rice and potatoes. He also responded to an increased dose of the GI anti-inflammatory Colazol.

He continued to have problems with seasonal exacerbation of allergies, which, in addition to triggering his rhinitis, would also exacerbate his negative behaviors.

He had significant problems with stims, but the stims decreased from the off-label use of the medications Namenda and low-dose naltrexone.

When he ran out of his Zithromax for about a month, his mother noticed that he became more obsessive. When he restarted it, she noted a decrease in his obsessiveness, and she reported that he was calmer.

The problems that remained were his hypersensitivity to sound, or hyperacusis, and some social difficulties. His mother noted, however, that he was moved into a resource program, and she said, "He is soaring. He is the best of all the resource kids." She said that she didn't believe any of the other kids were engaging in biomedical approaches.

During the last visit, he was calmer. He looked great. He was growing, thinning out, and he wasn't bloated, which had been prominent on previous exams. He was calmer and not as loud. He would say, "Hi, Dr. Bock," and answer my questions, but he still had some variable eye contact and some verbal repetition, or perseveration.

He is going to be changed to another delivery form of DMSA, to bypass his gut, because he has significant gut issues. He is also continuing to receive medication for the seasonal exacerbations of his allergies.

He is an example of a child whose verbalization had previously been very inappropriate. He had talked a mile a minute, but it had been all scripting, instead of communicative language.

His primary benefits were derived from treating his PANDAS with prophylactic antibiotics, putting him on appropriate programs of nutritional and supplementation therapy, treating him with GI anti-inflammatories, and treating him with IV-secretin.

He has made huge strides academically and behaviorally. He is so much more calm, attentive, interactive, and conversational.

Patient #3

This child was first seen when he was five years old. Now he is nine and a half. This young boy's neurological disorder consisted of auditory processing problems, Asperger's symptoms, language problems, inattentiveness, and anxiety. He had previously had more pronounced autism-spectrum symptoms, but had attained a higher level of function, consistent with that of Asperger's syndrome.

Comprehensive treatment included dietary modifications, regular methyl-B-12, and IV-glutathione every week or two. This resulted in huge, huge strides.

He still tended to have significant social gaps, however, and got along much better with younger children than his peers.

One of the biggest contributors to his improvement was heavy metal detoxification with DMSA. He had significant heavy metal overload, with high elevation of his red blood cell mercury, as well as huge amounts of mercury spill during treatment. He also excreted lead and arsenic during urine heavy metal testing.

He had evidence of impaired detoxification, linked to nutrient deficits, which required repletion.

He was also shown to be positive homozygous, for the A1298C mutation of the MTHFR gene, a genetic polymorphism which further hampered his detoxification capabilities.

He also needed to be repleted persistently with iron.

On his last follow-up, he had improved so much that he no longer had aides in his classroom. He was much more aware of the problems that had interfered with his social interaction. He loves his friends, and they appear to love him, despite his previous marked social gap.

He was started on a very small dose of methylphenidate, which, according to his mother, "transformed him." She reported increased attention, increased interaction, and much less impulsivity, with no adverse side effects. His mother noted that he was "more scattered" when the methylphenidate wore off.

The elements of the Healing Program that appeared to be of the most significant value were administration of DMSA, methyl-B-12, IV-glutathione, multiple nutritional supplements (especially selenium, iron, and zinc), and a small amount of a medication for lingering impulsivity and attentional problems.

His mother was very cooperative with treatment recommendations and follow-up.

Improvements noted during the last follow-up included further improvement of auditory processing, which had reached a level of essential normalcy. He still had some problems with the complicated semantics of language, but his teachers had noted huge improvements in his creativity, thinking, imagination, and verbalization. This child has changed so much. His interactions with adults have become completely normal, and only with his peers does he have some slight remaining difficulties. These difficulties, however, are normalizing at a rapid rate, and he is excelling at school, and in other situations.

He has moved out of the spectrum, and recovered. His last few quirks are in the process of being remediated.

This case indicates the benefit of sometimes adding a low dose of a medication to a comprehensive, integrative treatment program. This can help to bring a patient closer to normalcy, take the edge off of his or her behaviors, and improve the issues of focus and impulsivity.

Patient #4

First seen when he was twelve years old, he is now fifteen. He initially presented with symptoms of autism.

He had a history of recurrent infections, including sinusitis and bronchitis. He had evidence of immune deficiency, which improved with IV-gamma globulin.

He was also discovered to have PANDAS, characterized by facial tics, especially of his mouth. These were more pronounced when he had acute strep infections. In addition, he also had evidence of autoimmunity to his brain, as indicated by the presence of elevated levels of antimyelin basic protein antibodies.

As he responded to treatment, he was no longer in the autism spectrum, but still had significant problems with connectedness and focus, consistent with ADHD symptoms. He also still suffered from recurrent, chronic infections from the fall through the winter.

He had food sensitivities, including sensitivity to wheat, resulting in behaviors of acting silly, spacey, oppositional, and disconnected. He was placed on the gluten-free, casein-free diet, was administered supplements, and given IV-secretin.

He had previously been on IV-immunoglobulin, recommended by an immunologist, for his immune deficiency and recurrent infections. I reintroduced intravenous immunoglobulin as a treatment for several conditions, including his neuroimmune disorder, with its history of neurodevelopmental delays; hypotonia; regressive encephalopathy; PANDAS; and humoral immune deficiency, with recurrent infections (including otitis, sinusitis, bronchitis, and strep).

He also had evidence of bowel dysbiosis, and multiple food sensitivities. He had previously improved on both antifungals and antibiotics, and responded extremely well to IV-glutathione, coupled with IV-secretin. After these treatments, his mother would note a "big perk up." He was more engaged, and more verbal after IV-secretin and glutathione. She also noticed that his tics were helped by IV-immunoglobulin.

Methylcobalamin, or methyl-B-12, was added, and his mother noted that he was more alert and emotionally connected after this. Clonidine helped reverse his anxiety at school, and also helped with his occasional insomnia.

This child's improvement is an example of the balance that must be achieved during the administration of varying medications. His tics, which seemed to be related to bacterial infections and PANDAS, improved on antibiotics. However, the antibiotics triggered development of fungal dysbiosis, which was then treated with antifungals, including Sporanox and nystatin. The symptoms that seemed to respond to the antifungals included his oppositional behavior and his negativity.

Being a teenager, he would go through times in which he did not follow his wheat-free, yeast-free, and sugar-free diet, and his symptoms would return. The symptoms included increased acne, difficulties with his schoolwork, decreased attention, and oppositional behavior. However, when he returned to the dietary modifications, as well as to antifungals, it helped significantly. I frequently counseled the patient and his mother about some of the normal psychosocial issues of being a teenager, because these issues were often exacerbated by his health problems.

Methylcobalamin was consistently helpful, and when he ran out of it, his mother noticed a "big fall-off." When he stayed on it regularly, she noticed a big improvement in his emotional connectedness and his focus.

Additional improvement was noted after he began taking phosphatidylcholine. The improvements were in demeanor, focus, temperament, connectedness, responsiveness, and decreased oppositional/defiant behavior. His mother noted further improvement when the phosphatidylcholine was given intravenously.

By the time of his next-to-last visit, he was doing extremely well in school, with much harder classes. He was also doing well socially, playing school sports, remaining much healthier, and suffering no more recurrent infections.

He reported that he experienced increased focus when he took the nutritional supplement DMAE, which often helps with focus. His mother opposed administration of pharmaceutical medications for focus.

He was getting A's in school, was conversational, and was appropriate. His principal noted that his last year in high school was a great year for him. In addition to athletics, he also was doing very well in music.

This is a child who really blossomed on a Healing Program that included dietary modifications, especially restriction of yeast and allergenic foods (particularly wheat). Also critically important was supplementation therapy, including phosphatidylcholine and DMAE for his focus problems. His immune problems responded well to IV-gamma globulin. This remediated his immune deficiency, recurrent infections, PANDAS syndrome, and fungal dysbiosis. His overall school performance, both academically and socially, improved with methyl-cobalamin, IV-glutathione, IV-phosphatidylcholine, and IV-secretin.

I saw the patient again recently, and was tremendously impressed by him. He looks great, is healthy, is smart, and has become a fine young man.

Patient #5

First seen as a six-year-old, this boy, now ten and a half, had severe asthma. He had been hospitalized ten months prior to his first visit, due to asthma and failure to thrive. He had seen a number of doctors, including specialists, and had been treated with multiple medications, but his mother did not feel he was doing well.

He had allergies to cat and dog hair, and his asthma was triggered by colds, flu, cats, and sometimes dogs.

He had previously seen a naturopath, who had taken him off gluten. After this gluten restriction, he did begin gaining some weight, and eating somewhat more food. There was also some improvement in his chronic constipation.

He was very prone to recurrent upper respiratory infections, which frequently progressed to asthma. He tended to be chronically tired, had problems sleeping through the night, and had chronic anxiety. He had been treated with oral steroids, but his mother was not comfortable with that approach.

He had a family history of allergies and eczema, on both sides of his family.

His diagnoses from the pulmonary, asthma, and allergy specialists were allergic rhinitis, and asthma.

In the recent past, his family had experienced a flood in their basement after a hurricane, and he had become ill after this. This illness was suspected to have been triggered by molds, although the basement had been cleaned out, and the air-conditioning system had been cleaned and treated.

During the first visit, he was pale, and had allergic shiners. He had a tendency to cling to his mother, and was mildly whiny. He had evidence of keratosis pilaris (bilaterally), allergic rhinitis, and he had mildly enlarged anterior cervical lymph nodes.

He was taken off dairy, and started on various nutritional supplements, including zinc, vitamin C, cod liver oil, vitamin E, transfer factor, and probiotics. He responded extremely well to this nutritional and supplementation therapy, and stopped getting asthma attacks. He was actually able to stop all of his prescription medications.

A year later, his mother reported that he was "doing great." He was growing well, and had gained four and a half pounds. She said he rarely got sick, and if he caught a cold, it would no longer progress to wheezing. His bowels had become regular. He still had some mild problems with focus, which had improved with his nutritional therapy.

He continued to do very well over the next year, in terms of growth and weight gain, and did not have any problems with asthma. His mother noticed much improvement in his concentration and focus.

This is a good example of recovery in a child who was failing to thrive, was sickly, was not growing or gaining weight, and was often hospitalized for asthma, despite being treated with multiple medications. He responded very well to nutritional therapy, including the GF/CF diet, and to supplementation therapy, and environmental controls.

In addition to the previously noted supplements, he began taking calcium and magnesium (because he was off dairy), as well as querciplex and a homeopathic hay fever remedy during seasonal exacerbations. He also responded well to DMAE for his focus problems. At the first sign of an illness, he would increase his intake of transfer factor, and would take homeopathics, such as Thymactive and *Drosera homaccord*. Simultaneously, he would increase his vitamin C, for about a week. This eliminated the need for any asthma medications or antibiotics, except during one short illness. His parents are thrilled with his progress.

Patient #6

This case is a revealing example of the significant improvement that can occur in a short time period. This four-year-old boy was seen nine months ago at age three years, three months. He presented with extensive neurological disorder, with encephalopathy. He suffered from neurodevelopmental delay with PDD, with ADHD features. His exam revealed pronounced stimming, a chronic sideways glance, echolalia, babbling, decreased eye contact, moderate hyperactivity, and decreased focus.

He ate a very narrow range of foods, consisting mostly of dairy and wheat. He had chronic constipation, with hard stools. His evaluation showed evidence of multiple nutritional deficiencies, including iron deficiency, which had resulted in anemia. He also had low plasma sulfate. In addition, he had various metabolic imbalances, and dysbiosis.

He responded quite rapidly to nutritional therapy, including the GF/CF diet and the specific food reaction diet. Testing had revealed that he had multiple food sensitivities, including a soy reaction. He also eliminated *trans*-fats, which he had been consuming heavily.

His gut was treated with the appropriate antibacterial medications, and this was helpful with his bowels, and also improved his behavior. Methylcobalamin was also helpful. His mother noticed that he had increased attention, was more present, and was talking more. His teacher reported that, "He is getting much better." His teacher noted increased attention, much easier transitions, and more spontaneous speech.

He experienced more interest in a variety of foods, or increased palate, after starting the GF/CF diet, and restricting soy. He was also repleted with iron, for his iron deficiency anemia.

After these relatively limited treatments, he began interacting more with other kids at school, making increased eye contact, and using more spontaneous language. However, the stims continued, in a variable way.

He is soon going to be tested for heavy metal overload, and will start other treatments.

This boy's progress, in just nine months, indicates the possibility that exists of fairly rapid improvement, after only some basic changes. The changes included nutritional therapy, supplementation therapy, and administration of methyl-B-12.

Patient #7

This boy, three and a half years old, was referred by his mother's psychotherapist, whose son had been successfully treated here.

His mother noted that he had been normal until nine months of age, when she had weaned him abruptly from breast-feeding and had started feeding him adult foods. He developed allergic reactions to fruits, and had to be hospitalized. His mother was extremely stressed and overwhelmed at that point.

He alternated from hyperactive-impulsive behavior to spaced-out behavior, with decreased eye contact and decreased responsiveness. He had speech delay and fine motor delay, as well as some gross motor delay. He had been diagnosed with ADHD by his pediatrician but had never seen a developmental pediatrician or a pediatric neurologist. Because he suffered from defects in communication, eye contact, and social relatedness, and because he exhibited some repetitive behaviors, I felt he was in the autism spectrum, and referred him to a developmental pediatrician.

The boy had no history of having had any immunizations. His mother had a history of psoriasis, of severe yeast vaginitis, and she had a number of mercury amalgam dental fillings. She was also very stressed by her son's disorder.

His diet consisted of many starchy, high-gluten foods, and he craved sweets. He had a history of rapid mood shifts, during which he could get aggressive. He had been known to thrash restlessly in his crib as an infant.

His family lived in an old house, where there was extensive mold. In that house, he may also have been exposed to lead from old, chipped paint.

He also had frequent fatigue, cold extremities, was sluggish, tended to have bronchial congestion, had trouble falling asleep, and had a frequent cough. He had hypothyroid symptoms, and problems with concentration.

When first seen, he was a sweet, very quiet, three-year-old who lay on the couch sucking his thumb, appearing to have very low energy. He made minimal eye contact with me, and did not have any spoken words. He appeared to have some hand and eye stims when lying on the couch, and appeared to zone out. There was some degree of a sideways glance.

I suspected that he suffered from food allergies, fungal dysbiosis, fungal hypersensitivity, mold hypersensitivity, reactive hypoglycemia, and hypothyroidism. Contributing to his problems were some significant psychosocial factors.

He was started on the GF/CF diet, the antihypoglycemia diet, and supplementation therapy. I discussed environmental controls with his mother—especially mold avoidance.

Within approximately one year, the child had major, positive improvements with decreased hyperactivity, the acquisition of age-appropriate language, and a new ability to express many more thoughts, feelings, and ideas. His mother reported, "It's amazing." His mood became much more stable, and his mother noted that he had become "much more of a normal kid." His marked improvements resulted in great benefit to his mother's overall stress level.

At a follow-up visit he made good eye contact and responded conversationally to my questions.

Patient #8

This seven-year-old boy was first seen two and a half years ago. He presented with regressive encephalopathy and poor language development.

He had experienced regression in social contact between the ages of one and two, and had reportedly become much worse after his DTAP and polio vaccinations at eighteen months. He had been lethargic for three days after the vaccinations. He'd had his HIB and MMR three months earlier.

He had persistent fungal dysbiosis, and experienced significant improvement when he took the antifungals nystatin and Nizoral, with monthly follow-ups of liver function tests.

He also had a dramatic response to methyl-B-12, with increased alertness and increased eye contact. His teachers reported an "almost shocking improvement."

He had laboratory evidence of impaired detoxification, with low cysteine, low sulfate, and low glutathione, and he responded very nicely to IV-N-acetyl-cysteine, vitamin C, and magnesium sulfate.

He also responded well to phosphatidylcholine, with improved cognition. He achieved much better eye contact, and was no longer spacey.

He can occasionally get hyperactive but is now able to initiate appropriate, meaningful conversations. His mother reports that some days he seems like "a normal kid," and other days he still has moderate symptoms of variable eye contact, hyperactivity, and perseveration. Overall, however, he is very much improved.

Patient #9

This six-and-a-half-year-old boy was first seen three years ago, with symptoms consistent with those of the autism spectrum, including poor language development, lack of eye contact, impaired cognitive function, and behavioral difficulties.

He had regressed at twenty-six months, and had lost all words, and had become less expressive. He had then improved a few months later, and had started nursery school. Then he had regressed again, at the time of a move to an old house, which had been undergoing extensive renovation, and contained large amounts of mold.

He improved greatly with the anti-yeast diet, nystatin, and multiple nutritional supplements.

There was also some suspicion that he had experienced oxygen deprivation, or hypoxia, at birth. He is a twin, and was born an hour and a half later than his twin brother, who is not on the spectrum.

His family lives in England, and has a summer home in Rhinebeck. The Rhinebeck house is also an old home with a lot of mold, and he has regressed when he has been around this mold. He has progressed, and then regressed, on several occasions. Each time was in the summer and spring, when he came to Rhinebeck.

In the renovation of the house in England, he may have experienced exposure to lead, from old paint on the walls. He has shown evidence of heavy metal overload.

The anti-yeast diet, nystatin, supplementation therapy, and probiotics were significantly helpful, in terms of his bowel movements and abdominal complaints. This is important, because this child is a "gut-brain kid," whose behaviors seem to correlate with his GI dysfunctions, particularly diarrhea. I also discussed with his mother the importance of reducing exposure to mold, with environmental controls.

He has evidence of selenium and iron deficiencies, and elevation of the thyroid stimulating hormone. He has had a positive response to chelation therapy, as well as to IV-vitamin C, minerals, and B-complex.

At a follow-up visit, his mother stated that he had experienced the "best run of his life in the past two months."

He is also receiving phosphatidylcholine, which is helping him behaviorally and cognitively. He is still reported to be doing "great," with huge improvements in eye contact and speech. He is speaking to everyone.

Patient #10

This girl was first seen at five years old, and now is seven. Her diagnoses included PDD-NOS, sensory integration dysfunction, language and behavior problems, oral-motor dyspraxia, and ADHD features. She also had chronic nasal congestion and multiple food reactions, including IgE allergies.

She had regressed after her MMR at fifteen months, according to her mother.

Her initial lab work showed egg allergy; multiple nutritional deficiencies (including deficits of several minerals and vitamin E); immune deficiency, with decreased IgA and decreased IgG; and fungal dysbiosis.

She was initially placed on the anti-yeast diet, and antifungals. Her mother reported quick improvement. She said that her daughter's noncompliance in school had become "next to zero," and "she is already becoming a different kid."

Restricting eggs resulted in further significant improvement, including her being more responsive, being more present, doing even better in school, and learning new concepts more easily.

The patient had evidence of mild impairment of detoxification, indicated by mildly decreased glutathione, and mildly decreased cysteine and sulfate. She also had evidence of heavy metal burden. Therefore, she was treated with IV-glutathione, followed by treatment with DMSA.

At her most recent visit, she still had some remaining problems, but was continuing to experience improvements. She was becoming more conversational, her peer relations were improving, and she was listening more to other children.

We continued her detoxification with IV-glutathione and DMSA, administered nystatin, and continued her anti-yeast, egg-restricted diet.

Patient #11

This patient was first seen at age two. He was referred by a nurse, for consideration of heavy metal detoxification. The nurse, in consultation with a physician, had already begun dietary modifications and nutritional supplementation.

The boy had a history of autism-spectrum disorder, characterized by very minimal language development, poor social interaction, poor eye contact, impaired cognition, walking on his toes, and hyperactivity. He also had food allergies, chronic diarrhea, nutrient malabsorption, and dermatitis.

When he had received his second hepatitis B vaccination, he had developed colic, and had cried almost incessantly.

When he had been started on the GF/CF diet at age ten months, he had stopped toe-walking, and had become more attentive. When he had eaten corn, his ears had turned red, so corn had been discontinued. Administration of antifungals had resulted in more regular bowel movements, and improvements in neurobehavioral symptoms.

On initial testing, he showed evidence of heavy metal overload.

Upon examination, he showed some response to verbal prompting, and he attempted to mimic some of his father's words. He was mildly hyperactive at times.

His parents reported that he did "phenomenally" after being started on intravenous glutathione. Although he'd previously had no expressive language, he developed two-word combinations. He also demonstrated increased play skills. His parents later reported that he soon began "talking like crazy." They noted that, "He is so much more interactive." His therapist reported continuing progress, including "increased awareness, increased verbal skills, and increased interaction," since starting intravenous glutathione. He was also more relaxed.

Continued follow-up indicated that he was, according to his mother, "doing great." She said, "He is much more responsive to my verbal requests, makes eye contact, is affectionate, and is talking much more."

He was eventually started on methyl-B-12, and had continued improvements, including increased social interaction and the development of a good sense of humor. He achieved further positive response in these respects when TMG and folinic acid were added.

At his last visit, his mother showed me a speech evaluation that stated, "He is at level." His parents were planning to mainstream him in kindergarten, without an aide. He was swimming and playing soccer. He still had some mild gross motor problems, occasional hyperactivity, and mild attentional problems. On his last medical exam, however, he was initiating conversation, was so much more aware and present, and made much better eye contact.

Patient #12

This boy, first seen at ten years of age, suffered from epileptic disorder and the inattentive subtype of ADHD. He also had a history of eczema.

He had been given medications in the past, including Concerta, which had caused anger and aggressiveness. He'd received some benefit from Strattera, but his mother was not satisfied with a strictly pharmacologic approach. She brought him in for a comprehensive biomedical approach, including nutritional and supplementation therapy. She believed he might have food sensitivities, which appeared to trigger his focus and cognitive difficulties.

He had taken several antiseizure medicines in the past. His only current medication was Strattera, at a dosage of 40 mg. daily. He had mood swings and anxiety, which his mother felt were related to low blood sugar. He also had low energy, occasional headaches, impaired cognitive function, forgetfulness, obsessive traits, and frequent loose stools.

He had evidence of impaired detoxification, metabolic imbalance, dysbiosis, and multiple nutritional deficiencies, including low magnesium, zinc, fat-soluble vitamins, and essential fatty acids (especially omega-3).

He was started on oral medications and herbal antimicrobials for his bowel dysbiosis, including nystatin, vancomycin, and Advanced Biocidin. He was placed on the anti-yeast diet, the anti-hypoglycemia diet, and a diet that restricted chocolate. He was advised to take Epsom salt baths to remediate his magnesium and sulfate deficiencies, and to begin taking methyl-B-12. He had a positive response to these interventions, with reports of more alertness, increased attention and awareness, and better schoolwork.

However, he began to stray from his dietary recommendations. Even so, he was still taking nutritional supplements and methyl-B-12 shots, and his mother felt that these treatments were more effective than his ADHD medications. She stated that he wasn't angry, like he used to be. He seemed much happier.

He was also taking nystatin, but not following the antiyeast diet. His report card in school greatly improved.

After one year of treatment, the patient became resistant to taking nutritional supplements, and his mother and his teachers noted some negative changes. They said he was "slower, less focused, and more of a stargazer." He soon began to take his supplements again and his positive progress returned. His mother noted that he did best when he was on both methyl-B-12 and vitamin B-6. He was generally avoiding dairy, and he had no further eczema.

On examination in the office, he was much calmer, and much more engaged in conversations with me and his mother.

This is an example of a child with ADHD who responded nicely to supplementation therapy, nutritional therapy, improved methylation and detoxification with methyl-B-12, and the appropriate medications.

Patient #13

This child was two years old when he was first seen, three and a half years ago. He was on the autism spectrum, with symptoms of poor speech and language development, stims, poor eye contact, hypotonia, moodiness, inappropriate social behavior, and motor delay. He also had a history of asthma, eczema, and food allergies, as well as a family history of autoimmunity.

During pregnancy, his mother had broken a mercury thermometer and had cleaned it up.

On first examination, he said no words, except once, when he was prompted to say "Hi." He could make some sounds, generally high-pitched. His stims included hand flapping, and he made no significant eye contact, but instead engaged in a sideways glance. He was happy, but had some inappropriate giggling. He showed some mild pallor on exam, some mild to moderate allergic shiners, and hypotonia. He was found to have fungal and bacterial dysbiosis, as well as a low level of carnitine, multiple food sensitivities, and impaired detoxification.

He was placed on an individualized Healing Program, which included treatment of his fungal and bacterial dysbiosis, avoidance of reactive foods, and administration of *N*-acetyl-carnitine. He returned in six months to pursue further evaluation and treatment. At this visit, his mother noted that TMG was helpful in regard to his mood and sensitivity.

He was started on methyl-B-12 and had an excellent response.

At a subsequent visit his mother reported that, "He is doing great." His progress report from his preschool was by far the best it had ever been. He was now initiating conversations, was very interested in social interactions, was more confident and not as skittish. His mother reported huge benefits from methyl-B-12, and from other elements of his supplementation therapy, which included vitamin C, quercitin, magnesium taurate, liquid iron, liquid selenium, calcium, magnesium, amino acids, and probiotics (including *S. boulardii*). He still had some persistent stims, particularly hand flapping, as well as hyperacusis. On exam, he was happy and talkative, and he responded to verbal requests with appropriate answers and articulate language, except for mixing up some pronouns. He had a good sense of humor, made jokes, initiated conversations with myself and his mother, and he stated, "I am feeling good."

This is an example of a child who had a very positive response to supplementation therapy, including administration of methyl-B-12.

Patient #14

This seven-year-old boy on the autism spectrum was first seen three years ago, as a four-year-old. He was referred by a pediatrician, to pursue possible heavy metal detoxification. This boy had classic symptoms of the autism-spectrum disorders. He had regressed at age one-year, and by the time he was two, he had many stereotypical autistic behaviors. By age three, he had difficulty with relating to others.

He had a significant degree of fungal dysbiosis, which was treated effectively with antifungals, especially nystatin. He improved with DMSA initially, but this therapy appeared to increase the problems with his dysbiosis. Therefore, he had to be treated with prophylactic courses of nystatin while on DMSA.

He had impaired detoxification, with low plasma glutathione, low cysteine, low sulfate, and also an increase in lipid peroxides, indicative of increased oxidant stress.

He improved with DMSA, intravenous and transdermal glutathione, methyl-B-12, and nystatin.

At his last visit, his mother and his ABA therapist reported that he was doing "incredible" at summer camp. He was using more spontaneous language, and was having conversational interactions with kids for the first time. His ABA therapist felt that he did not stand out at camp. He was learning to swim, and he was really enjoying playing with kids in the playground. For the first time, he had cried when he'd had to leave the playground. He was asking more questions. He was still engaging in some stims, such as pacing while he played with a toy. However, he was the most relaxed and conversational he had ever been with me.

This is an example of a case in which a father was initially quite skeptical about biomedical intervention, including chelation therapy for heavy metal overload. However, after the father observed positive changes and improvement in his child, the father became convinced of the efficacy of this approach. The child's changes have been noted not only by his ABA therapist and parents, but by all of his family members, his teachers, and others who knew him prior to biomedical treatment.

Patient #15

This child was first seen when he was five years, four months old, and was on the autism spectrum.

At two and a half to three years old, he began withdrawing from people, as well as scripting. At around three years, he became hyperactive, with excessive bouncing and running back and forth. He also suffered from constipation.

One of his problems was that he had hypoglycemic symptoms, which consisted of him needing to eat every hour. If he didn't, his mother said, "His metabolism would run out," and he would experience meltdowns, with a combination of listlessness, low energy, tantrums, and aggressive behavior.

He had a history of recurrent otitis media, and on three occasions had been treated with antibiotics. There was a family history of hypoglycemia and allergies. Laboratory testing showed evidence of IgE reactivity to eggs. He had a history of an elevated lead level, of 10 mcg. per deciliter, at two years old, which had been treated with iron.

I recommended a glucose tolerance test, because I suspected reactive hypoglycemia, but his mother did not want to do this test, so the hypoglycemia was treated empirically.

He had a significant response to the anti-hypoglycemia diet, which consisted of frequent feedings, increased protein, and avoidance of refined carbohydrates. His improvements included increased calm, increased focus, and improved social skills, as well as decreased meltdowns, tantrums, and aggressive behaviors.

He later began the GF/CF diet, and responded positively.

Because he had reactive hypoglycemia, I provided functional support with supplements, including zinc, magnesium, chromium, and biotin.

He was also advised to avoid eggs, because of his egg allergy.

He had evidence of several low minerals, as well as a deficiency of his fat-soluble vitamins.

He had previously had an endoscopy and colonoscopy by an experienced pediatric gastroenterologist, and apparently there had been a motility disorder present, which responded extremely well to the secretin challenge that was performed during the endoscopy. The secretin also appeared to affect his mood. His mother reported that he was "so relaxed, and very calm." The next day he continued to be much less tense and much more relaxed.

The behavioral therapy of Auditory Integration Training was helpful for his hypersensitivity to sound, or hyperacusis.

Follow-up lab tests showed evidence of a fungal dysbiosis that was sensitive to the antifungal Sporanox, so he was treated with Sporanox. He had a very positive response, resulting in regularity of his bowel movements. His liver function was monitored while he was on Sporanox, and it remained within normal limits.

He began to interact with his peers, which had been one of his biggest problems. That began to improve after the fungal dysbiosis was treated, and after he received IV-glutathione. Antifungals included Sporanox and nystatin, and eventually his laxative medication, MiraLax, was able to be tapered.

His mother stated, "He is doing great, and his teachers can't believe it." She said his teachers had noticed so much improvement that they were requesting that I come to his school to speak, because they had so many other kids whom they thought would be helped by this approach.

He was seen recently, and seemed to be doing extremely well. He attended two local camps and his mother said he did "fabulous." No one there knew he had a history of problems. He made friends, was liked by the other kids, and his parents were thrilled that no one knew "anything was amiss." He took swimming, piano, and boating lessons. He interacted very well with visitors, including his grandparents, other family members, and his peers. He could even sit and watch a movie, whereas in the past, that level of stimulation would have been problematic.

He was placed in a regular class, and continued receiving occupational therapy and physical therapy once per week.

This is a child whose improvement was so marked that he is now off the spectrum, in a regular class. He has experienced resolution of severe constipation, extreme behavioral meltdowns, and significant problems with social interaction. This was achieved with treatment of reactive hypoglycemia and fungal dysbiosis, and with the administration of proper medications, nutritional therapy, behavioral therapy, and supplementation therapy.

We continued his anti-hypoglycemia diet, GF/CF diet, restriction of eggs, his supplementation therapy, and administration of the medication Rhinocort for allergic rhinitis.

The last time I spoke to his mother was just after they had traveled to England for a long vacation. His mother reported, "I couldn't even have dreamed two years ago that something like that could happen. He even spent a night alone with his grandparents, which allowed my husband and I to have a little time for ourselves." I was gratified to hear that, because although the primary goal of the biomedical approach is to heal children, when this occurs, it also heals families. Helping whole families to once again center their lives around their love for one another, rather than around the daily routine of medical necessities, is the final, fullest goal of the Healing Program.

AFTERWORD

A NEWER WORLD

And so we are at the end of one exploration and the beginning of another.

At end now are the stories of some brave children who grasped their own lives with the feeblest of grips but would not let go: Paul Avram, Kyle Olson, Brian Dunn, Alisa Winters, Aniyka Usman, Teia O'Connor, and all the others. They alchemized medical history out of the power of their own hearts.

Beginning now is the new story of your *own* child's life.

What will that story be?

Have faith, and let the story unfold.

It has been said that faith is the bird that feels the light, and sings while the dawn is still dark. That now must be your mission: To *feel* the light, and to see, despite the current darkness, the saving grace within your child that can be seen only through the eyes of mothers and fathers.

You, and you alone, will be able to see this, because only mothers and fathers can see their children through the most insightful of eyes: the eyes of love.

These eyes bring a clarity that supersedes reality and creates new worlds.

The eyes of love hold an idea, not an image. It is the idea of what can be.

Long ago, Alfred Tennyson wrote of the epic voyage of the exiled Ulysses, who in his journey home overcame the dark forces of inertia, fear, betrayal, confusion, and despair.

Ulysses was separated from those he loved for what seemed to be forever. But his journey home was guided always by the light of those he held most dear.

Your journey with your own child, cloaked in earthbound routine, will be no less epic than that of Ulysses. You will at times be lost in the darkness. But you will continue, illumined by love, because at journey's end lies a new world for your child.

Your days will be long and you will have doubt. But your faith in your child will heal your hurt, and bring you finally home to your child's heart.

As Tennyson wrote, "... The long day wanes, the slow moon climbs, the deep moans 'round with many voices. Come, my friends, 'tis not too late to seek a newer world."

So, in closing, I say this to you: Come, my fellow parent, my fellow medical detective, my friend—let *our* journey begin.

On this journey, your child will be your mission, your beacon, and your blessing. And now I leave you and your child with this blessing of my own: May the love of your family, made eternal by each new generation, remain undefeated by epidemic, and even by death, as it heads toward the horizon of time.

APPENDIX #1

A SAFER VACCINATION SCHEDULE

Vaccinations can generally be administered within reasonable boundaries of safety. Therefore, I recommend that parents vaccinate their children. However, it is critically important that this be done in as safe a manner as is absolutely possible.

Furthermore, parents should know that no vaccination is completely free of risk. There is always at least a very small chance of adverse effects. Within the entire population of all children who are vaccinated, these adverse reactions are relatively rare, but they do occur. Particularly if you have had a child with a 4-A disorder, or an older child that appeared to have an adverse reaction to vaccination, you should discuss these guidelines with your pediatrician, who can adapt them to your family's needs and history.

Adverse reactions are far more likely to occur, however, if vaccinations are administered in an unsafe manner. Unfortunately, I believe that some of the standard practices of vaccine administration are at least moderately unsafe. For example, it is standard practice to vaccinate children with flu vaccines that contain thimerosal, but in my opinion this is unsafe. It's also standard practice to vaccinate newborn babies with the hepatitis-B vaccine on the first day of their lives, but I believe that this is also unsafe.

Safety can be greatly increased by following a few practical guidelines. Safety can also be increased by administering the vaccinations on a somewhat slower schedule than the standard schedule.

The following safety guidelines are the general rules that apply to virtually all children. Many of these guidelines were first described by Stephanie Cave, M.D., in her excellent book, *What Your Doctor May Not Tell You About Children's Vaccinations*.

General Safety Guidelines

1. Administer vaccinations only to abundantly healthy children. Postpone the vaccinations if your child is ill, has a fever, was ill within the past week or two, or appears to possibly be coming down with an illness. Any condition that compromises immunity can lead to adverse reactions.

2. Be certain that your child is not receiving one of the older varieties of vaccinations that contain thimerosal. This is now quite unlikely to occur, but it has happened. The best way to check on the contents of the vaccine is to look at the package insert that comes with the vaccine.

Also, do not give your child a flu vaccination that contains thimerosal, as many do. The risks outweigh the benefits.

Furthermore, if you should happen to be traveling or living abroad at the time of a vaccination, be especially vigilant about not receiving a vaccine containing thimerosal, because many vaccines with thimerosal were sold abroad after their use was discontinued in America.

3. If your child is old enough to take supplements, and has no history of reactions to supplements, give him or her vitamins C and A, zinc, and transfer factor. Start the supplements one to two weeks before the vaccination. Also give them on the day of the vaccination and for one to two weeks after. At a minimum, give them the day before, and on the day of the vaccination, and the day after. Dosage should be appropriate to age, size, and other indications. Be especially sure not to give an excess of vitamin A. Vitamin A should preferably be given as cod liver oil.

4. Try to have all vaccinations administered one at a time, in single-dose vials. This will reduce the risk of overwhelming the immune system.

5. After the immunization is given, monitor your child carefully for adverse reactions, such as symptoms similar to those of a minor illness. If these symptoms occur, contact your doctor immediately, and be especially proactive about helping your child overcome the symptoms, with rest, extra fluids, a healthy diet, and moderate intake of appropriate supplements. The symptoms could be an indication that your child is responding unfavorably to the vaccination.

6. If your child appears to have an adverse reaction to a vaccination, be very cautious about administering further vaccinations. It may be wise to postpone the vaccinations until your child is older, and has a more fully developed immune system.

7. If your child is experiencing a notable allergic response at the time of the vaccination, such as a seasonal allergy, postpone the vaccination until allergic symptoms have cleared.

8. Do not agree to administration of the hepatitis-B shot on your child's day of birth, or shortly thereafter. This vaccination is appropriate on the day of birth only when the mother is hepatitis-B-positive.

9. Do not have your child vaccinated with vaccines that contain substances that you suspect your child may be allergic to, such as yeast in the hepatitis-B vaccination.

10. If possible, breast-feed your infant, to confer added immunity.

11. Make sure your child's diet is healthy and rich in nutrients before, during, and after all vaccinations.

Proposed Schedule of Vaccinations

Hepatitis-B
- First dose: shortly before starting day care. If your child does not attend day care, postpone the vaccination until the year before kindergarten.
- Second dose: one to two months after the first dose.
- Third dose: four to six months after the second dose.

HIB (*Haemophilus influenzae*); IPV (polio); DTaP (diphtheria, tetanus, pertussis):

- HIB: first dose at four months old.
- IPV: first dose at four months old.
- DTaP: first dose at five months.

- HIB: second dose at six months.
- IPV: second dose at six months.
- DTaP: second dose at seven months.

- HIB: third dose at eight months.
- DTaP: third dose at nine months.

- HIB: fourth dose at seventeen months.
- IPV: third dose at seventeen months.
- DTaP: fourth dose at eighteen months.

- DTaP: booster at four to five years old.
- IPV: booster at four to five years old.

Pneumococcal

- One dose, at two years old.

Varicella (chicken pox)

- One dose, at four to five years old, if mandated by state law, and if your child does not show evidence of immunity to chicken pox on a blood test.

MMR (measles, mumps, rubella)

- Vaccinations should be given separately, rather than in one combined injection.
- Measles: at fifteen months old.
- Rubella: six to twelve months after measles.
- Mumps: six to twelve months after rubella.
- Boosters, given separately: at age four to five. Check titers of measles, mumps, and rubella prior to receiving boosters, and if they show evidence of immunity, you do not need to receive a booster.

APPENDIX #2

RESOURCES FOR HELP

Autism Informational Agencies and Websites

Defeat Autism Now! DAN offers a doctor referral service, video presentations, audio files, and an extensive website. Highly recommended site. www.autismwebsite.com/ARI/index.htm

Autism Research Institute. This is the sponsoring group of Defeat Autism Now. The ARI conducts research and disseminates information. Highly recommended site. (619-281-7165) www.autismwebsite.com/ARI/index.htm

Healing-Autism. This is Dr. Bock's own website, with updates, newsletter information, and news of ongoing research and resources. Very helpful for 4-A parents. www.healing-autism.com

4-A Healing.com. This is Dr. Bock's other website. It covers all of the 4-A disorders, including autism. Highly recommended for all parents. www.4-Ahealing.com

American College for Advancement in Medicine. This is one of the finest organizations of integrative physicians, and it offers a doctor referral service. www.acam.org

Safe Minds. Founded by parents of autistic children. Focuses on heavy metal links to autism. Well-researched, good credibility. www.safeminds.org

Autism Society of America. Major, long-established autism organization. Strong advocacy for autistic children. www.autism-society.org

Rhinebeckhealth.com. This is the website of Dr. Bock's health centers, located in New York State, which have been at the forefront of integrative medicine, and particularly the biomedical treatment of the 4-A disorders, for many years. (845-876-7082) www.rhinebeckheath.com

First Signs, Inc. Focuses on early intervention. Strongly recommended. This site is well-informed, insightful, practical, and empathetic. www.firstsigns.org

Autism Speaks. Influential informational and assistance organization. Important organization, with excellent resources. (212-332-3580) www.autismspeaks.org

Cure Autism Now. Supports autism research. Progressive, scientifically sound perspective. www.canfoundation.org

Doug Flutie Jr. Foundation for Autism. Information, help, and other resources. Caring and responsible. www.dougflutiejrfoundation.org

The Deidre Imus Environmental Center for Pediatric Oncology. Offers not only important information on childhood cancers, but also on autism and environmental toxins. www.dienviro.com

Floortime Foundation. Offers information on one of the most popular and effective behavioral therapies. (443-738-0807) www.floortime.org

M.I.N.D. Institute. A medical collaborative center for research. Good scientific investigational resource. (916-703-0280) www.ucdmc.uc-davis.edu/mindinstitute

Unlocking Autism. International organization of parents. Great networking site. (566-366-3361) www.unlockingautism.org

Organization for Autism Research. Focuses solely on applied research. (703-351-5031) www.researchautism.org

Parents Action for Children. Targets parents' roles in therapy. www.parentsaction.org

ABA Resources. Provides information on behavioral therapies. www.rsaffran.tripod.com/aba.html

Center for Autism Related Disorders (CARD). It is one of the world's largest organizations that helps autistic children, primarily with ABA Therapy. www.centerforautism.com

Center for the Study of Autism. Associated with ARI. Excellent understanding of the biomedical approach. www.autism.org

ADHD Informational Agencies and Websites

Ritalindeath.com. Offers information about the risks of ADHD medication. Powerful message, delivered frankly. Very helpful to involved, responsible parents. www.ritalindeath.com

Fraud of Attention Deficit Hyperactivity Disorder. Essays and articles on possible misdiagnosis of ADHD. A neurologist presents emerging trends in ADHD treatment. Informative alternative perspective. www.adhdfraud.org

National Foundation for Gifted and Creative Children. Explores the common element of giftedness among the ADHD population. Encouraging and inspiring. www.nfgcc.org

4-A Healing.com. Dr. Bock's own website, focusing on each of the 4-A disorders, contains information on ADHD, and practical help for parents. www.4-Ahealing.com

Focus Adolescent Services. Provides information on alternatives to conventional ADHD treatment. www.focusas.com/attentionaldisorders.html

Children and Adults with ADHD. Offers information on ADHD therapies. (800-233-4050) www.chadd.org

Attention Deficit Disorder Help Center. Support for parents, and new ideas. www.add-adhd-help-center.com

Asthma and Allergy Informational Agencies and Websites

Allergy and Asthma Network/Mothers of Asthmatics, Inc. Provides information and support. Good site for current research.

4-A Healing.com. Dr. Bock's own site, focusing on each of the 4-A disorders, contains information on asthma and practical help for parents. www.4-Ahealing.com

Asthma and Allergy Foundation of America. Information about new treatments. www.aafa.org

Food Allergy and Anaphylaxis Network. Offers research information and support. www.foodallergy.org

The Allergy Report. Latest trends in treatment. www.acaai.org

Immune.com: Allergy Discussion Group. Self-care and new approaches. www.immune.com

Pecanbread.com. Information on the Specific Carbohydrate Diet. www.pecanbread.com

GF/CF Diet Page. Role of food reactions in autism, edited by early autism author Karyn Seroussi. In association with the Autism Network for Dietary Intervention. www.autismdiet.com

Books

The following are some of the best resources to learn more about the biomedical approach to autism, ADHD, asthma, and allergies.

All of these books will probably be readily available from Internet sources, including Amazon.com. If not, they may be available from various organizations, such as Defeat Autism Now.

Autism: Effective Biomedical Treatments, by Jon Pangborn, Ph.D., and Sidney MacDonald Baker, M.D. A highly detailed account of biomedical therapies for autism, focused upon supplementation therapy. An extraordinary compilation, highly recommended.

The Defeat Autism Now Conference Proceedings. These are written accounts of the presentations by doctors and others at DAN conferences. They are published twice per year. To receive them, contact DAN. These highly detailed accounts offer the best overview of current research and clinical findings. Strongly recommended.

Could It Be Autism?, by Nancy D. Wiseman. A mother's moving, inspiring, and helpful story of successful early intervention. Highly recommended.

Children with Starving Brains, by Jaquelyn McCandless, M.D. An early classic, documenting the need for biomedical intervention. A must-read for proactive parents.

The Vaccine Guide, by Randall Neustaedter, O.M.D. A practical guide to the risks and benefits of vaccination, extremely well researched.

What Your Doctor May Not Tell You About Children's Vaccinations, by Stephanie Cave, M.D., and Deborah Mitchell. Dr. Cave was one of the first physicians to document harm from vaccinations. Powerful and insightful information.

Unraveling the Mystery of Autism and Pervasive Developmental Disorder, by Karyn Seroussi. One of the first and best books on autism. Well-informed and very readable. Strongly recommended.

Evidence of Harm, by David Kirby. The most well-documented account of vaccination risks. Excellent science, objective presentation. An important book.

Thinking in Pictures, by Temple Grandin. A personal story by one of America's most successful autistic people. A superb account of how autism feels.

Building Wellness with DMG, by Roger Kendall, Ph.D., with Adena Therrien. A very detailed description of the important nutritional approach of DMG supplementation.

Enzymes for Autism and Other Neurological Conditions, by Karen DeFelice. A good account of enzyme use in supplementation therapy.

Special Diets for Special Kids, by Lisa Lewis, Ph.D. Has menu plans and practical advice for parents of autistic children.

A Shot in the Dark, by Harris L. Coulter and Barbara Loe Fisher. An indictment of careless vaccination procedures.

Diet Intervention and Autism, by Marilyn LeBreton. A well-researched, scholastic account.

Autism Spectrum Disorders, by Chantal Sicile-Kira. Important information, well presented by a caring mother of an autistic child.

Embracing the Sky, by Craig Romkema. Poems by a young autistic man, some of them brilliant, that reveal the inner world of the autistic experience.

A Parent's Guide to Asperger's Syndrome and High-Functioning Autism, by Sally Ozonoff, Ph.D., Geraldine Dawson, Ph.D., and James McPartland. Appropriate informational choice for parents of kids with Asperger's.

The Autism Sourcebook, by Karen Siff Exkorn. A helpful overview.

The Myth of the A.D.D. Child, by Thomas Armstrong, Ph.D. One of the first about the new perspectives on ADHD.

The ADHD-Autism Connection, by Diane M. Kennedy. A book that shows how the two disorders are linked.

The Great Misdiagnosis: ADHD, by Julian Stuart Haber, M.D. An unbiased, innovative point of view on ADHD.

The Road to Immunity, by Kenneth Bock, M.D., and Nellie Sabin. A highly detailed, impeccably researched, and practical guide to building and modulating immunity, which is one of the key elements in overcoming the 4-A disorders.

Say Good-bye to Allergy Related Autism, by Devi Nambudripad, Ph.D., D.C. One of the more promising new approaches to allergy treatment.

Natural Relief for Your Child's Asthma, by Steven Bock, M.D., Kenneth Bock, M.D., and Nancy Pauline Bruning. One of the first books on the integrative approach to asthma. Highly recommended to parents of asthmatic children. Detailed and specific.

The Asthma Sourcebook, by Francis V. Adams, M.D. A general account of asthma treatment and resources.

Alternative Answers to Asthma and Allergies, by Barbara Rowlands. This *Reader's Digest* publication has interesting new ideas.

All About Asthma, by Irwin Polk, M.D. Good overview of the subject.

Family Guide to Asthma and Allergies, by the American Lung Association Asthma Advisory Group, with Norman H. Edelman, M.D. A general summary of existing treatment.

Brain Longevity, by Dharma Singh Khalsa, M.D., and Cameron Stauth. The first book to document the success of the biomedical approach to cognitive impairment. Detailed but clear and readable.

APPENDIX #3

CLINICAL SIGNS OF AUTISM AND ADHD

- **Is Your Child on the Autism Spectrum?**
- **Does Your Child Have ADHD?**

This section contains the diagnostic criteria that establish the presence of the autism spectrum disorders, and also ADHD.

These criteria have primarily been extrapolated from the standard diagnostic reference guide that is employed by the medical profession to determine the presence of all psychological, psychiatric, and neuropsychiatric disorders, the *Diagnostic and Statistical Manual of Mental Disorders, Fourth Edition,* which is commonly referred to as DSM-IV.

These standard criteria are generally good indicators that problems do exist. If your child meets these criteria–based upon your own observations and opinions, or the opinion of your child's pediatrician or family practitioner, it would be wise to consult a developmental pediatrician, a pediatric neurologist, or a pediatric neuropsychologist, for possible confirmation of a suspected disorder.

However, even though I believe that the symptomatology described by these criteria can be meaningful in making a diagnosis, I do not place primary value in the various diagnostic labels. You have probably noticed that I used these diagnostic labels very sparingly in the book. In my opinion, the various diagnostic categories are adequate descriptors of behaviors, but they reflect very little about the root causes of these behaviors.

The most effective way to use these diagnostic measures, I believe, is to identify disordered behaviors from them, and to then address these disorders on not merely the behavioral level, but also the biomedical level.

Following are the five different disorders that comprise the autism spectrum.

All of the five disorders on the autism spectrum are Pervasive Developmental Disorders.

The Autism Spectrum
Pervasive Development Disorders

1. Autistic Disorder.
2. Asperger's Disorder.
3. Rett's Disorder.
4. Childhood Disintegrative Disorder.
5. Pervasive Developmental Disorder–Not Otherwise Specified.

Autistic Disorder

A. Diagnosis is established by a total of at least six characteristics from categories 1, 2, and 3, with at least two from 1, and one each from 2 and 3.

1. Impairment in social interaction, as indicated by two or more of the following:
   (a) Significant impairment in multiple nonverbal behaviors, including eye-to-eye gaze, facial expression, body language, and gestures that express social interaction.
   (b) Failure to develop peer relationships appropriate to age and developmental level.
   (c) Lack of spontaneous sharing of enjoyment, interests, or achievements.
   (d) Lack of social or emotional sharing and interaction.

2. Impairments in communication, as indicated by at least one of the following:
   (a) Delay in, or total lack of, the development of spoken language, with little attempt to compensate with gestures.
   (b) Impairment in the ability to initiate or sustain a conversation.
   (c) Frequent repetition of language, or perseveration; or idiosyncratic use of language.
   (d) Lack of varied, spontaneous imaginative play, or social imitative play, appropriate to age.

3. Repetitive and stereotypical patterns of behavior, interests, and activities, as indicated by at least one of the following:
   (a) Preoccupation with one or more interests that are abnormal in intensity or focus.
   (b) Inflexible engagement in specific, nonfunctional routines or rituals.

(c) Stereotypical and repetitive motor mannerisms, including hand or arm flapping, twisting, or whole-body movements.

(d) Persistent preoccupation with individual parts of objects.

B. Delays or abnormal functioning in at least one of the following areas, with onset prior to age three:

1. Social interaction;

2. Communicative language; or

3. Imaginative play.

C. Clinical determination that the disturbance is not a reflection of Rett's Disorder, or Childhood Disintegrative Disorder.

Asperger's Disorder

A. Impairment in social interaction, as indicated by at least two of the following:

1. Significant impairment in the use of multiple nonverbal behaviors, such as eye-to-eye gaze, facial expression, body language, and gestures that express social interaction.

2. Failure to develop peer relationships that are appropriate to age and developmental level.

3. Lack of spontaneous sharing of enjoyment, interests, or achievement.

4. Lack of social or emotional sharing and interaction.

B. Restricted, repetitive, and stereotypical patterns of behavior, interests, and activities, as indicated by at least one of the following:

1. Preoccupation with one or more interests that are abnormal in intensity or focus.

2. Inflexible engagement in specific, nonfunctional routines or rituals.

3. Stereotypical and repetitive motor mannerisms, including hand or arm flapping, twisting, or whole-body movements.

4. Persistent preoccupation with individual parts of objects.

C. The disturbance causes clinically significant impairment in social, recreational, or other important areas of functioning.

D. There is no clinically significant, general delay in language. Single words are used no later than age two, and communicative phrases are used by no later than age three.

E. There is no clinically significant delay in cognitive development, development of age-appropriate self-help skills, adaptive behaviors, or interests.

F. Diagnostic criteria do not apply for another specific Pervasive Developmental Disorder, or schizophrenia.

Rett's Disorder

A. All of the following are applicable:
    1. Apparently normal prenatal and perinatal development.
    2. Apparently normal psychomotor development, through the first five months after birth.
    3. Normal head circumference at birth.
B. Onset of all of the following, occurring after the period of normal development.
    1. Deceleration of head growth, between the ages of five months and four years.
    2. Loss of previously acquired hand skills, between the ages of five months and thirty months, with the subsequent development of stereotypical hand movements, such as hand-wringing, or obsessive hand washing.
    3. Loss of social engagement in early childhood, followed in some cases by appropriate development at a later age.
    4. Poorly coordinated gait, or awkward movements.
    5. Severely impaired expressive and receptive language development, with severe psychomotor impairment.

Childhood Disintegrative Disorder

A. Apparently normal development until at least age two, as indicated by age-appropriate verbal and nonverbal communication, social relationships, play, and adaptive behaviors.
B. Clinically significant loss of previously acquired skills, before the age of ten, in at least two of the following areas:
    1. Expressive or receptive language.
    2. Social skills, or adaptive behaviors.
    3. Bowel or bladder control.
    4. Play.
    5. Motor skills.

C. Abnormalities of functioning in at least two of the following areas:
   1. Impairment in social interaction, including failure to develop peer relationships and lack of social or emotional sharing and interaction.
   2. Impairments in communication, including a delay or lack of spoken language, inability to initiate or sustain a conversation, stereotypical and repetitive use of language, or lack of varied imaginative play.
   3. Restricted, repetitive, and stereotypical patterns of behavior, interests, and activities, including movements and mannerisms.
D. Clinical determination that the disturbance is not a reflection of another Pervasive Developmental Disorder, or schizophrenia.

Pervasive Developmental Disorder– Not Otherwise Specified

This category applies when there is a severe and pervasive impairment in the development of reciprocal social interaction, or communication skills. Stereotypical behaviors, interests, and activities are present, but the criteria are not met for another Pervasive Developmental Disorder, schizophrenia, Schizotypal Personality Disorder, or Avoidant Personality Disorder. Symptoms do not meet the criteria for Autistic Disorder because of late age of onset, atypical symptomatology, or mild symptomatology.

Information extrapolated and paraphrased from several sources including the *Diagnostic and Statistical Manual of Mental Disorders,* Fourth Edition, text revision. Copyright 2000 American Psychiatric Association.

Modified Checklist for Autism in Toddlers

Many parents and doctors also identify negative symptoms of neurobehavioral and cognitive development with a questionnaire called the Modified Checklist for Autism in Toddlers. This questionnaire was compiled by Diana Robins, Deborah Fein, and Marianne Barton, and was first published in the *Journal of Autism and Developmental Disorders*.

The following is a paraphrased extrapolation of that questionnaire, which is often referred to as the M-CHAT questionnaire.

Checklist for Toddlers

If the following behavior has occurred only once or twice, or occurs quite rarely, mark "No." If it has occurred regularly, or on a number of occasions, mark "Yes."

	YES	NO
1. Does your child enjoy physical play with you, such as bouncing on your knee?	✓	
2. Does your child show interest in other children?	✓	
3. Does your child like climbing, including climbing up stairs?	✓	
4. Does your child enjoy playing peekaboo and hide-and-seek?	✓	
5. Does your child engage in imaginative play?	✓	
6. Does your child point with his or her index finger to ask for something?	✓	
7. Does your child point with his or her index finger to indicate interest in something?	✓	
8. Does your child play imaginatively with small toys, rather than just handle them?	✓	
9. Does your child show you or bring you things?	✓	
10. Does your child make sustained eye contact?		✓
11. Is your child exceptionally sensitive to noise?		✓
12. Does your child smile in response to your smile?	✓	
13. Does your child imitate your expressions or gestures?	✓	
14. Does your child respond to his or her name?	✓	
15. If you point at something across the room, does your child look at it?	✓	
16. Can your child walk?	✓	
17. Does your child look at things you are looking at?	✓	
18. Does your child make unusual hand or finger movements, especially near his or her face?	✓	

19. Does your child try to attract your attention to his or her own activity?   ✓   ____

20. Have you ever wondered if your child has hearing loss, due to poor response to you?   ____   ✓

21. Does your child understand receptive language?   ✓   ____

22. Does your child sometimes stare at nothing, or wander with no purpose?   ____   ✓

23. Does your child look at your face to monitor your reactions?   ✓   ____

Scoring the Questionnaire

The answers that indicate abnormal development are:

1. No	9. No	17. No
2. No	10. No	18. Yes
3. No	11. Yes	19. No
4. No	12. No	20. Yes
5. No	13. No	21. No
6. No	14. No	22. Yes
7. No	15. No	23. No
8. No	16. No	

Results. Indication of a possible disorder is characterized by: two or more inappropriate answers to questions number 2, 7, 13, 14, and 15. Or: three or more inappropriate answers to any of the questions.

Diagnosing ADHD

The following diagnostic criteria have also been derived and paraphrased from the DSM-IV, and other sources.

Similar to the criteria for diagnosing the autism-spectrum disorders, these criteria are meaningful, but they mostly just describe behaviors, instead of indicating the probable causes of these behaviors.

If these criteria accurately describe your child, it would be wise to consult with a developmental pediatrician, a pediatric neurologist, or a pediatric neuropsychologist.

However, I strongly believe that if this doctor does diagnose your child with ADHD, you should not confine your therapeutic efforts to just medication. Many doctors apply only standard ADHD medications to this disorder, but in my opinion this is a limited therapeutic approach, and might never solve the underlying root causes of the negative behaviors.

The Diagnostic Criteria of ADHD

Following are the characteristics and behaviors that result in a diagnosis of ADHD, in four different categories: Inattentive Subtype; Hyperactive Subtype; Combined Subtype; and ADHD–Not Otherwise Specified.

A. A diagnosis of ADHD is confirmed if there has been a persistent pattern of inattention and/or hyperactivity-impulsivity that is displayed more frequently, or is more severe, than that which is typically observed in individuals at a comparable level of development. The individual must meet criteria for either Category 1 or Category 2.

Category 1. Six or more of the following symptoms of inattention have persisted for at least six months, and are maladaptive, and inconsistent with age and development level:

(a) Often fails to pay close attention to details. Makes careless mistakes in schoolwork, work at home, or other activities.

(b) Often has difficulty sustaining attention in tasks or in play.

(c) Often fails to listen when spoken to.

(d) Often fails to follow through on instructions, and fails to finish schoolwork, chores, or other duties.

(e) Often has difficulty organizing tasks and activities.

(f) Often avoids or dislikes tasks that require sustained mental effort.

(g) Often loses things.

(h) Is often easily distracted.

(i) Is often forgetful.

Category 2. Six or more of the following symptoms of hyperactivity-impulsivity have persisted for at least six months and are maladaptive, and inconsistent with age and developmental level:

Hyperactivity:

(a) Often fidgets or squirms in seat.

(b) Often leaves seat in classroom, or in other situations.

___ (c) Is often physically active or boisterous in situations in which it is inappropriate.

⌐ (d) Often has difficulty quietly engaging in leisure activities.

⌐ (e) Is often excessively active, or seems to be driven.

⌐ (f) Often talks excessively.

Impulsivity:

⌐ (g) Often blurts out answers before questions have been completed.

⌐ (h) Often has difficulty awaiting turn.

⌐ (i) Often interrupts or intrudes on others.

⌐ B. Some hyperactive-impulsive or inattentive symptoms, which caused impairments, were present before age seven.

⌐ C. Some impairment due to the symptoms is present in two or more settings, such as school or home.

⌐ D. There is clear evidence of clinically significant impairment in social, academic, or recreational functioning.

⌐ E. The symptoms are not associated with Pervasive Developmental Disorder, schizophrenia, or other mood or mental disorders.

These diagnostic criteria for ADHD can result in the following diagnoses:

ADHD, Inattentive Subtype. Diagnosis is confirmed if the criteria of Category 1 have applied for six months or longer, but not those of Category 2.

ADHD, Hyperactive-Impulsive Subtype. Diagnosis is confirmed if the criteria of Category 2 have applied for six months or longer, but not those of Category 1.

ADHD Combined Subtype. Diagnosis is confirmed if the criteria of both Category 1 and Category 2 have applied for six months or longer. This subtype is also referred to as Mixed Subtype.

ADHD–Not Otherwise Specified. Diagnosis is confirmed in this subtype if children do not meet the classic criteria of the other three types, but still have certain qualities and characteristics of ADHD.

Information extrapolated and paraphrased from the *Diagnostic and Statistical Manual of Mental Disorders,* Fourth Edition, text revision. Copyright 2000. American Psychiatric Association. Information was also derived from other related sources.

GLOSSARY

Acetylcholine: The neurotransmitter that is the primary carrier of thought and memory, which is often low among autistics, and sometimes people with ADHD.

ADHD: Attention deficit hyperactivity disorder, a variable neurobehavioral condition generally characterized by inattentiveness and/or hyperactivity and impulsivity.

Adjuvant: A chemical, such as aluminum, added to vaccines to promote antibody response.

Adrenaline: A hormone released during times of stress by the adrenal glands that can relax bronchial tubes. Also known as epinephrine.

Airway twitchiness: A sign of asthma indicating that the airways are prone to inflammation and hyperreactivity from exposure to an asthma trigger.

Allergen: A substance that causes an allergic reaction, such as dust, pollen, animal dander, chemicals, or foods.

Allergy: A condition in which the immune system responds in an inappropriate or exaggerated way to certain normally harmless substances.

Amino acids: The building blocks, or individual components, of proteins.

Amygdala: The brain's primary fear center, which is often overactive among autistics. It is part of the brain's limbic system, which governs memory and emotion.

Anaphylaxis: A severe, sometimes fatal allergic reaction, which affects the entire body.

Antibody: A protein produced by the white blood cells in response to an allergen, or other foreign body, such as a virus. Although many types of antibodies are protective, inappropriate or excessive formation of antibodies may lead to illness.

Antidepressant: A drug most commonly used to prevent or treat depression.

Antihistamine: A substance that reduces the effects of histamine, a chemical made by the body in response to foreign substances, including allergens.

Anti-inflammatory: A nutrient, herb, or drug that inhibits the inflammatory reaction.

Antioxidant: A molecule made by the body, or eaten as a food or supplement, which prevents oxidation of cells by free radicals.

Aphasia: Loss of ability to use or understand language.

Applied Behavior Analysis (ABA): A behavioral treatment based on the theories of operant conditioning originated by B. F. Skinner.

Asthma: A chronic lung condition resulting from bronchial tubes that are obstructed because of muscle constriction, excess mucus, or swelling and inflammation.

Atopic: A predisposition to allergy, such as atopic eczema or atopic asthma.

Autism: A pervasive developmental disorder that includes symptoms such as speech difficulties, lack of eye contact, cognitive impairment, social impairment, and repetitive stereotypic movements.

Autism-Spectrum Disorders: The following five disorders: Autistic Disorder, Asperger's Disorder, Childhood Disintegrative Disorder, Rett's Disorder, and Pervasive Developmental Disorder–Not Otherwise Specified.

Autistic savant: An autistic person who possesses extraordinary mental abilities, often in the fields of numerical calculation, art, or music.

Autoimmune response: An antibody attack by the body against its own tissues or cells.

Basal ganglia: A region located at the base of the brain that is responsible for involuntary movements and cognitive processes. This area is sometimes dysfunctional among people with ADHD.

Bipolar disorder: A depressive disease that involves cycles of depression and elation, or mania.

Bowel dysbiosis: The existence of abnormal intestinal flora that have harmful effects, due to putrefaction, fermentation, deficiency, or sensitization. It can cause widespread effects, including neurological problems.

Bronchioles: The small air passages that branch off from the bronchi.

Bronchitis: Inflammation of the mucus membranes of the lungs.

Bronchoconstriction: Airflow limitation due to contraction of airway smooth muscle.

Bronchodilator: A substance used to open up the air passages in order to prevent and treat asthma symptoms.

Candida albicans: A form of yeast normally found in the body. In excess, it can cause yeast overgrowth, sometimes affecting the neurological system, and other systems.

Candidiasis: An infection or overgrowth caused by candida.

Casein: The most common of several proteins found in milk, accounting for 80 percent of all milk protein.

Chelation therapy: A medical treatment that can help remove heavy metals from the body.

Cognitive: The process of remembering, reasoning, understanding, and using judgment.

Co-morbid disorders: Conditions that often occur in conjunction with autism-spectrum disorders, including mood disorder, and physical disorders, such as bowel dysbiosis.

Controller medications: Medications taken daily, on a long-term basis, that are useful in controlling persistent asthma.

Corticosteroids: Drugs that reduce inflammation, because they are similar to hormones produced by the adrenal gland.

Creatine: An amino acid particularly important in muscle tissue health, growth, and energy production.

Cytokines: Messenger molecules produced by cells of the immune system.

D-4 dopamine receptor: A key neuronal receptor in allowing the arousing neuro-transmitter dopamine to enter brain cells. This receptor is often dysfunctional among people with ADHD.

Dander: Microscopic scales from the skin, feathers, or fur of animals.

Decongestants: A class of drugs used to reduce mucus and congestion.

Depression: A mood disorder that negatively affects the way a person functions, feels, and thinks.

Differential diagnosis: The process of weighing the probability of the existence of one disease versus that of other diseases.

DMG (dimethylglycine): Glycine, with two attached methyls, that can aid in the detoxification process of methylation.

Dopamine: A neurotransmitter associated with a positive mood, energy, and physical grace, which is often disordered among people with autism and ADHD.

Encephalitis: An inflammatory response in the brain.

Endocrine system: The system of glands and organs that secrete hormones, which affect mood, health, and energy. People with autism and ADHD sometimes have endocrine disorders.

Environmental controls: Actions that reduce exposure to asthma triggers, such as mold and dander, in the home, school, and work environments.

Enzyme: A substance that increases the speed of a chemical reaction, such as the digestion of food.

Executive function: The cognitive ability to control impulses and to act rationally.

Flavonoids: Plant chemicals that are helpful in many essential body functions, including protection from free radicals.

Free radical: An unstable molecule that harms the cells, including those of the immune system and nervous system.

Frontal lobe: The area of the brain, behind the forehead, that is a primary center of higher thought and cognition.

Fungi: Mold plants that lack stems, and provoke asthma and allergy attacks.

GABA: Gamma aminobutyric acid, a calming neurotransmitter that is often low among people with autism and ADHD.

Gastrointestinal: Referring to or affecting the stomach and intestines.

Glutathione: A protein tripeptide, made from glutamic acid, cysteine, and glycine. It is critical for binding and detoxifying heavy metals, and is the main cellular antioxidant.

Gluten: Proteins found in wheat, oats, barley, rye, and triticale. They often cause food reactions, which can result in neurological symptoms.

Heavy metals: Mercury, lead, cadmium, arsenic, tin, and aluminum. They cannot be metabolized by the body and, if accumulated, can cause toxic effects, and can impair natural detoxification.

Helper T-cells: White blood cells that patrol the bloodstream, recognize antigens, and alert other components of the immune system, to amplify their response.

Histamine: A compound released as part of the immune response to a foreign body, causing inflammation, increased blood flow, and mucus production.

Hyperactivity: A higher than normal level of activity, often accompanied by impulsivity.

Hypoglycemia: Low blood sugar, which often results in cognitive and mood dysfunction.

IgE: Immunoglobulin E, an antibody involved in allergy.

IgG: Immunoglobulin G, an antibody involved in food sensitivities, and the immune response to pathogens.

Immune system: A complex system of cells and proteins that protects the body from infection. It plays a role in the control of cancer and other diseases, but also is involved in allergies, hypersensitivity, and asthma.

Impulsivity: An inclination to act on impulse rather than thought.

Intolerance: A food reaction that is not caused by the immune system.

Leaky Gut Syndrome: Excessive intestinal permeability that can allow unwanted substances to enter the system.

Leukocytes: White blood cells.

Limbic system: A network of brain structures that governs memory and emotion. Its function is sometimes impaired among people with autism and ADHD.

Low-Oxalate Diet: A diet that restricts the common food component oxalate, which sometimes improves health and cognitive function.

Lymphocytes: Certain types of white blood cells that include T-cells and B-cells that arise from the lymph glands.

Mast cells: Cells that release histamine and other inflammatory mediators.

Meningitis: Inflammation of the membranes of the brain or spinal cord.

Mercury: A toxic heavy metal that can cause mental, emotional, and physical distress.

Methionine: An essential amino acid that supplies sulfur and other compounds required by the body for normal metabolism, growth, and detoxification.

Methylation: The transfer of a methyl group to another molecule. It can enable the body to detoxify itself, particularly from heavy metals.

Methylcobalamin: A particular form of vitamin B-12 that is uniquely helpful in detoxification and neurological disorders.

Methylphenidate: The most common class of ADHD drugs, including Ritalin.

Mirror neuron: A particular type of brain cell, closely associated with empathy, which is often disordered in autistic people.

Mites: Microscopic insects that exist in house dust, human and animal skin, and feathers.

MMR: Measles, mumps, and rubella vaccine.

Mold: A type of fungus that produces microscopic spores, often triggering allergy.

Myelin: The sheath surrounding a nerve, made of fats and protein.

Nebulizer: A device that turns liquid medicine into a mist.

Neocortex: The most advanced areas of the brain, including the frontal lobes, which are responsible for most thought and memory. It is sometimes impaired among people with autism and ADHD.

Neuron: A nerve cell in the brain or peripheral nervous system.

Neurotransmitter: Substances in the brain that carry messages from one brain cell to the next. They are sometimes dysfunctional among people with autism and

ADHD. They include serotonin, acetylcholine, dopamine, GABA, and norepinephrine.

Norepinephrine: A stimulating hormone, and a neurotransmitter, associated with a positive mood and the creation of long-term memory, also known as noradrenaline.

Opioids: Substances that are derived from the opium poppy plant, contain opium, or have opium-like effects.

PANDAS: Pediatric Autoimmune Neuropsychiatric Disorder Associated with Streptococcal Infection, an inflammatory brain condition that can create neuropsychiatric symptoms, including tics, OCD, anxiety, intermittent rage, and symptoms similar to those of ADHD.

Pollen: Microscopic spores from plants, which cause an allergic reaction in some people when inhaled.

Pseudo-morphines: Substances created by some people during the metabolism of common food substances, most notably gluten and casein, that can mimic the effects of morphine or endorphins.

RAST: A blood test used to determine levels of antibodies, indicating the existence of allergies.

Reliever medications: Short-acting bronchodilating medications that act quickly to relieve airflow limitation.

Reticular activating system: A network of brain connections that governs attention, and is often dysfunctional among people with ADHD.

Rhinitis: Inflammation of the lining of the nose.

Rhinovirus: The type of virus that causes most colds.

Secretin: A neurohormone that controls digestion, and can affect mood and cognition.

Serotonin: A neurotransmitter associated with contentment, often dysfunctional among people with autism and ADHD.

Specific Carbohydrate Diet: A diet very low in most forms of carbohydrate, specifically disaccharides, which sometimes improves health, including gastrointestinal health and cognitive function.

Sulfation: A common, natural form of detoxification.

Thalamus: An information-sorting center in the brain, often dysfunctional among people with autism and ADHD.

Thimerosal: A mercury-containing preservative used in some vaccines.

TMG (trimethylglycine): Glycine, with three attached methyls, that can aid in the detoxifying metabolic process of methylation.

Wheal: A small, round, red, raised area that develops after a positive allergy skin test.

Wheezing: A hissing or whistling sound caused by bronchiole obstruction.

Sources: DAN Syllabus 2006, *Natural Relief for Your Child's Asthma*, *The Bantam Medical Dictionary*.

BIBLIOGRAPHY AND RESEARCH

Autism Sources

Adolphs, R., "Is the Human Amygdala Specialized for Processing Social Information?" *Ann N.Y. Acad Sci,* 2003; 985, 326.

Adolphs, R., et al., "Amygdala Damage Impairs Recognition of Social Emotions from Facial Expressions," *J Cogn Neurosci,* 14: 1, 2002.

Allen, Arthur, "The Not-So-Crackpot Autism Theory." *New York Times Magazine,* Nov. 10, 2002.

Amaral, D. G., "The Primate Amygdala and the Neurobiology of Social Behavior: Implications for Understanding Social Anxiety," *Biol Psychiatry,* 2002; 51: 11.

Ames, B. N., et al., "High-Dose Vitamin Therapy Stimulates Variant Enzymes with Decreased Coenzyme Binding Affinity: Relevance to Genetic Disease and Polymorphisms," *Am J Clin Nutr,* 75: 616–58, 2002.

Aschner, M., et al., "The Neuropathogenesis of Mercury Toxicity," *Molecular Psychiatry,* Supp. 2. 2002; 7: S40–41.

Asperger, H., "Problems of Infantile Autism," *Communication,* 1979; 13: 45–52.

Ballas, N., et al., "The Many Faces of REST Oversee Epigenetic Programming of Neuronal Gene," *Curr Opin Neurobiology,* Oct. 15, 2005.

Baron-Cohen, S., et al., "The Amygdala Theory of Autism," *Neurosci Biobehav,* 2000; rev. 24: 355.

Baron-Cohen, S., et al., "Autism Occurs More Often in Families of Physicists, Engineers, and Mathematicians," *Autism,* 1995; 2: 296–301.

Bauman, M. I., et al., "Structural Brain Anatomy in Autism: What Is the Evidence?" in: Bauman, M.I., et al. *The Neurobiology of Autism.* Johns Hopkins Press, Baltimore, MD. 2004: 119–45.

Bernard, S., et al., "Autism: A Novel Form of Mercury Poisoning," *Medical Hypotheses,* 2001; 56: 462–71.

Bernard, S., et al., "The Role of Mercury in the Pathogenesis of Autism," *Molecular Psychiatry,* 2002; 7: S42–43.

Bernard, Sallie, "Letter to the editor," *Journal of the American Medical Association,* 2004; 291(13): 180.

Bernard, Sallie, "Re: Safe Mind's Response to Frist Bill," Statement from Safe Minds. July 2002.

Bettelheim, B. *The Empty Fortress: Infantile Autism and the Birth of Self.* New York: Free Press, 1967.

Boddart, N., et al., "Temporal Lobe Dysfunction in Childhood Autism: A PET Auditory Activation Study," abstract *Pediatr Radiol,* 2001; 31–53.

Bradstreet, J., et al., "A Case-Control Study of Mercury Burden in Children with Autistic Spectrum Disorders," *Journal of American Physicians and Surgeons.* 2003; 8(3): 76–79.

Bradstreet, Jeffrey, et al., "Detection of Measles Virus RNA in Cerebrospiral Fluid of Children with Regressive Autism: Results of Three Cases," *JAPS,* 2004; 9(2): 38–45.

Bradstreet, J. J. et al., "Spironolactone might be a desirable immunologic and hormonal intervention in autism spectrum disorders," *Medical Hypotheses,* Nov. 2006, in press.

Brasic, J. R., et al., "Clomipramine Ameliorates Adventitious Movements and Compulsions in Prepubertal Boys with Autistic Disorder and Severe Mental Retardation," *Neurology,* 1994; 44: 1309–12.

Burton, Dan, Representative, Letter to Walter Orenstein, Assistant Surgeon General, Director of National Immunization Program, July 28, 2001.

Carpenter, D. O., et al, "Understanding the Human Health Effects of Chemical Mixtures," *Environ Health Perspect,* Feb. 2002.

Chauhan, A., et al., "Oxidative Stress in Autism: Increased Lipid Peroxidation and Reduced Serum: Levels of Ceruloplasmin and Transferrin–the Antioxidant Proteins," *Life Sci,* Oct. 2004; 8: 75(21): 2539–2549.

Chicago Tribune, "The Mercury Menace," Dec. 12, 2005.

Chopra, D. *Perfect Health–The Complete Mind/Body Guide.* New York: Harmony Books. 1991.

Corrigan, Sue, "Former Science Chief: MMR Fears Coming True," *London Daily Mail,* Feb. 5, 2006.

Dales, L., et al., "Time Trends in Autism and in MMR Immunizations Coverage in California," *Journal of the American Medical Association,* 2001; 285(9): 1183–85.

Deplancke, B., et al., "Redox Control of the Transsulfuration and Glutathione Biosynthesis Pathways," *Curr Opin Clin Nutr Metab Care,* 2002; 5: 85–92.

Dolske, M.C., et al., "A Preliminary Trial of Ascorbic Acid as Supplemental Therapy for Autism," *Prog Neuropsychopharmacol Biol Psychiatry,* Sep. 1993; 17(5): 765–74.

Dourson, M. L., et al., "Uncertainties in the Reference Dose for Methylmercury," *Neurotoxicology,* 2001; 22(5): 677–89.

Duk-Hee, Lee, "Graded Associations of Blood Lead and Urinary Cadmium Concentrations with Oxidative Stress Related Markers in the U.S. Population," *Environmental Health Perspectives,* Mar. 2006.

Dunn-Geier, J., et al., "Effect of Secretin on Children with Autism: A Randomized Controlled Trial," *Dev Med Child Neurol,* 2000; 42: 796–802.

Eigsti, I. M., et al., "A Systems Neuroscience Approach to Autism: Biological, Cognitive, and Clinical Perspectives," *Ment Retard Dev Disabil Res Rev,* 2003; 9: 205–15.

El-Dahr, Jane M., "Thimerosal-Containing Vaccines and Neurodevelopmental Outcomes," National Academy of Sciences, Institute of Medicine, Immunization Safety Review Committee, July 16, 2001.

Ellaway, C., et al., "Rett Syndrome: Randomized Controlled Trial of L-Carnitine," *J Child Neurol.,* 1999; 14: 162–67.

Filipek, D., "Relative Carnitine Deficiency in Autism," *Journal of Autism and Developmental Disorders,* Dec. 2006.

Finkelstein, J. D., "Methionine Metabolism in Mammals," *J Nutr Biochem,* 1990; 1: 228–37.

Finkelstein, J. D., "The Metabolism of Homocysteine: Pathways and Regulation," *Eur J Pediatr,* 1998; 157: S40–4.

Fischer, Douglas, "Chemical Mixtures More Toxic than Their Parts," *Oakland Tribune,* Jan. 2006.

Garber, H. J., et al., "Clomipramine Treatment of Stereotypic Behaviors and Self-Injury in Patients with Developmental Disabilities," *Journal of the American Academy of Child and Adolescent Psychiatry,* 1992; 31: 1157–60.

Geier, D. A., et al., "A Review of the Vaccine Adverse Event Reporting System Database," *Expert Opin Pharmacother,* 5: 691–98, 2004.

Geier, D.A., et al., "A Comparative Evaluation of the Affects of MMR Immunization and Mercury Doses from Thimerosal-Containing Childhood Vaccines on the Population Prevalence of Autism," *Med Sci Monit,* 2004; 10: P133–39.

Geier, D.A., et al., "An Assessment of the Impact of Thimerosal on Childhood Neurodevelopmental Disorders," *Pediatr Rehabil,* Apr–Jun 2003; 6(2): 97–102.

Geier, M. R., et al., "Thimerosal in Childhood Vaccines, Neurodevelopment Disorders, and Heart Disease in the United States," *J Amer Phys Surg,* 2003; 8(1): 6–11.

Geier, M.R., et al., "Neurodevelopment Disorders after Thimerosal-Containing Vaccines: A Brief Communication," *Exp Biol Med,* 228: 660–64, 2003.

Georgetown University Medical Center, "Commonly Used Antidepressants May Also Affect Human Immune System," *Science Daily,* Jan. 2006.

Goldberg, Carey, "The Human Brain's Source of Empathy May Also Play a Role in Autism," *Boston Globe,* Dec. 12, 2005.

Gordon, C. T., et al., "A Double-Blind Comparison of Clomipramine, Desipramine, and Placebo in the Treatment of Autistic Disorder," *Archives of General Psychiatry,* 1993; 50: 441–47.

Gordon, N., "The Therapeutics of Melatonin: A Pediatric Perspective," *Brain & Development,* June 2000; 22(4): 213–17.

Goth, S., et al., "Uncoupling of ATP-Mediated Calcium Signaling and Dysregulated IL-6 Secretion in Dendritic Cells by Nanomolar Thimerosal," *Environmental Health Perspectives,* Mar. 2006.

Grandjean, P., et al., "Milestone Development in Infants Exposed to Methylmercury from Human Milk," *Neurotoxicology,* 1995; 16: 27–33.

Gyory, I., et al., "Epigenetic Regulation of Lymphoid Specific Gene Set," *Biochem Cell Biol,* June 2005.

Haley, B. E., Letter to Committee on Immunization Safety Review, Institute of Medicine, May 14, 2001.

Hansen, P. R. et al., "Spiromelactone inhibits production of proinflammatory cytokines by human mononuclear cells," *Immunology Letters,* 2004; 91: 87–91.

Hashimoto, T., et al., "Development of the Brainstem and Cerebellum in Autistic Patients," *J Autism Dev Disord,* 1995; 25: 1–18.

Heeley, A. F., et al., "A Study of Tryptophan Metabolism in Psychotic Children," *Dev Med Child Neurol.,* 1966; 8: 708–718.

Hill, A., et al., "Stability and Interpersonal Agreement of the Interview-Based Diagnosis of Autism," *Psychopathology,* 2001; 34(4): 187–91.

Holmes, A. S., et al., "Reduced Levels of Mercury in First Baby Haircuts of Autistic Children," *Intl J Toxicology,* 22(4): 277–85, 2003.

Holmes, A., et al., "Open Trial of Chelation of Children with Autism," Presentation at the International Meeting for Autism Research, 2002.

Horvath, I., et al., "Autistic Disorder and Gastrointestinal Disease," *Curr Opin Pediatr,* 2002; 14: 583–87.

Horvath, K, et al., "Gastrointestinal Abnormalities in Children with Autistic Disorder," *J Pediat.* 1999; 135:559–563.

Horvath, K., et al., "Improved Social and Language Skills after Secretin Administration in Patients with Autistic Spectrum Disorders," *J Assoc Acad Minor Phys,* 1998; 9: 9–15.

James, S. J., et al., "Metabolic Biomarkers of Increased Oxidative Stress and Impaired Methylation Capacity in Children with Autism," *Am J Clin Nutr,* 2004; 80: 1611–17.

James, S. J., et al., "Thimerosal Neurotoxicity Is Associated with Glutathione Depletion. Protection with Glutathione Precursors," *Neurotoxicology,* January, 2005.

Kanner, L., "Autistic Disturbances of Affective Contact," *Nervous Child,* 1943; 2: 217–50.

Keller, F., et al., "The Neurobiological Context of Autism," *Mol. Neurobiol,* 2003; 28: 1–22.

Kennedy, Robert Jr., "Deadly Immunity," *Rolling Stone,* June 20, 2005.

Kidd, P. M., "Autism, an Extreme Challenge to Integrative Medicine, Part 1, The Knowledge Base," *Altern Med Rev,* 2002; 7: 292–316.

Landrigan, P. J., et al., "Chronic Effects of Toxic Environmental Exposures on Children's Health," *Journal of Toxicology–Clinical Toxicology,* 2002; 40(4): 449–56.

Landrigan, P., et al., "Neurologic Disorders Following Measles Virus Vaccinations," *JAMA,* 1973: 233: 1459.

Lathe, Richard. *Autism, Brain, and Environment.* Jessica Kingsley Publishers, London, 2006.

Lelord, G., et al., "Effects of Pyridoxine and Magnesium on Autistic Symptoms–Initial Observations," *J Autism Deve Disord,* 1981; 11: 219–30.

Madsen, K. M., et al., "Thimerosal and the Occurrence of Autism: Negative Ecological Evidence from Danish Population-Based Data," *Pediatrics,* 2003; 112: 604–06.

McDougle, C. J., et al., "Clomipramine in Autism: Preliminary Evidence of Efficacy," *Journal of the American Academy of Child and Adolescent Psychiatry,* 1992; 31: 746–50.

Megson, M. N., "Is Autism a G-Alpha Protein Defect Reversible with Natural Vitamin A?" *Med Hypotheses,* 2000; 54: 979–83.

Olivieri, G., et al., "The Effects of Beta-Estradiol on SHSY5Y Neuroblastoma Cells During Heavy Metal Induced Oxidative Stress, Neurotoxicity, and Beta-Amyloid Secretion," *Neuroscience,* 113: 849–55, 2002.

Olmsted, Dan, "The Age of Autism," United Press International, Dec. 7, 2005.

Ostrea, E. M., et al., "Prevalence of Fetal Exposure to Environmental Toxins as Determined by Meconium Analysis," *Neurotoxicology,* 2002; 23: 329–39.

Palomo, T., et al., "Brain Sites of Movement Disorder: Genetic and Environmental Agents in Neurodevelopmental Perturbations," *Neurotoxological Research,* 2003; 5(1–2): 1–26.

Pangborn, J. B., and Baker, S. M. *Biomedical Assessment Options for Children with Autism and Related Problems.* San Diego, CA: Autism Research Institute, 2005.

Patterson, J. E., et al., "Mercury in Human Breath from Dental Amalgams," *J Den Res,* 1981; 60: 1668–71.

Pelton, Tom, "Teflon Chemical Found in Infants," *Baltimore Sun.* Feb. 6, 2006.

Pfeiffer, S. I., et al., "Efficacy of Vitamin B6 and Magnesium in the Treatment of Autism: A Methodology Review and Summary of Outcomes," *J Autism Dev Disord,* 1995; 25: 481–93.

Piaget, J. *The Construction of Reality in the Child.* New York: W. W. Norton, 1962.

Purdon, S. E., et al., "Risperidone in the Treatment of Pervasive Developmental Disorder," *Canadian Journal of Psychiatry,* 1994; 39: 400–405.

Rapin, I., et al., "Neurobiology of Autism," *Ann Neurol,* 1998; 43: 7–14.

Realmuto, E. M., et al., "Clinical Effect of Buspirone in Autistic Children," *Journal of Clinical Psychopharmacolog,* 1989; 9: 122–25.

Redwood, Lyn, Safe Minds, Letter to Committee on Immunization Safety Review, Institute of Medicine, June 8, 2001.

Reichelt, K. I, et al., "Gluten, Milk Proteins and Autism: Dietary Intervention Effects on Behavior and Peptide Secretion," *J Appl Nutr,* 1990; 42: 1–11.

Rimland, B., "Controversies in Treatment of Autistic Children: Vitamin and Drug Therapy," *J Child Neurol,* 1988; 3: S68–72.

Rimland, B., "Dimethylglycine (DMG), a Nontoxic Metabolite, and Autism," *Autism Research Review International,* 1990; 4: 2.

Rimland, B. *Infantile Autism: the Syndrome and Its Implications for a Neural Theory of Behavior.* New York: Appleton Century Crofts, 1964.

Rimland, B., "The Autism Epidemic, Vaccinations, and Mercury," *J Nutr Environ Med* 2000; 10: 261–66.

Rimland, B., et al., "The Effects of High Doses of Vitamin B6 on Autistic Children. A Double-Blind Crossover Study," *American Journal of Psychiatry,* 1978; 135: 472–75.

Rossignol, D. A., "Hyperbaric Oxygen Therapy Might Improve Certain Pathophysiological Findings in Autism," *Medical Hypotheses,* Dec. 2006, in press.

Rothlein, J., et al., "Organophosphate Pesticide Exposure and Neurobehavioral Performance in Agricultural and Non-Agricultural Hispanic Workers," *Environ Health Perspect,* Jan. 2006.

Rubin, M., "Use of Atypical Antipsychotics in Children with Mental Retardation, Autism, and Other Developmental Disabilities, *Psychiatric Annals,* 1997; 27: 219–21.

Safe Minds, Denmark Study on Autism and MMR Vaccine Shows Need for Biological Research, Letter to *New England Journal of Medicine* and press release, Nov. 6,
2002.

Sanchez, L. E., et al., "A Pilot Study of Clomipramine in Young Autistic Children."
Journal of the American Academy of Child and Adolescent Psychiatry, 35, 1996;
537–44.

Sargent, J. D., et al. "The Association between State Housing Policy and Lead Poisoning in Children," *American Journal of Public Health,* 1999; 89(11): 1690–1695.

Schulz, J. B., et al., "Glutathione, Oxidative Stress and Neurodegeneration," *Eur J
Biochem,* 2000; 267: 4904–911.

Science News, "Empathy Related Neurons May Turn Off in Autism," Dec. 10, 2005.

Seroussi, K. *Unraveling the Mystery of Autism and Pervasive Developmental Disorder: A
Mother's Story of Research and Recovery.* New York: Simon and Schuster, 2000.

Shattock, P., et al., "Role of Neuropeptides in Autism and their Relationships with
Classical Neurotransmitters," *Brain Dysfunct,* 1990; 3: 328–45.

Simeon, J. G., et al., "Risperidone Effects in Treatment-Resistant Adolescents: Preliminary Case Reports," *Journal of Child and Adolescent Psychopharmacolog,* 1995; 5:
69–79.

Srikameswaran, Anita, "CDC Says 2 Deaths Caused by Chelation Drug Errors," *Pitts-
burgh Post-Gazette,* Mar. 3, 2006.

Stehr-Green, P., et al., "Autism and Thimerosal-Containing Vaccines: Lack of Consistent Evidence for an Association," *Am J Prev Med,* 2003; 25: 101–106.

Stokes, L., et al., "Neurotoxicity Among Pesticide Applicators Exposed to Organo-
phosphates," *Occup Environ Med,* 52: 648–53, 1995.

Thornton, I. M., "Out of Time: A Possible Link between Mirror Neurons, Autism, and
Electromagnetic Radiation," *Med Hypotheses,* Mar. 9, 2006.

Vela, Susan, "Arsenic: How Much Is Too Much?" *Lansing State Journal,* Jan. 8, 2006.

Vojdani, A., et al., "Infections, Toxic Chemicals and Dietary Peptides Binding to Lymphocyte Receptors and Tissue Enzymes Are Major Instigators of Autoimmunity
in Autism," *Intl J Immunopath and Phar,* 2003; 16: 189–199.

Wakefield, A. J., Letter to the Editor, *Lancet,* 1998; 355–379.

Wakefield, A. J., et al., "Illeal-Lymphoid Nodular Hyperplasia, Non-specific Colitis,
and Pervasive Developmental Disorder in Children," *Lancet,* Feb. 28, 1998; 351:
9103.

Wakefield, A. J., et al., "Enterocolitis in Children with Developmental Disorders," *Am
J Gastroenterol,* 2000 Sep.; 95(9): 2154-6.

Walter, P. B., et al., "Iron Deficiency and Iron Excess Damage Mitochondria and Mitochondrial DNA in Rats," *Proc Natl Acad Sci USA,* Feb. 2002.

Weaver, I., "Reversal of Maternal Programming of Stress Responses in Adult Offspring
through Methyl Supplementation," *The Journal of Neuroscience,* Nov. 23, 2006.

Weisman, Jonathan, "In Massive Bill, Someone Buried a Clause to Benefit Drug Maker
Eli Lilly," *Washington Post,* Nov. 28, 2002.

Weldon, Dave, Representative, "Something Is Rotten, But Not Just in Denmark. Re-
marks at Autism One Conference, Chicago, May 29, 2004.

Whiteley, P., et al., "A Gluten Free Diet as Intervention for Autism and Associated Disorders Preliminary Findings," *Autism: Intl J Res Pract,* 1999; 3: 45–65.

Zilbovicius, M., et al., "Temporal Lobe Dysfunction in Childhood Autism: A PET Study. Positron Emission Tomography," *Am J Psychiatry,* 2000; 157: 1988–93.

Zuddas, A., et al., "Clinical Effects of Clozapine on Autistic Disorder," letter, *American Journal of Psychiatry,* 153: 1996; 738.

ADHD Sources

American Academy of Pediatrics. *Clinical Practice Guidelines: Diagnosis and Evaluation of the Child with ADHD.* Oct. 27, 2000.

American Academy of Pediatrics. *Clinical Practice Guidelines: Diagnosis and Evaluation of the Child with Attention Deficit/Hyperactivity Disorder.* 2000; 105(5): 8.

Armstrong, T. *The Myth of the ADD Child: Fifty Ways to Improve Your Child's Behavior and Attention Span Without Drugs, Labels, or Coercion.* New York: Dutton, 1995.

August, G., et al., "Comorbidity of ADHD and Reading Disability Among Clinic-Referred Children," *Journal of Abnormal Child Psychology,* 8(1): 29–45, 1990.

Axelrod, J. C., et al., "Interactions between Pesticides and Components of Pesticide Formulations in an In-Vitro Neurotoxicity Test," *Toxicology,* May 2002.

Barkley, R. *ADHD and the Nature of Self-Control.* New York: Guilford Press, 1997.

Barkley, R., "*Shift in Perspective Offers Insights into Biological Nature of ADHD,*" *AAP News,* Apr. 1999; 38.

Barkley, R. *Taking Charge of ADHD.* New York: Guilford Press, 2000.

Bateman, B., et al., "The Effects of a Double-Blind, Placebo Controlled, Artificial Food Colorings and Benzoate Preservative Challenge on Hyperactivity in a General Population of Preschool Children," *Arch Dis Child,* Jun. 2004.

Biederman, J., et al., "Gender Differences in a Sample of Adults with Attention Deficit Hyperactivity Disorder," *Psychiatry Research,* 1994; 53: 13–29.

Biederman, J., et al., "Influence of Gender on Attention Deficit Hyperactivity Disorder in Children Referred to a Psychiatry Clinic," *American Journal of Psychiatry,* 2002; 159: 36–42.

Biederman, J., et al., "Pharmacotherapy of Attention Deficit Hyperactivity Disorder Reduces Risk for Substance Use Disorder," *Pediatrics,* 104(2): 20, 2002.

Blakemore-Brown, L., "Weaving the Tapestry of ADD and Asperger Syndrome," in *A World of Understanding ADHD Issues & Answers.* New York: CHADD, 1998; 394.

Bornstein, R., et al., "Plasma Amino Acids in Attention Deficit Disorder," *Psychiatry Research,* 1990; 33(3): 301–306.

Bridges, A., "FDA to Examine New Ways to Study ADD Drugs," *Associated Press,* Jan. 4, 2006.

Brucker-Davis, F., "Effects of Environmental Synthetic Chemicals on Thyroid Function," *Thyroid,* 1998; 8: 827–56.

Burn, Cull, et al., "Reward Deficiency Syndrome," *American Scientist,* Mar.–Apr. 1996; 143.

Cantwell, D., et al., "Association between Attention Deficit Hyperactivity Disorder and Learning Disorders," *Journal of Learning Disabilities,* 24(2): 88–95, 1991.

Carter, C., et al., "Effects of a Few-Food Diet in ADHD," *Archives of Disease in Childhood,* 69:564.568, 1993.

Davidson, P. W., et al., "Evaluation of Techniques for Assessing Neurobehavioral Development in Children," *Neurotoxicology,* 2000; 21: 957–72.

Dunn, J. T., et al., "Neurotoxic Complaint Base Rates of Personal Injury Complaints," *Journal of Clinical Psychology,* 41: 577–84, 1995.

Evancoe, J., et al. *What Causes Autism, Attention-Deficit Hyperactivity Disorder, & Bipolar Disorder?* Harrisonburg, VA: James Madison University, 1999.

Explosive Children. Found at http//.www.Oprah.com, Feb. 2000.

Fitzgerald, S., "Hidden Danger is Coming into Focus–Celiac Disease Was Once Thought Rare," *Philadelphia Inquirer,* Jan. 4, 2006.

Goodman, R., et al., "A Twin Study of Hyperactivity," *Journal of Child Psychiatry,* 1989; 30(5): 671–709.

Grandin, T. *Thinking in Pictures.* New York: Doubleday, 1996; 68.

Greene, R. W. *The Explosive Child.* New York: HarperCollins, 1998.

Haber, J., "Medication in Hyperactive Children," *Pediatrics,* 80(5): 758–60.

Hagberg, H., et al., "Effect of Inflammation on Central Nervous System Development and Vulnerability," *Current Opinion in Neurology,* 2005; 18: 117–23.

Hallowell, E. M., et al. *Driven to Distraction.* New York: Pantheon, 1994; 282.

Haslam, R., "Is There a Role for Megavitamin Therapy in the Treatment of ADHD?" *Advances in Neurology,* 58: 303–10.

Hauser, P., et al., "Attention Deficit Hyperactivity Disorder in People with Generalized Resistant Thyroid Hormone," *New England Journal of Medicine,* 1993; 328(14): 997–1003.

Heilprin, J., "Tap Water Contains Hundreds of Chemicals," Associated Press, Dec. 12, 2005.

Hunt, R., et al., "Clonidine Benefits Children with ADD and Hyperactivity," *Journal of the American Academy of Child and Adolescent Psychiatry,* 24: 617–29.

Hynd, G., et al., "Corpus Callosum Morphology in ADHD," *Journal of Learning Disabilities,* 24: 141–46, 1991.

Kamel, F., et al., "Association of Pesticide Exposure with Neurologic Dysfunction and Disease," *Environ Health Perspect.,* 112: 750–758.

Levy, F., "A Study of Twins in Australia: Genetics Plays an Important Role in ADHD Comorbidity," *Pediatric News,* Feb. 1998; 30.

Lewis, L., *Special Diets for Special Kids.* Arlington, TX: Future Horizons, 1998.

Lubar, J., et al., "Evaluation of EEG Neurofeedback Training for ADHD," *Biofeedback and Self-Regulation,* 20: 83–99, 1997.

McConnell, H., "Catecholamine Metabolism in Attention Deficit Disorder: Implications for the Use of Amino Acid Precursor Therapy," *Medical Hypotheses,* 1985; 17(4): 305–11.

Mocarelli, P., et al., "Paternal Concentrations of Dioxin and Sex Ratio of Offspring," *The Lancet,* 355: 1858–63, 2000.

MTA Cooperative Group, "A Fourteen Month Randomized Clinical Trial of Treatment Strategies for Attention-Deficit/Hyperactivity Disorder," *Archives of General Psychiatry,* 1999; 56.

National Institute of Mental Health. *Interdisciplinary Research on Attention Deficit Hyperactivity Disorder.* Washington, D.C., 2000.

Nemzer, E., et al., "Amino Acid Supplementation as Therapy for Attention Deficit Disorder," *Journal of American Academy of Child and Adolescent Psychiatry.* 1986; 25(4): 509–13.

Nissen, S., M.D., "ADHD Drugs and Cardiovascular Risk," *The New England Journal of Medicine,* Apr. 6, 2006.

Osborne, L., "The Little Professor Syndrome," *New York Times Magazine,* Jun. 18, 2000.

Palanza, P., et al., "Prenatal Exposure to Endocrine Disrupting Chemicals Effects on Behavioral Development," *Neurosci Biobehav.,* 1999; Rev 23: 1011–27.

Pelham, W., et al., "Sustained Release and Standard Methylphenidate Effects on Cognitive and Social Behavior in Children with ADD," *Pediatrics,* 80: 491–501.

Pliska, S., "Tricyclic Antidepressants in the Treatment of Children with an ADHD Disorder," *Journal of the American Academy of Child and Adolescent Psychiatry,* 26: 127–33.

Rapport, M. D., "Bridging Theory and Practice: Conceptual Understanding of Treatments for Children with Attention Deficit Hyperactivity Disorder (ADHD), Obsessive-Compulsive Disorder (OCD), Autism, and Depression," *Journal of Clinical Child Psychology,* 2001; 30(1): 3–7.

Ratey, J., "The Biology of ADD," *First Annual National ADDA Adult ADD Conference,* Merrillville, Ind., Apr. 1995; 20–22.

Richardson, W., M.A., "LMFCC ADHD, Alcoholism and Other Addictions," *ADD Resources,* Feb. 10, 2006; 1

Robin, A. L. *ADHD in Adolescents.* New York: Guilford Press, 1998.

Rucklidge, J. J., et al., "Psychological Functioning of Women Identified in Adulthood with Attention-Deficit/Hyperactivity Disorder," *Journal of Attention Disorders,* 1997; 2: 167–76.

Sargent, J. D., et al., "The Association between State Housing Policy and Lead Poisoning in Children," *American Journal of Public Health.,* 1999; 89(11): 1690–1695.

Silver, L. B., M.D. *ADHD: Attention Deficit-Hyperactivity Disorder and Learning Disabilities.* Summit. NJ: Ciba-Geigy Corporation, Pharmaceuticals Division, 1995; 9.

Silverman, J., "Thirteen Percent of Oregon Public School Children in Special Ed," Associated Press, Feb. 16, 2006.

Simon, H., M.D. "What Is Attention Deficit Disorder?" Found at CBS Health-Watch, 1998.

Spencer, T., et al., "ADHD and Thyroid Abnormalities: A Research Note," *Journal of Child Psychology,* July, 36(5): 879–85, 1995.

Stanley, J. A., Ph.D., "In Vivo P Spectroscopy Evidence of Altered Membrane Phospholipid Metabolites in Children with Attention-Deficit/Hyperactive Disorder," *WPIC Research Day,* Jan. 18, 2006; 12.

Wasowicz, L., "The Skinny on ADHD Contributors," *U.P.I.,* Mar. 16, 2006.

Weinberg, W., et al., "The Myth of the Attention Deficit Hyperactivity Disorder: Symptoms Resulting from Multiple Causes," *Journal of Child Neurology,* 7(4): 431–45, 2000.

Weiss, R., "Legion of Little Helpers in the Gut Keeps Us Alive," *Washington Post,* Jun. 5, 2006.

Wetry, J. S., "Pharmacological Treatments of Autism, Attention Deficit Hyperactivity Disorder, Oppositional Defiant Disorder, and Depression in Children and Youth." *The Journal of Clinical Child Psychology,* Mar. 2001; 30: 110–13.

Zametkin, A., et al. Cerebral Glucose Metabolism in Adults with Hyperactivity of Childhood Onset. *New England Journal of Medicine,* 323(20):1351–1366, 1990.

Asthma Sources

Agata, H., et al., "Comparison of the MAST Chemiluminescent Assay System with RAST and Skin Tests in Allergic Children," *Annals of Allergy,* 1993; 70: 153–57.

Ballard, R. D., "Nocturnal Asthma: Potential Mechanisms and Current Therapy," *Clinical Pulmonary Medicine,* 1(5): 271–78.

Barnes, P. J., "A New Approach to the Treatment of Asthma," *The New England Journal of Medicine,* 1995, 332(13): 868–75.

Bener, A., et al., "Genetics and Environmental Risk Factors Associated with Asthma in Schoolchildren," *Allerg Immunol* (Paris), May 2005; 37(5): 163–68.

Britton, J. I., et al., "Dietary Magnesium, Lung Function, Wheezing, and Airway Hyperreactivity in a Random Adult Population Sample," *Lancet.* 344: 357–62, 1994.

Brody, J., "Steroids Interfere with Both Calcium and Hormones," *New York Times,* May 14, 1997.

Brown, A., "Fish Oil Can Prevent Airway Constriction in Asthma," *Reuters Health,* Jan. 9, 2006.

Check, W. A., et al., "Pharmacology and Pharmacokinetics of Topical Corticosteroid Derivatives Used for Asthma Therapy," *American Review of Respiratory Disease,* 141: S44–51.

Christen, K., "Arsenic Treated Wood May Have a Long Toxic Legacy," *Science,* Dec. 21, 2005.

Cohet, C., et al., "Infections, Medication Use, and the Prevalence of Symptoms of Asthma, Rhinitis, and Eczema in Childhood," *Journal of Epidemiology and Community Health,* Oct. 2004; 59(10); 852–57.

Cone, M., "Cancer Study Cites Hazards of Indoor Air for N.Y., L.A. Teens," *Los Angeles Times,* June 22, 2006.

Cornell University, "Rise in Asthma May Be Due to Fetal Exposure to Toxins," www.news.cornell.edu. 2006.

Cumming, R. G., et. al., "Use of Inhaled Corticosteroids and the Risk of Cataracts," *The New England Journal of Medicine,* Jul. 3, 1997; 337(1).

Dennis, S. M., et. al., "Regular Bronchodilators Worsen Asthma Control," *The Lancet,* 1990; 336: 1391.

Environmental News Service, "Newborns Exposure to Toxins May Trigger Asthma and Allergies," Oct. 10, 2005.

Erbas, B., et al., "Air Pollution and Childhood Asthma Emergency Hospital Admissions: Estimating Intra-City Regional Variations," *Int J Environ Health Res,* Feb. 2005; 15(1):11–20.

Gergen, P. J., et al., "National Survey of Prevalence of Asthma Among Children in the United States 1976–1980," *Pediatrics,* 1988; 81:1–7.

Greene, L. S., "Asthma and Oxidant Stress: Nutritional, Environmental, and Genetic Factors," *Journal of the American College of Nutrition,* Aug. 1995; 14(4): 317–24.

Hersoug, L. G., "Viruses as the Causative Agent Related to 'Dampness' and the Missing Link between Allergen Exposure and Onset of Allergic Disease," *Indoor Air,* Oct. 15, 2005.

Huggins, C., "Study Links Bad Asthma with Bad Behavior," Reuters Health. *Pediatrics,* Feb. 2006.

Hurwitz, E. L., et al., "Effects of Diphtheria-Tetanus-Pertussis or Tetanus Vaccination on Allergies and Allergy-Related Respiratory Symptoms Among Children and Adolescents in the US," *Journal of Manipulative and Physiological Therapeutics,* 2000: 318(7192): 1173–76.

"Inhaled and Nasal Glucocorticoids and the Risks of Ocular Hypertension or Open-angle Glaucoma," *Journal of the American Medical Association,* Mar. 5, 1997; 277: 722–27.

Janson, C., et al., "Anxiety and Depression in Relation to Respiratory Symptoms and Asthma," *American Journal of Respiratory and Critical Care Medicine,* 149: 930–34, 1994.

Johnson, P. R., et al., "Fine Particulate Matter and National Ambient Air Quality Standards: Public Health Impact on Populations in the Northeastern United States," *Environ Health Perspect,* Sep. 2005; 113(9): 1140–47.

Kemp, T., et al., "Is Infant Immunization a Risk Factor for Childhood Asthma or Allergy?" *Epidemiology,* 1997; 8: 678.

Kikuchi, Y., et al., "Chemosensitivity and Perception of Dyspnea in Patients with a History of Near-fatal Asthma," *The New England Journal of Medicine,* 330: 1329–34.

Kim, J. H., et al., "Effects of Air Pollutants on Childhood Asthma," *Yonsei Med J,* Apr. 30, 2005; 46(2):239–44.

Lantner, R. R., et al., "Emergency Management of Asthma in Children: Impact of NIH Guidelines," *Annals of Allergy, Asthma and Immunology,* 1995; 74: 188–91.

Lewis, T. C., et al., "Air Pollution-Associated Changes in Lung Function Among Asthmatic Children in Detroit," *Environ Health Perspect,* Aug. 2005; 113(8): 1068–75.

Li, J., et al., "Clinical Evaluation of Asthma," *Annals of Allergy, Asthma and Immunology,* 1996; 76: 1–10.

"Magnesium and Bronchial Asthma," *International Journal of Alternative and Complementary Medicine,* Feb. 1996; 14.

Maier, K., "The Allergy-Asthma Link," *Energy Times,* Sep. 2005.

Martinez, F. D., et al., "Asthma and Wheezing in the First Six Years of Life," *New England Journal of Medicine,* 1995; 332(3): 133–39.

Mazzarella, G., "Th-1/Th-2 Lymphocyte Polarization in Asthma," *Allergy,* 2000; 55(61): 6–9.

Mickleborough, T. D., et al., "Dietary Polyunsaturated Fatty Acids in Asthma and Exercise Induced Bronchoconstriction," *Eur J Clin Nutr,* Dec. 2005.

Mittelstaedt, M., "Asthma Now Hits 1 in 10 Children," *Boston Globe,* Jan. 27, 2006.

MMWR Weekly, "Asthma Mortality and Hospitalization Among Children and Young Adults, U.S., 1980–1993," May 3, 1996.

National Institutes of Health, "Environmental Roots of Asthma," Nih.gov, 2005.

National Institutes of Health, "Even Olympians Get Exercise Induced Asthma," *Medline Plus,* Feb. 8, 2006.

National Institutes of Health, "Rheumatoid Arthritis Drug Could Fight Problem Asthma," *Medline Plus,* Mar. 18, 2006.

Norton, A., "Childhood Depression Tied to Adult Asthma, Obesity," *Int J Obesity,* Feb. 21, 2006.

Noverr, M. C., et al., "Role of Antibiotics and Fungal Microbia in Driving Pulmonary Allergic Responses," *Infectious Immunology,* Sep. 2004; 72(9): 4996–5003.

Nygaard, U. C., et al., "The Allergy Adjuvant Effect of Particles–Genetic Factors Influence Antibody and Cytokine Responses," *BMC Immunol,* Jun. 21, 2005; 6: 11.

Odent, M. R., et al., "Letter to the Editor. Pertussis Vaccination and Asthma: Is There a Link?" *JAMA,* 1994; 272: 592–93.

Preidt, R., "Little Progress Made in Closing Asthma Gap," NIH, *Medline Plus,* Feb. 13, 2006.

Raloff, J., "Fruits and Veggies Limit Inflammatory Protein," *Science News,* Jan. 2005.

Rapp, D. *Is This Your Child?* New York: William Morrow and Company, 1991.

Rauscher, M., "Prenatal Vitamin D May Protect Child from Asthma," NIH, *Medline Plus,* Mar. 6, 2006.

Sampson, H. A., "Number of people with food allergies on the rise," Presentation at the American Medical Association media briefing on nutrition, Sep. 18, 1997.

Scarfone, R. J., et al., "Controlled Trial of Oral Prednisone, in the Emergency Department Treatment of Children with Acute Asthma," *Pediatrics.* 1993; 42(4): 513–518.

Shirakawa, T., et al., "Association between Atopy and Variants of the B Subunit of the High-Affinity Immunoglobulin E Receptor," *Nature Genetics.* 7(2): 125–29, 1994.

Spector, S. L., "Leukotriene Inhibitors and Antagonists in Asthma (Part 1)," *Annals of Allergy, Asthma and Immunology,* 1995; 463–96.

Triche, E. W., et al., "Low-Level Ozone Exposure and Respiratory Symptoms in Infants," *Environ Health Perspect,* Dec. 2005.

Turkeltaub, P. C., "Deaths Associated with Allergenic Extracts," *FDA Medical Bulletin,* 24(1):7, 1994.

Varner, A. E., et al., "Inflammation in Asthma: Why Is It So Important?" *Journal of Respiratory Diseases,* 1966; 17(7):605–616.

Vedal, S., et al., "Acute Effects of Ambient Inhalable Particles in Asthmatic and Nonasthmatic Children," *American Journal of Respiratory and Critical Care Medicine,* 1998; 157:1034–43.

Warner, J., "Toxins in Dust Raise Risk of Asthma," *WebMD Medical News,* Dec. 1, 2005.

Weil, A. *Health and Healing–Understanding Conventional and Alternative Medicine.* Dorling Kindersley, 1995.

Allergy and Other Childhood Epidemics Sources

Atherton, D., "Role of Diet in Treating Atopic Eczema–Elimination Diets Can Be Beneficial," *British Medical Journal,* 297: 1458–60.

Bazar, K. A., et al., "Obesity and ADHD May Represent Different Manifestations of a Common Environmental Oversampling Syndrome: A Model for Revealing Mechanistic Overlap Among Cognitive, Metabolic, and Inflammatory Disorders," *Medical Hypotheses,* 2006; 66: 263–69.

Becker, E., "White House Undermined Chemical Tests, Report Says," *The New York Times,* Apr. 2, 2004; C2.

Bernstein, J. M., "The Role of IgE-Mediated Hypersensitivity in Otitis Media with Effusion," *Otolaryngology,* 89: 874, 1993.

Burns, C., et al., "Pesticides and Neurologic Symptoms," *Agricultural Health Study,* Monsanto Co. 2005.

Campbell, M. B., "Neurological Manifestations of Allergic Disease," *Annals of Allergy,* 31: 485–98, 1973.

Colborn, T., "A Case for Revisiting the Safety of Pesticides: A Closer Look at Neurodevelopment," *Environ. Health Perspect,* 2006; 114: 10–17.

Cone, M., "A New Alarm Sounds for Amphibians," *Los Angeles Times,* Jan. 25, 2006.

Cugini, P., et al., "Anxiety, Depression, Hunger and Body Composition: III. Their Relationships in Obese Patients," *Eat Weight Disord,* 1999; 4(3): 1307–10.

Dandona, P., et al., "Inflammation: The Link between Insulin Resistance, Obesity and Diabetes," *Trends in Immunology,* Jan. 2004; 25(1).

Del Prete, G. F., et al., "Allergen Exposure Induces the Activation of Allergen-Specific Th-2 Cells in the Airway Mucosa of Patients with Allergic Respiratory Disorders," *Eur J Immnol,* 1993: 23: 1445–49.

Dell'Amore, C., "Gene Found for Severe Allergic Disease," U.P.I., Feb. 2, 2006.

Duncan, B. B., et al., "Low-Grade Systemic Inflammation and the Development of Type 2 Diabetes: the Atherosclerosis Risk in Communities Study," *Diabetes,* 2003; 52: 1799–1806.

Eklind, S., et al., "Bacterial Endotoxin Sensitizes the Immature Brain to Hypoxic–Ischemic Injury," *Eur J Neurosci,* 2001; 13: 1101–06.

El-Sherif, Y., et al., "Melatonin Regulates Neuronal Plasticity in the Hippocampus," *J Neurosci Res,* 2003; 72(4): 454–60.

Esposito, K., et al., "Inflammatory Cytokines Concentrations are Acutely Increased by Hyperglycemia in Humans: Role of Oxidative Stress," *Circulation,* 2002; 106: 2067–72.

FactSheet. *National Cancer Institute Research on Childhood Cancers: 1.* May 10, 2006.

"Food Intolerance in Patients with Angioedema and Chronic Urticaria," *European Journal of Allergy and Clinical Immunology,* 1995; 50:26.

Gerschwin, M. E., M.D. *Taking Charge of Your Child's Allergies.* New York: Berkley Books, 1998.

Gordon, N., "The Therapeutics of Melatonin: A Pediatric Perspective," *Brain & Development,* Jun. 2000; 22(4): 213–17.

Gregus, Z., et al., "Effect of Lipoic Acid on Biliary Excretion of Glutathione and Metals," *Toxicology & Applied Pharmacology,* May 1992; 114(1): 88–96.

Grosse, S. D., et al., "Economic Gains Resulting from the Reduction in Children's Exposure to Lead in the United States," *Environmental Health Perspectives,* Jun. 2002; 110(4): 563–69.

Haas, E., M.D. *The Detox Diet.* Berkeley, CA: Celestial Arts Publishing, 1996.

Hagberg, H., et al., "Effect of Inflammation on Central Nervous System Development and Vulnerability," *Current Opinion in Neurology,* 2005; 18: 117–23.

Hattevig, G., et al., "Clinical Symptoms and IgE Responses to Common Food Proteins and Inhalants in the First 7 Years of Life," *Clin Allergy,* 1987; 17: 571–78.

Hirano, T., "Interleukin 6 and Its Receptor Ten Years Later," *Int Rev Immunol,* 1998; 16: 249–84.

Holt, P. G., et al., "Effect of Influenza Virus Infection on Allergic Sensitization to Inhaled Antigen in Mice," *Int Arch Allergy Appl Immunol,* 1998; 86: 121–23.

Karkalainen, J., "A Bovine Albumin Peptide Is a Possible Trigger of Insulin-Dependent Diabetes," *New England Journal of Medicine,* 1992; 327: 302.

Khalsa, D. S., M.D., and Cameron Stauth. *Brain Longevity.* New York: Warner Books, 1997.

Kleinfield, N. R., "Diabetes and Its Awful Toll Quietly Emerge as a Crisis," *New York Times,* Jan. 9, 2006.

Krohn, J., M.D. *Allergy Relief and Prevention.* Point Roberts, WA: Hartley & Marks, 1996.

Landrigan, P. J., et al. *Pesticides in the Diets of Infants and Children* Washington, D.C.: National Academy Press, 1993; 9.

Leerdam, C. M., et al., "Recurrent Parotitis of Childhood," *J Pediatric Child Health,* Dec. 2005.

Lourdes, S., et al., "Reduced Intellectual Development in Children with Prenatal Lead Exposure," *Environmental Health News,* 2005.

Maggi, E., et al., "Accumulation of Th-2-Like Helper T-Cells in the Conjunctiva of Patients with Vernal Conjunctivitis," *J Immunol,* 1991; 146: 1169–74.

Mangano, J. J., "A Rise in the Incidence of Childhood Cancer in the United States," *Int J Health Serv,* 2000; 30(2): 373–77.

McDowell, M., M.D., "Appetite Controls: An Addiction-Like Component in Overeating and Its Cure," *Obesity and Bariatric Medicine,* 1980; 9.

Milburn, L. J., et al., "Corticosteroids Restore the Balance between Locally Produced Th-1 and Th-2 Cytokines and Immunoglobulin Isotypes to Normal in Sarcoid Lung," *Clin Exp Immunol,* 1997; 188: 105–13.

Miller, E. I., et al., "Synthesis of IgE by the Human Conceptus," *J Allergy,* 1973; 52: 182–88.

Miller, G. E., et al., "Pathways Linking Depression, Adiposity, and Inflammatory Markers in Healthy Young Adults," *Brain Behav Immun,* 2003; 17: 276–85.

Mishima, H., et al., "CD4+ T-Cells Can Induce Airway Hyperresponsiveness to Allergen Challenge in the Brown Norway Rat," *Am J Respir Crit Care Med,* 1998: 158:1863–70.

Mitchell, E., "The Childhood Food Allergy Mystery," *Newsday,* Feb. 21, 2006.

Monje, M. L., et al., "Inflammatory Blockade Restores Adult Hippocampal Neurogenesis," *Science,* 2003; 302: 1760–85.

Montague, T., "Environmental Toxicants and Developmental Disabilities," *Rachel's Environment & Health News,* Jul. 7, 2005; 821.

Mosman, T. R., et al., "The Expanding Universe of T-Cell Subsets," Th-1, Th-2 and More," *Immunol Today,* 1996; 17: 138–46.

Nguyen, M. D., "Innate Immunity: The Missing Link in Neuroprotection and Neurodegeneration?" *Nat Rev Neurosci,* 2002; 3: 216–27.

Noble, E. P., "The DRD2 Gene in Psychiatric and Neurological Disorders and Its Phenotypes," *Pharmacogenomics,* 2000; 1(3): 309–33.

Nori, M., et al., "Ebastine Inhibits T-Cell Migration, Production of Th-2-Type Cytokines and Proinflammatory Cytokines," *Clin Exp Allergy,* 2001; 33: 1544–54.

Ohta, N., "Analysis of Th-1, Th-2, Tc-1 and Tc-2 Cells in Patients with Allergic Rhinitis," *Clin Exp All Rev,* 2005; 5: 68–71.

Padgett, D. A., et al., "How Stress Influences the Immune Response," *Trends Immunol,* 2003; 24: 444–8.

Patterson, J. E., et al., "Mercury in Human Breath from Dental Amalgams," *J Dental Res,* 1981; 60: 1668–71.

Perry, V. H., "The Influence of Systemic Inflammation on Inflammation in the Brain: Implications for Chronic Neurodegenerative Disease," *Brain Behav Immun,* 2004; 18: 407–13.

Pincus, S., "Potential Role of Infections in Chronic Inflammatory Diseases," *ASM News,* 2005; 71: 11.

Pirkle, J. L., et al., "The Decline in Blood Lead Levels in the United States," *Journal of the American Medical Association,* Jul. 27, 1994; 272(4): 284–91.

Poulos, A., "What Is In Our Water?" *The Epoch Times,* Jan. 4, 2006.

Pradhan, A. D., et al., "C-Reactive Protein, Interleukin 6, and Risk of Developing Type-2 Diabetes Mellitus," *JAMA,* 2001; 286: 327–34.

Reuters Health, "Allergies Reach Epidemic Levels in Europe," Mar. 31, 2006.

Robinson, D. S., et al., "Predominant Th-2-Like Bronchoalveolar T Lymphocyte Population in Atopic Asthma," *New Engl J Med,* 1992; 326: 298–304.

Romagnani, S., "Regulatory T-Cells: Which Role in the Pathogenesis and Treatment of Allergic Disorders?" *Allergy,* 2006; 61: 3–14.

Romagnani, S., et al., "An Update on Human Th-1 and Th-2 Cells," *Int Arch Allergy Immunol,* 1997; 223: 153–56.

Ross, R., "Atherosclerosis–An Inflammatory Disease," *N Engl J Med,* 1999; 340: 115–26.

Royal, F. F., M.D., "Food Allergy Addiction in a Bariatric Practice," *Obesity and Bariatric Medicine,* 1978; 7: 45.

Sahashi, K., et al., "Significance of Interleukin 6 in Patients with Sarcoidosis," *Chest,* 1994; 106: 156–60.

Saloga, J., et al., "Does Sensitization Through the Skin Occur?" *Allergy,* 2000; 55: 905–909.

Sears, B., Ph.D. *The Anti-Aging Zone.* New York: ReganBooks, 1999.

Seeman, B., "American Kids Are Increasingly Allergic to Peanuts and Scientists Don't Know Why," *Newhouse News Service,* Dec. 19, 2005.

Sheehan, C., "Kids' Food Allergies Skyrocket," *The Chicago Tribune,* Jun. 8, 2006.

Shi, H.Z., et al., "CD4+ CD25+ Regulatory T Lymphocytes in Allergy and Asthma," *Allergy,* 2005; 60:936–95.

Spalter, A. R., et al., "Thyroid Function in Bulimia Nervosa," *Biological Psychiatry,* Mar. 15, 1993; 408–14.

Stannegard, O., "Early Sensitization to Food Antigens–When and How?," *Pediatric Allergy and Immunology,* 2001; Suppl 14: 20–23.

Sternberg, S., "To Head Off Allergies, Expose Your Kids to Pets and Dirt Early," *USA Today,* Mar. 20, 2006.

Taylor, P.C., et al., "Immunotherapy for Rheumatoid Arthritis," *Curr Opin Immunol,* 2001; 13: 611–16.

Till, S. J., et al., "Immunological Responses to Allergen Immunotherapy," *Clin Allergy Immunol,* 2004; 18: 85–104.

Vela, S., "Arsenic: How Much Is Too Much?," *Lansing State Journal,* Jan. 8, 2006.

Weiner, H. L., "Oral Tolerance: Immune Mechanisms and Treatment of Autoimmune Diseases," *Immunol Today,* 1997; 18: 335–41.

Weisberg, S. T., et al., "Obesity is Associated with Macrophage Accumulation in Adipose Tissue," *The Journal of Clinical Investigation,* Dec. 2003; 112(12).

Wellen, K. E., "Obesity-Induced Inflammatory Changes in Adipose Tissue," *The Journal of Clinical Investigation,* Dec. 2003; 112(12): 1785.

Wong, C. K., "Proinflammatory Cytokines (IL-17, IL-6, IL-18 and IL-12) and Th Cytokines (IFN-y, IL-4, IL-10 and IL-13) in Patients with Allergic Asthma," *Clin Exp Immunol,* 2001; 125: 177–83.

Woosley, R. I., "Cardiac Actions of Antihistamines," *Annu Rev Pharmacol Toxicol,* 1996; 36: 233–52.

Wucherpfennig, K. W., "Mechanisms for the Induction of Autoimmunity by Infectious Agents," *J Clin Invest,* 2001; 108: 1097–1104.

Xu, H., et al., "Chronic Inflammation in Fat Plays a Crucial Role in the Development of Obesity-Related Insulin Resistance," *The Journal of Clinical Investigation,* Dec. 2003; III(12).

Young, D., et al., "Chronic Bacterial Infections: Living with Unwanted Guests," *Nature Immunol,* 2002; 3: 1026–32.

INDEX

ABOUT THE AUTHORS

Kenneth A. Bock, M.D.

Kenneth Bock, M.D., an internationally known innovator in the treatment of autism, has created one of the world's first comprehensive biomedical treatment programs for autism, which has been applied in approximately 1,000 cases over the past seven years.

Dr. Bock was also one of the first American physicians to note the clinical similarities among the causative factors, symptomatology, and treatment of autism, ADHD, asthma, and allergies. He designed a Healing Program that encompasses treatment of all four of these new childhood epidemics, which he now refers to as the 4-A Disorders.

For the past several years, Dr. Bock has spoken extensively about autism in the media, in physicians' councils, and at conferences of groups such as Defeat Autism Now. He has appeared on *The Today Show,* Fox News Network, Global Television of Canada, and ABC National Radio, and has been published in magazines such as *Psychology Today,* and in medical journals that include *The Journal of Neuroimmunology, American Journal of Medical Genetics, American Journal of Public Health,* and *Expert Review of Anti-Infective Therapy.*

President of the American College for the Advancement of Medicine, he is the author of three books, including the acclaimed *The Road to Immunity.* Dr. Bock is the co-founder and co-director of both the Rhinebeck Health Center in Rhinebeck, New York, and The Center for Progressive Medicine, in Albany, New York. These facilities now receive patients from all around the nation and the world.

He is a clinical instructor in the Department of Family Medicine at Albany Medical College and is a Fellow of the American College of Nutrition, and the American Academy of Family Physicians. He is a Certified Nutrition Specialist, and has practiced integrative medicine for 23 years.

Cameron Stauth

For more than two decades, Cameron Stauth has been at the forefront of health and healing literature, and he has earned widespread critical praise for his literary nonfiction. His books have been published in eleven languages and eighteen countries, and *The New York Times* has hailed him as "a tireless reporter and a talented and graceful writer."

A prolific author with a wide range of expertise, he has written 22 prior books in the varied fields of biography, medicine, narrative nonfiction, business, psychology, fitness, diet, and professional sports.

Two of his books, *The New Approach to Cancer* (the first book on integrative medical care for cancer), and *Brain Longevity* (the first report on multidisciplinary treatment of Alzheimer's disease), have had an impact upon medical treatment in America and abroad.

Stauth has appeared on over 500 television and radio programs, co-founded the natural health products firm Quantum Inc., and has written over 100 articles for publications including *The New York Times Magazine, Esquire, The Saturday Evening Post,* and *Prevention.*

Former Editor in Chief of *The Journal of Health Science* and *The Journal of the Nutritional Academy,* he has been a columnist for *Natural Health, American Film,* and *California Business.*

He was Executive Producer and Story Editor of two films: *Because Mommy Works,* the first media presentation of the issue of working mothers losing custody of their children, and *Prison of Secrets,* which contributed to prison reform for female inmates in Hawaii.

ABOUT THE TYPE

This book was set in Caslon, a typeface first designed in 1722 by William Caslon. Its widespread use by most English printers in the early eighteenth century soon supplanted the Dutch typefaces that had formerly prevailed. The roman is considered a "workhorse" typeface due to its pleasant, open appearance, while the italic is exceedingly decorative.